Sexually Transmitted Diseases

CURRENT ◊ CLINICAL ◊ PRACTICE

NEIL S. SKOLNIK, MD • SERIES EDITOR

Sexually Transmitted Diseases

A Practical Guide for Primary Care

Edited by

Anita L. Nelson, MD

Harbor/UCLA Medical Center
Torrance, CA

JoAnn Woodward, RNC, BSN, NP

Health Care Partners, Redondo Beach, CA
and
Harbor/UCLA Nurse Practitioner Program,
Torrance, CA

Foreword by

Susan Wysocki, RNC, NP, FAANP,

President and CEO
National Association of Nurse Practitioners in Women's Health
Washington, DC

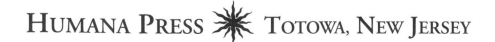

HUMANA PRESS ✳ TOTOWA, NEW JERSEY

3/13/08

© 2006 Humana Press Inc.
999 Riverview Drive, Suite 208
Totowa, New Jersey 07512

humanapress.com

Due diligence has been taken by the publishers, editors, and authors of this book to assure the accuracy of the information published and to describe generally accepted practices. The contributors herein have carefully checked to ensure that the drug selections and dosages set forth in this text are accurate and in accord with the standards accepted at the time of publication. Notwithstanding, as new research, changes in government regulations, and knowledge from clinical experience relating to drug therapy and drug reactions constantly occurs, the reader is advised to check the product information provided by the manufacturer of each drug for any change in dosages or for additional warnings and contraindications. This is of utmost importance when the recommended drug herein is a new or infrequently used drug. It is the responsibility of the treating physician to determine dosages and treatment strategies for individual patients. Further it is the responsibility of the health care provider to ascertain the Food and Drug Administration status of each drug or device used in their clinical practice. The publisher, editors, and authors are not responsible for errors or omissions or for any consequences from the application of the information presented in this book and make no warranty, express or implied, with respect to the contents in this publication.

This publication is printed on acid-free paper. ∞
ANSI Z39.48-1984 (American Standards Institute) Permanence of Paper for Printed Library Materials.

Production Editor: Amy Thau

Cover design by Donna Niethe

For additional copies, pricing for bulk purchases, and/or information about other Humana titles, contact Humana at the above address or at any of the following numbers: Tel.: 973-256-1699; Fax: 973-256-8341; E-mail: orders@humanapr.com; or visit our Website: www.humanapress.com

Photocopy Authorization Policy:

Printed in the United States of America. 10 9 8 7 6 5 4 3 2 1

eISBN 13 978-1-59745-040-9

eISBN 1-59745-040-5

Library of Congress Control Number: 2007926689

Dedication

Sexually Transmitted Diseases: A Practical Guide for Primary Care is a collaboration of physicians and advanced practice nurses who share a deep appreciation for the tremendous contributions made by Felicia H. Stewart, MD.

Dr. Stewart was an adjunct professor in the Department of Obstetrics, Gynecology, and Reproductive Services and co-director of the Center for Reproductive Health Research and Policy at the University of California, San Francisco. She had done it all. She was in private practice, made public policy, and taught generations of women and their providers about reproductive health. As deputy assistant secretary for population affairs for the US Department of Health and Human Services, she oversaw and redefined the Title X Family Planning Program. As director of reproductive health programs for the Henry J. Kaiser Foundation, she pioneered new ways to communicate with adolescents. She wrote a number of groundbreaking and influential books. As the lead author of *My Body, My Health: The Concerned Women's Guide to Gynecology*, she helped enable women to become informed consumers and to assert their rights to knowledge and decision making about their reproductive health. Both the original and its revision *Understanding Your Body* were Book of the Month Club selections. Dr. Stewart was an author of 11 editions of *Contraceptive Technology*. She championed access to contraception and emergency contraception, as well as to sexually transmitted infection services. As an activist, she was uniquely sensitive to the social responsibility of scientists and the ethical responsibility of policymakers to make evidenced-based decisions. She demanded moral clarity and integrity in a field that is often driven by short-term political forces.

Dr. Stewart was the recipient of numerous honors, including the Carl S. Shultz Award from the American Public Health Association, the Irvin M. Cushner Memorial Lectureship presented by the Association of Reproductive Health Professionals, the Distinguished Service Award from the American College of Obstetricians and Gynecologists, and the Olivia Schieffelin Nordberg Award for excellence in writing and editing in the population sciences.

We thank Dr. Stewart for her dedication, her vision, and for the significant impact that she had on reproductive health and on the reproductive rights of women in this country and around the world. We hope that in these pages we have upheld the spirit of practicality, clarity, and excellence that she always represented.

Anita L. Nelson, MD
JoAnn Woodward, RNC, BSN, NP

Series Editor Introduction

Sexually Transmitted Diseases: A Practical Guide for Primary Care, edited by Dr. Anita Nelson and JoAnn Woodward, is a superb book that skillfully balances detailed yet concise overviews of the important sexually transmitted infections that patients encounter. Sexually transmitted diseases (STDs) account for 5% of all outpatient office visits in the United States, and are primarily taken care of by family doctors, internists, obstetrician-gynecologists, and emergency room physicians. These are a set of diseases that require a great deal of knowledge, as well as sensitivity to individual patients needs in order to provide excellent care. This textbook covers the fascinating history of sexually transmitted infections in the Western world and current epidemiology, as well as diagnosis and treatment algorithms, including the latest recommendations from the Centers for Disease Control.

This text is clearly written by physicians who are attuned to the finer points of patient care. In addition to giving diagnostic and treatment algorithms, the authors also provide advice on how to openly and honestly discuss these often charged personal topics in a sensitive and culturally appropriate manner with patients. Honest, practical, intelligent recommendations discussed in *Sexually Transmitted Diseases: A Practical Guide for Primary Care* address both the organization of an integrated public health approach to STDs as well as individual clinician education. Each chapter is organized for ease of use and includes "fast facts," history, epidemiology, etiology, clinical manifestations, and mode of transmission, diagnosis, and treatment.

In summary, *Sexually Transmitted Diseases: A Practical Guide for Primary Care* is an excellent book for both the practicing clinician who wants to learn more about STDs and for those primary care physicians who have a special interest in STDs and STD education.

Neil S. Skolnik, MD

vii

Foreword

At the risk of sounding old, when I first became a nurse practitioner, sexually transmitted diseases (STDs) were called venereal disease. The sexually transmitted infections (STIs) we most commonly think of today, with the exception of gonorrhea, were either not named or not recognized. In the clinic I worked for back then, we screened for gonorrhea and, occasionally, syphilis. We diagnosed and treated vaginal infections. Chlamydia was generically identified as mucupurulent cervicitis (MPC). We did not screen for MPC or classify it as an STI. I remember first hearing about herpes from a *Time Magazine* cover and asking whether anyone had seen it at our clinic site. We all wrongly assumed this was only something we would see from the merchant marines a few towns away. The role of human papillomavirus (HPV) in cervical dysplasia was not recognized. Human immunodeficiency virus (HIV) did not exist. And I am not that old.

It is a new day in terms of STDs, and this is one of the many reasons why clinicians need to read *Sexually Transmitted Diseases: A Practical Guide for Primary Care*. Few, if any, clinicians can afford not to know about STIs. These infections do not discriminate. They affect all ages, races, and socioeconomic classes. They affect the educated and the noneducated. The infections can even affect babies. One in 10 Americans will have an STI sometime in their lifetime.

Occasionally, I hear someone say that their patients do not have STIs or are not at risk. This is usually followed by a description of the location of their practice—usually not the big cities—or a description of their clientele (generally middle to upper-middle class). A friend of mine has a term for this: *ophthalmic diagnosis*. In other words, if a patient looks well-dressed and respectable, he or she is not at a high risk for infection. Perhaps this perception is going away because most clinicians see STIs on a frequent basis, whether it is related to an abnormal Pap smear or another presentation.

Some clinicians feel awkward asking questions related to STIs because it involves asking personal questions that we are generally not familiar with in polite conversation. However, these questions can be asked in a careful, nonjudgmental manner that will not offend. The clinician's office generally is not the first place that an individual will hear about STDs. In general, patients want to be asked those questions rather than having to bring the subject up themselves. It is far easier for the patient to answer some questions presented in the usual history taking than to figure out the way to bring up the topic. Furthermore, perhaps they too do not think that their risk is great, even if their behavior is.

Sexually Transmitted Diseases: A Practical Guide for Primary Care covers the diagnosis and treatment of STDs and other information critical to patient care in the new millennium. Here, readers will learn not only how to identify and manage these infections, but they will also obtain information about preventing these infections. Preventing, where possible, the sequelae of these infections is also critical to patient care. The reader will find resources for patients as well as clinicians.

Written by clinicians, many of whom have been diagnosing, treating, and counseling patients since the days of venereal disease, this book is packed with evidence-based information steeped in these clinicians' years of practice.

The more information clinicians have, the better they can educate their patients, whether it is information about preventing new or recurring infections or preserving health with those STIs that have no cure. This book is an excellent resource.

Susan Wysocki, RNC, NP, FAANP,
President and CEO
National Association of Nurse Practitioners
in Women's Health

Preface

As a group, primary care providers treat most of the people who are infected with sexually transmitted infections (STIs); however, each individual health care provider may not see enough cases to keep current with new information about the clinical presentations of or the diagnostic tests or treatments needed for these infections. JoAnn Woodward envisioned a book that would meet the special needs of providers awash in the demands of a busy practice. The purpose of *Sexually Transmitted Diseases: A Practical Guide for Primary Care* is to give primary office-based physicians, nurse practitioners, physician assistants, and certified nurse midwives, relevant practical and interesting-to-read information about each of the STIs.

Experts in each of the specific infections succinctly reviewed clinical pearls about the presentation, diagnosis, and treatment of each infection. To give readers a perspective on the scope of the problem and the impact pregnancy may have on diagnosis and treatment, that information is included in each chapter. The most recent CDC treatment recommendations are summarized in separate tables, which can be easily updated with any future change in those guidelines.

However, the editors and authors recognize that STIs are very special infections. STIs have a rich and sometimes shocking history. They have helped to define the need for subjects in research studies to have informed consent, they have shaped public policy, and they have demonstrated egregious gender inequities. These important, but not necessarily medical, impacts of STIs are highlighted in the overview chapter. STIs also raise issues and challenges that are not often encountered with other disease states. Felicia Guest was kind enough to share her wisdom and advice about how to break the news of an STI to the infected patient. Linda Dominguez provided insight on how to communicate with people from different cultural backgrounds. Penelope Bosarge reviews the scientific evidence about the role that barrier methods may play in reducing the spread of various STIs. Finally, Patricia Lohr brings the hope of new STI preventions by vaccination in advance of exposure and by microbicides that could be used at the time of coitus to reduce the risk of acquiring a variety of STIs.

The editors want to express their heartfelt gratitude to LeRoy Nelson who provided the structure for this project. His research, fact checks, coordination, editing, and compilation made this book possible. For all intents and purposes he functioned as an editor, but has declined that title. The editors also want to thank each of the authors for contributing their expertise and practical knowledge in each of the chapters. Others who helped us process the text include Andrew Park, Delores Thomas, and Joanna Benavidez. We thank them for their hard work and dedication.

Finally, the editors want to thank Richard Lansing at Humana Press for his patience and belief that *Sexually Transmitted Diseases: A Practical Guide for Primary Care* could make a significant contribution not only to Humana's outstanding collection of primary care books, but also to the health of sexually active men and women and their offspring.

Anita L. Nelson, MD
JoAnn Woodward, RNC, BSN, NP

Contents

Contributors

PENELOPE M. BOSARGE, RNC, MSN, CRNP • *Coordinator Women's Health Nurse Practitioner Option, University of Alabama School of Nursing, Birmingham and Clinical Practice, Planned Parenthood of Alabama, Birmingham, AL*

LINDA DOMINGUEZ, RNC, BSN, WHNP • *Assistant Medical Director, Planned Parenthood of New Mexico, Clinician, Southwest Women's Health, Albuquerque, NM*

FELICIA GUEST, MPH, CHES • *Director of Training, Southeast AIDS Training and Education Center, Emory University School of Medicine, Atlanta, GA*

MICHELLE L. GELLER, MD • *Assistant Clinical Professor of Medicine, David Geffen School of Medicine at UCLA, Section Head, Women's Health Section, Division of General Internal Medicine, Department of Medicine, Harbor-UCLA Medical Center, Torrance, CA*

LINDA GOLDMAN, RN, MSN, FNP • *Family Nurse Practitioner, Women's Health Care Nurse Practitioner, School of Nursing, College of Health & Human Services, California State University Dominguez Hills, Carson, CA; Harbor UCLA Medical Center, Women's Health Care Nurse Practitioner Program, Torrance, CA; and Nurse Practitioner, Obstetrics and Gynecology Office, Axminster Medical Group, Inglewood, CA*

JEREMY R. HERMAN, MD • *Department of Medicine, Harbor-UCLA Medical Center, Torrance, CA*

FRANCES E. LIKIS, DrPH, NP, CNM • *Coordinator of Graduate Education, Frontier School of Midwifery and Family Nursing, Nashville, TN*

PATRICIA A. LOHR, MD • *Department of Obstetrics and Gynecology, Harbor-UCLA Medical Center, Torrance, CA*

ANNE MOORE, RNC, MSN, FAANP • *Professor of Nursing, Women's Health Nurse Practitioner, Vanderbilt University, Nashville, TN*

ANITA L. NELSON, MD • *Associate Professor of Obstetrics and Gynecology, Harbor/UCLA Medical Center, Torrance, CA*

GENE PARKS, MD • *Assistant Clinical Professor, Department of Obstetrics and Gynecology, David Geffen School of Medicine at UCLA, Los Angeles, CA*

ALBERT JOHN PHILLIPS, MD, FACOG • *Clinical Professor of Obstetrics and Gynecology, University of Southern California, School of Medicine, Santa Monica, CA*

GUNTER RIEG, MD • *Assistant Clinical Professor of Medicine, David Geffen School of Medicine at UCLA, Harbor-UCLA Medical Center, Torrance, CA*

CAROLYN SUTTON, RN, MS, WHNP, RNC, FAANP • *Faculty Associate, Department of Obstetrics and Gynecology; Associate Director of Clinical Services, Division of Community Women's Health Care, University of Texas Southwestern Medical Center at Dallas, Dallas, TX*

JOANN WOODWARD, RNC, BSN, NP • *Certified Nurse Practitioner, Health Care Partners, Redondo Beach, CA; and Consulting Faculty, Harbor/UCLA Nurse Practitioner Program, Torrance, CA*

Companion CD

The companion CD contains all color versions of images in the text.

1

Introduction to Sexually Transmitted Infections

A View of the Past and an Assessment of Present Challenges

Anita L. Nelson

According to the Centers for Disease Control and Prevention (CDC), sexually transmitted infections (STIs) are a group of contagious diseases most commonly transmitted "from person to person by close, intimate contact." Although most of this contact has traditionally been sexual intercourse, many categories of sexual practices permit transmission from "person to person." Vertical transmission from mother to newborn is also possible. The *means of transmission* unite these diseases—not etiologies, symptoms, or clinical consequences.

The pathogens causing STIs represent a wide spectrum of microorganisms: spirochetes, bacteria, protozoans, viruses, and obligate intracellular organisms. STIs infect the mucosal surfaces of the genitourinary tract. The World Health Organization (WHO) has identified more than 20 pathogens that are transmissible through sexual intercourse (1). The CDC discussed 24 conditions in its 2006 Sexually Transmitted Disease (STD) Treatment Guidelines (Table 1) that meet these criteria (2). The Sexuality Information and Education Council of the United States (SIECUS) and the Institute of Medicine (IOM) reported that more than 25 infectious organisms are primarily spread through sexual activity (3).

Some of these infections are life threatening (human immunodeficiency virus [HIV], syphilis), others predispose to malignancy (hepatitis B, human papillomavirus [HPV], HIV), and others destroy fertility (gonorrhea, chlamydia). The WHO points out that STIs are a major global cause of acute illness, infection, long-term disability, and death, with severe medical and psychological consequences for millions of men, women, and infants. In the United States, STIs are among the most common infections; of the 10 most frequently reported infections, 5 are STIs (4).

From: *Current Clinical Practice: Sexually Transmitted Diseases:
A Practical Guide for Primary Care*
Edited by: A. L. Nelson and J. A. Woodward © Humana Press, Totowa, NJ

Table 1
Sexually Transmitted Diseases, Centers
for Disease Control and Prevention 2006

Diseases characterized by genital ulcers
- Chancroid
- Genital herpes simplex virus infections
- Granuloma inguinale (donovanosis)
- Lymphogranuloma venerum
- Syphilis

Diseases characterized by urethritis and cervicitis
- Chlamydial infections
- Gonococcal infections
- Nongonococcal infections
- Mucopurulent cervicitis

Diseases characterized by vaginal discharge
- Bacterial vaginosis
- Trichomoniasis
- Vulvovaginal candidiasis

Pelvic inflammatory disease

Epididymitis

Human papillomavirus infection
- Genital warts

Vaccine-preventable sexually transmitted infections
- Hepatitis A
- Hepatitis B
- Hepatitis C

Proctitis, proctocolitis, and enteritis

Ectoparasitic infection
- Pediculosis pubis
- Scabies

Human immunodeficiency virus

The history of STDs provides fascinating insight into the evolution of science and human attitudes toward sexuality. These types of infections were recognized relatively easily as being spread by sexual contact, as implied in the term *venereal disease*, which was named after the Greek goddess of love, Venus. One of the first recognized STIs emerged in the 1490s and was called the "French disease" (Morbus Gallicus) because it first appeared in great numbers with the French invasion of Naples, Italy in 1495. After its introduction, the highly contagious infection spread rapidly through Europe, making its way in large numbers to Scotland within 3 years. The infection was ultimately named syphilis after a poem written by an Italian pathologist named Girolamo Fracastoro in 1530 about a mythical shepherd named Syphilus who developed buboes and spread the disease. Another name for syphilis was the "Great Pox." Syphilis was considered at least as terrifying as the other scourge of the time—small pox. It is most telling that one of the strongest curses of the day was to wish "a pox on you." What they were wishing on the target of their enmity was syphilis, not small pox.

As Nance describes the impacts of syphilis, "this new infection covered the body with abscesses and racked it with pain. Eventually the malady filled the streets with beggars, for, unlike the plague, it killed slowly. It changed medicine, leading to new ideas and institutions, producing a quantity of medical literature second only to that of the plague" *(5)*. Authorities of the time agreed that this infection originated with some group other than their own: the Italians blamed it on the French in Spain, the French blamed it on the denizens of northern Italy, others blamed it on the Moslems and Jews expelled from Spain in 1492. However, for most of history, blame was placed on the natives in the new world because syphilis appeared about the time Columbus and his crew returned from their Caribbean exploration. Today, the most accepted explanation for the origin of syphilis is a mutation that occurred in the spirochete that caused a leprosy-like condition (Yaws). Leper houses were very common in the outskirts of towns in the Middle Ages. In the 15th century, decreases in population (because of the cold weather of the prior century and the plague) and more textile production permitted more per capita fuel and personal clothing. In addition, temperatures rose late in the 15th century. People did not have to huddle together at night for warmth. For survival, this spirochete is thought to have mutated to target mucosal cells of the genitalia instead of squamous cells *(6)*. Mucosal cells are generally exposed only during coitus, an activity for which people persisted in huddling together.

In a stirring parallel to initial political reaction to the emergence of HIV infection, it has been noted that with syphilis, the "stench of the diseased beggars aroused as much disgust as charity in contemporaries and led to a hardening of official attitudes toward the poor during the Renaissance, particularly since this illness could be closely associated with sexual immorality and prostitution" *(5)*.

For three centuries after its appearance in Europe, gonorrhea and syphilis were considered by most experts to be different forms of inoculation with the same poison or "liver." In the mid-18th century, there emerged so-called "dualists" who claimed that gonorrhea and syphilis were two different infections. However, in 1767, when the famous surgeon John Hunter injected his penis with pus from a patient with apparent gonorrhea (but who was silently co-infected with syphilis) and developed symptoms of syphilis, the dualists suffered a setback *(7)*. It was not until the 1830s that it became more widely accepted that there were two infections. This was conclusively verified when Albert Neisser isolated *Neis-*

seria gonococcus in 1879 and Fritz Schaudinn and Erich Hoffman identified the spirochete *Treponema pallidum* in 1905.

However, the story does not end there. These two infections helped to define the US approach to treatment for STIs for the next century. After World War I, veterans returned to American shores in large numbers with undiagnosed infections, which they then spread to their partners and offspring. The Chamberlain-Kahn Act was passed in 1918 requiring premarital serology testing for syphilis infection. Although not thoroughly appreciated at the time, the false-positive rate for that test was 25%, which undoubtedly upset many nuptial plans. Syphilis was epidemic. In 1937, the US surgeon general estimated that 10% of Americans would be infected with syphilis during their lives *(8)*. Case findings for gonorrhea and syphilis were introduced in most states in the 1930s as an attempt to curb their spread. With the discovery and mass production of penicillin, the war on each of those infections was thought to have been won. However, as the following chapters on each of those pathogens describe, gonorrhea, in particular, has returned many times and still presents considerable challenges to modern medicine.

Before the 1960s, syphilis and gonorrhea were the only major recognized STIs. It was not until the 1970s that *Chlamydia trachomatis* was recognized to have an important role in urethritis, cervicitis, and salpingitis. In the 1970s–1980s, the spread of herpes simplex virus type 2 (HSV-2) infection was noted. In 1981, acquired immune deficiency syndrome (AIDS) was identified, and later the human immunodeficiency virus was isolated. Genital warts were first recognized to be sexually transmitted in the 1950s *(9)*, but the involvement of HPV in squamous cell dysplasia and carcinoma was not recognized until the 1980s *(10)*.

The history of STIs reflects the influence of scientific understanding on ignorance and mysticism. However, in some countries today, we see a rejection of the scientific method as accepted criteria in favor of more obtuse explanations. In 2002, a senior official in the governing party of South Africa claimed that "HIV does not exist and cannot be spread through sexual intercourse, that AIDS drugs are deadly and that the epidemic itself is a fiction created by multinational drug companies hoping to boost their profits by forcing poor countries to buy AIDS drugs and by financing researchers to terrorize the public with lies about AIDS" *(11)*.

The scientific community is not immune to discomfort in discussing sexual issues. I remember once moderating a local group of clinicians who gathered along with similar groups across the nation to hear a panel of experts on HSV-2 and to discuss new advances in its treatment via satellite. During the question-and-answer period, the only question my group asked was how HSV-1 ever got "below the belt?" The response of this expert panel was astonishing; every panelist broke eye contact with the camera and had an overwhelming urge to straighten papers. One of them finally mumbled (without moving his lips), "I don't know." If we, as health care professionals cannot comfortably discuss oral–genital sexual practices or any of the other ways couples pleasure each other sexually, how can we ever effectively communicate with our patients about the STI risks associated with their sexual practices? How will our patients ever feel comfortable discussing their practices with us or asking important questions to protect their health?

The impact STIs have on world health is staggering. In many countries, STI surveillance systems exist, but the data are not always complete or reliable. The accuracy depends on the availability of STI services, the extent to which patients seek health care, the completeness of the reporting system, and the influence social stigmas associated with an STI impact on patients seeking diagnosis and treatment *(12)*. Even within the United States, not all states and territories provide information to the CDC about reportable diseases. In 1999, only 33% of the 58 diseases and conditions on the list for national surveillance (which includes STIs) were actually reportable in each of the 53 US states and territories *(13)*. The natural history of the infection also affects reporting, because many infections are asymptomatic.

At the end of 2005, an estimated 40.3 million individuals, including 2.3 million children younger than 15 years of age, were living with HIV worldwide. An estimated 4.9 million new infections developed during that year, representing 14,000 new infections each day—the greatest number in any 1 year since the beginning of the epidemic. Also in that year, 3.1 million people died as a result of HIV/AIDS-associated illnesses, including an estimated 570,000 children younger than 15 years *(14)*. In the United States in 2006, the CDC estimated that more than 1 million people were living with HIV infection; one-fourth of infected women were unaware of their infection *(15,16)*. Approximately 40,000 new cases of HIV infection occur each year in the United States, half of them in individuals younger than 25 years of age *(16,17)*.

Problems of other STIs are also growing, even in the face of effective therapies and programs designed to reduce the spread of infection. The WHO estimated that in 1999, 340 million new cases of syphilis, gonorrhea, chlamydia, and trichomoniasis occurred worldwide in men and women aged 15–49 years. By pathogen, the incidence (the number of new cases) of infection worldwide in 1999 was as follows:

- Chlamydia   92 million
- Gonorrhea   62 million
- Syphilis   12 million
- Trichomoniasis   174 million

The WHO noted many troubling patterns. In general, the prevalence of STIs tends to be higher in urban residents, unmarried individuals, and young (15–35 year old) adults. STIs tend to occur at a younger age in females than in males. Not all new cases were treated; the prevalence in 1999 of curable STIs among repro-

Table 2
Number of Cases of Sexually Transmitted Diseases Reported
by State Health Departments, United States 2004

Chlamydia	929,462
Gonorrhea	330,132
Acquired immunodeficiency syndrome	44,108
Syphilis	34,583

Source: Centers for Disease Control and Prevention. Summary
of notifiable diseases—United States, 2004. Published April 22,
2005, for MMWR 2003;52 (No. 54). From ref. *18*.

ductive-aged adults was estimated to be 116.5 million cases. In some regions, such as sub-Sahara Africa, the prevalence rate is 119 cases per 1000 adults; in Latin American and the Caribbean, that rate is 71 per 1000; and in South and Southeast Asia, the rate is 50 per 1000; at any one time, 5–12% of the population is infected.

In the United States, more than 65 million people are currently living with an incurable STI *(18)*. Rates of curable STIs in the United States are the highest in the developed world, and are higher than in some developing countries. One in 10 Americans will have an STI at some time during his or her life. The annual direct medical care costs of treating major STIs (excluding HIV) are approximately $13 billion. The IOM pointed out that the cost is shared by all Americans through higher health care costs and taxes. An additional 15 million people become infected with one or more STIs each year. Corey et al. reported in 2000 that 22% of the US population (45 million) had serological evidence that they had already been infected with HSV-2. This estimate does not include the millions who have HSV-1 genital herpes *(19)*. Infected individuals are often undiagnosed, whether they are asymptomatic or not. They serve as a large reservoir for spreading the infection. HSV has potentially serious consequences. It increases the infected individual's susceptibility to HIV infection. The infection can also be spread to the newborn *(20)*. The CDC National STD hotline receives about 60,000 herpes-related calls each year, almost as many as for all the other STIs combined *(21)*.

In the United States, nearly half of all STIs occur in people age 15 to 24. Weinstock et al. estimated that this most vulnerable group acquired 9.1 million new cases of STIs in 2002 (Table 3). This represents one-fourth of the ever-sexually active population aged 15–49 *(22)*. In a parallel study, Miller et al. tested 14,322 young adults aged 18–26 years and found that 4.19% had chlamydia and 0.43% were infected with gonorrhea with wide differences between ethnic group and genders (Table 4) *(23)*. The reported gonorrhea rate in the United States remains the highest of any industrialized country; it is about 50 times higher than

Table 3
Estimated Incidence of Selected STIs
Among 15- to 24-Year-Olds, United States 2000

Chlamydia	15 million
Gonorrhea	431,000
Syphilis	8200
Genital herpes	640,000
Humanpapilloma virus	46 million
Hepatitis B	7500
Tichomoniasis	19 million
Human immunodeficiency virus	15,000

From ref. 22.

Table 4
Prevalence of Chlamydia and Gonorrhea,
US Young Adults (18–26) 2001–2002

	Chlamydia (%)	Gonorrhea (%)
Overall prevalence	4.19	0.43
Women (all)	4.74	0.42
Men (all)	3.67	0.44
Women (Black)	13.95	1.91
Men (Black)	11.12	2.36
Women (White)	2.52	0.13
Men (White)	1.38	0.07
Women (Latino)	4.42	0.13
Men (Latino)	7.24	0.27

From ref. 23.

Sweden and 8 times that of Canada (18). One percent of the US population at any moment has external genital warts, but that is just the tip of the HPV iceberg; an estimated 20 million Americans have evidence of HPV infection. An additional 5.5 million people in the United States become infected each year with HPV.

Women, adolescents, and people of color are disproportionately affected by STIs and their consequences. Of women with gonorrhea or chlamydia, 10–20% will develop pelvic inflammatory disease; far fewer men develop upper genital tract involvement. Women are much more likely to develop cervical cancer from HPV infection than men are to develop penile carcinoma. Women are also more likely to develop health problems, such as infertility, ectopic pregnancy, and chronic pelvic pain from STIs. Half of all female infertility is the result of STIs (24). Herpes is more common in women (25%) than men

(20%). Only HIV and syphilis currently infect more men than women in the United States. Worldwide, HIV is equally prevalent in both genders. In developing countries, STIs and their complications are among the top five disease categories for which adults seek health care. In women of childbearing age, STIs (excluding HIV) are second only to maternal factors as cause of disease, death, and healthy life lost *(25)*.

Younger women are more likely to become infected with HPV and chlamydia if exposed to these agents than older women are, because younger women are biologically more vulnerable. Chlamydia preferentially infects the columnar cells of the cervix, which are found in abundance in the ectropion on the younger woman's cervix. In older women, the ectocervix has undergone squamous metaplasia and the columnar cells are sequestered much higher in the endocervical canal. Similarly, HPV infects rapidly dividing cells. Coital trauma is more frequent in newly sexually active women, so external genital warts are more likely to develop. The process of squamous metaplasia, which ultimately protects the cervix from chlamydia, requires more cellular division on the ectocervix in young women, which renders their cervices more vulnerable to acquiring HPV infection. Younger women are socially more vulnerable to infection because they may be more likely to have multiple sexual partners, unprotected intercourse, and they may select partners at higher risk—especially relatively older, experienced partners. In a Kaiser Family Foundation and *Seventeen Magazine* survey of adolescents, half of those who were sexually active said they knew someone with an STI *(26)*.

STIs have been pivotal in the development of infectious disease as a subspecialty. More recently, the role of sexually transmitted viral infections has been important to oncology, because cervical carcinoma has been found to require integration of fragments of high-risk human papilloma viral genome into the host DNA. HIV has shed light on the body's ongoing battle against transcription errors in everyday life as many HIV-infected, immunocompromised patients develop very uncommon malignancies.

Shameful experiments conducted on patients with STIs in the name of science helped highlight the need to recognize the rights of all human subjects who agree to participate in medical trials. The Tuskegee Syphilis Study was conducted by the US Public Health Service from 1932 to 1972 to determine the natural history of untreated syphilis in black American men. It was designed to see if cardiovascular disease was a more common sequelae of syphilis than neurological damage and to see if the outcomes were different in African-American men than in white men. The study was originally designed to last 6–9 months. Altogether, 412 infected subjects and 204 uninfected men were recruited; all were local poor African-American sharecroppers. Not one of the subjects was told that he had syphilis or even that he had a STI. Instead, the men were told they had "bad blood," which only later became a popular expression for syphilis. Prevailing treatment was offered (arsenic, bismuth, mercury). However, when that failed to produce results, treatment was stopped. The study was redesigned to follow the subjects until they died. Even when penicillin became available in the 1940s, antibiotic treatment was denied to the subjects for 25 years, during which time an estimated 100 of the men died of tertiary syphilis. The study ended when it was exposed in the *Washington Star*. The government settled a class action suit for $10 million. The case prompted Congress to pass legislation to require the creation of institutional review boards to review all studies involving human subjects.

It is important for the practicing clinician to be aware of the almost ubiquitous nature of STIs and the unspoken issues that exist (from the past and present), which may act as barriers to their detection, treatment, and, most importantly, prevention. This book provides solid clinical advice about the symptoms, clinical presentation, appropriate tests, and treatments for each of the individual STIs, and highlights the interaction between those infections. But it goes beyond more traditional discussions to offer information about some of the larger but often intangible challenges clinicians face in the office—how to obtain an accurate and thorough sexual history and how to deal with STIs in different cultural and ethnic groups. A glimpse of the hopeful future is provided in discussions of vaccines and microbicides.

Before these pathogen-specific chapters, it may be helpful to look at an overview of the challenges facing us today; there are human, technical, and organizational challenges. The human challenges include a lack of resources for health care, unsustainable population growth, risk-taking behaviors, and the low status of women.

In some of the sub-Saharan countries, where STI rates are highest, the per capita health care expenditures are only a few dollars a year. In the face of such abject poverty, STI testing and treatment are virtually impossible. Unfortunately, this poverty is often coupled with low literacy, so mass education programs to modify behaviors to prevent STI spread are not easily introduced. Population-based treatments may be helpful. Studies of monthly antibiotic therapy for female sex workers in Nairobi, Kenya found that such therapy lowered the incidence of STIs but did not reduce the incidence of HIV-1, which was already highly prevalent in the population *(27)*.

The rapid increase in worldwide population is important for several reasons. First, it demonstrates the staggering frequency of unprotected intercourse. Conception can happen only a few days during a woman's cycle, but transmission of infection can occur at any time. It is possible for STIs to spread more rapidly than *Homo sapiens* can procreate. Secondly, the rapid explosion in the number of human beings alters the world's demographics. Although there is a concern about the aging of America, the world population is now young, and it is the younger adults who are most vulnerable to acquiring and spreading STIs. Weinstock et al.

found that 48% of the 18.9 million new cases of STIs in the United States in 2001 were among persons aged 15–24, demonstrating that the burden of STIs is on younger people *(22)*. Based on the numbers of births in the last decade, it would be reasonable to expect a tremendous increase in STIs in the coming years.

The lack of recognition of risk and misinformation contribute to the spread of STIs. Lack of recognized risk is frequently cited as a reason for not using condoms. STIs are more apt to infect younger women because they have the least knowledge about reproductive health, the least skills in communicating with their partners about safer sex practices, and barriers to access to health services. In a survey of 500 sexually active African-American teenage girls from "high-risk, low-income" neighborhoods, 50% of respondents thought that all STIs were curable and that douching after sex could protect against STIs. Slightly less than one-half thought oil-based lubricants would reduce their HIV risk when used with condoms. One-third said they thought they "could always tell" if a partner had an STI *(28)*.

Risk-taking behaviors are an ever-present human element that we must acknowledge. Under the passion of the moment, people can make unwise decisions. Safer sex is not always the most enjoyable sex. Rapid worldwide travel spreads STIs, not only because it permits organisms to travel over international borders, but also because sexual inhibitions may be loosened in exotic lands. With the threat of AIDS, men who have sex with men (MSM) radically altered their behaviors in the 1980s and 1990s. As a result, the spread of HIV, as well as the spread of other STIs, dramatically slowed. However, with the introduction of antiretroviral agents, that threat has seemingly been reduced, and the safer sex message is being less well heeded. As a result, rates of syphilis and gonorrhea have increased markedly in MSMs *(29,30)*.

Unstable social conditions, marked by unrest and upheaval, such as those associated with war and population dislocation, are classically the situations in which STIs spread the most rapidly. This is the result of sexual risk-taking and the lack of available protection. Refugee camps with extraordinary poverty, overwhelming human suffering, rampant violence, and little long-term hope are also sites with high STI prevalence.

The low status of women in many cultures prevents women from protecting themselves from STIs. Lack of education and career opportunities forces a woman into one of two life paths—wife or prostitute. In South Africa, commercial sex workers have been beaten for requesting that their customers wear condoms. In areas of Southeast Asia, daughters are sold at a young age to groups pandering to HIV-infected tourists who believe that having sex with a virgin will cure their HIV infections. Those women who select marriage face other challenges to their health. Some young South Asian women have been reported to be at risk for violence in the form of suicide and "dowry murder"— the killing of a bride whose dowry has been found lacking *(31)*. In Kenya, STI prevalence among 20- to 24-year-olds is three times higher among women than men. Researchers report that the young women's physiological susceptibility and sexual relationships with older men contribute to their increased risk of infection; 12–25% of young women have partners more than a decade older than they are ("sugar daddies") *(32)*. In general, women with a history of forced sex are significantly more likely to practice higher-risk sex: a greater number of sexual partners and alcohol or drug use at last sex. Screening for past abuse may help identify high-risk women *(33)*.

At the microbiological level, we face organisms that are able to mutate and develop antibiotic resistance faster than we can develop new antibiotics to combat them. More than 10% of *Neisseria gonorrhoeae* specimens from the Pacific Islands, Hawaii, and California are resistant to quinolones and it is expected that resistance will rapidly spread. Growing numbers of strains of *Trichomonas vaginalis* are resistant to metronidazole. Cocktails of antiretroviral drugs are prescribed to slow the inevitable development of viral resistance in HIV infections.

At a technical level, we are hindered in our ability to detect infection. Recent studies have found that existing technologies for detecting Chlamydia infections (although better than prior tests) are still shockingly insensitive. In a recent study of nine different tests, specimen sources, and collection methods for screening of genital *C. trachomatis* infection in young women, the best tests had sensitivities of only 52–63%; some tests detected only 22% of cases *(34)*. Traditional microscopic evaluation of vaginal smears (the "wet mount") detects only 62% of women infected with trichomonas *(35)*. There are problems with clinicians who fail to perform appropriate microscopy testing to make correct diagnosis, and both over diagnosis (false-positive rate of about 50%) and missed diagnosis (sensitivity of about 50%) with current microscopic techniques. Ledger et al. observed that training in microscopy is inadequate ("at times, the high-power lens becomes only an effective tool for breaking cover slips") and there is inadequate reimbursement for those important services (which reduces the clinician's incentive to perform a test that is already made difficult by Clinical Laboratory Improvement Act regulations) *(36)*.

Even if perfect tests were available, surveys show that the use of tests is inadequate. Although the evidence is clear that routine screening of all sexually active women under age 26 for *C. trachomatis* prevents pelvic inflammatory disease and is cost effective, adherence to those practice guidelines is suboptimal *(23)*. HIV testing is rarely offered in emergency rooms or urgent care settings, where many at-risk individuals access health care services *(37)*. The introduction of over-the-counter (OTC) treatment for vulvovaginal candidiasis has lead to inappropriate and inadequate treatments. Ferris et al. found that of 95 women who had purchased OTC antifungal medication to treat self-diagnosed infections, only 33.7% were correct in their assessment *(38)*.

Even if infections are diagnosed correctly, patients do not always complete the course of treatment prescribed. For example, it is believed that one of the most significant reasons that *T. vaginalis* is developing resistance to metronidazole is that people rarely complete the recommended 7-day treatment course. One study found that only 25% of patients diagnosed with *C. trachomatis* took the 7-day course of doxycycline as directed, the same number took no medication at all, and 51% used some intermediate amount of medication. The author suggested that this behavior contributes to the persistence of infection *(39)*.

In 1996, the IOM published its report on prevention and control of STDs in the United States *(3)*. More than a decade ago, the IOM characterized STDs as hidden epidemics in the United States with tremendous health and economic consequences. The IOM concluded that an effective system to control and prevent STIs does not exist in the United States. Most STI programs are run by local health departments, which provide access primarily for patients with bacterial STIs (gonorrhea, syphilis) who need sex partner(s) notification and treatment. Little investment is made in networking with the many independent clinicians who care for the index patients. Even fewer resources are spent on community-based prevention programs.

We also need to reassess our case management approach to STI treatment. The focus should not only be on single-contact tracking, but should also evolve to identify the sexual networks that constitute the reservoir of infection responsible for recurrent and new infections *(40)*.

The US government funding and oversight is handled separately for family planning, STIs, and HIV. There are unexpected negative effects of single focus campaigns, such as the one aimed at AIDS. The message of condom use is important to reduce the spread of HIV. However, surveys done in 1994 and 1998 showed that many women abandoned their more effective contraceptive methods to rely on condoms, rather than adding condoms to their first method, because the concern for AIDS was not integrated into a pregnancy prevention program *(41)*.

The loss of support for the safer sex education programs in favor of the abstinence-only message does not protect young people *(42)*. Teens who pledge to remain virgins until marriage have the same rates of STIs as those who do not pledge abstinence *(43)*. Similarly, US AIDS policy internationally has dramatically altered recently to focus on the "ABC" message for adolescents and unmarried individuals. The message is "A" for abstinence; "B" for being faithful (for married individuals or those in committed relationships); and "C" for condom use (for individuals who engage in behavior that puts them at risk for HIV). Reflecting a shift away from prevention and toward treatment, no more than 20% of funding can be spent for HIV prevention programs. Moreover, according to the law, prevention funds may be appropriated to organizations that are not required to "endorse, utilize or participate in prevention method or treatment program" to which it has a religious or moral objection—such as condoms. The importance of birth control in slowing STI epidemics was highlighted by Reynolds et al., who demonstrated that at the same level of funding, a contraceptive strategy averts 26.8% more HIV-positive births than nevirapine for the prevention of mother-to-child HIV transmission *(43a)*.

There have been some hopeful developments in efforts to detect, treat, and prevent the spread of STIs. Technologically, there are new tests for many STIs, which are easier to administer. Urine-based testing for chlamydia and gonorrhea enables the screening of larger numbers of adolescents and pregnant women *(44)*. This is important for screening in settings in which exam rooms are not available, such as correctional facilities and schools. There are new office-based (but not Clinical Laboratory Improvement Act-waived) tests for bacterial vaginosis and trichomonas that do not rely on microscopy *(45)*. New rapid tests for HIV using saliva samples provide accurate information when the test is negative, but require confirmation with serum Western blot if positive. Rapid HIV testing has made major contributions to management of women in labor *(46)*, care given in the emergency room, determination of the need for therapy for the victims of needle-stick injuries, and effective counseling about a positive HIV test result. Patients appear more motivated to return for test results and effectively deal with their infection status if they have time to prepare themselves for bad news. Serological testing for HSV-2 infections may help identify those pregnant women who are at risk for acquiring infection in pregnancy and those who might benefit from suppressive therapies in the third trimester.

Newer treatment agents have helped reduce the spread of infection and the consequences of infection for the individual. Single-dose therapies have been helpful in reducing noncompliance. Gonorrhea, chlamydia, and trichomonas all have single-dose treatment options. Reducing the re-infection of the patient and the spread of STIs require that the sex partners of infected patients be treated epidemiologically and tested for other STIs. Some progress has been made in this area. New patterns of treatment delivery have proven helpful. In California, a law was passed allowing clinicians to prescribe single-dose azithromycin for the genital chlamydia-infected individual to deliver to one's partner(s) with instructions, in cases in which the expectation is that the partner would not seek recommended care *(47)*. New antiretroviral cocktails have rapidly reduced viral loads in HIV-infected people and slowed the progression to AIDS. Topical therapies that boost the immune system locally to identify and destroy cells infected with HPV (e.g., Imiquimod™) have reduced recurrence rates (and, potentially, contagiousness) *(48)*. The introduction of tinidazole to treat trichomonal infections will aid, at least temporarily, in the treatment of that protozoan *(49)*.

In the future, there is genuine hope that we will develop vaccines to prevent many STIs. Current STI vaccine research lags behind vaccines targeted against pathogens that infect other mucosal regions, such as the respiratory tract, but STI vaccine development has been slowed by an array of technical challenges, such as incomplete attenuation (HSV-2), accentuated immunopathology (*C. trachomatis*), poor immunogenicity (*T. palladium*), and broad antigenic heterogeneity (*N. gonorrhoeae*) (50). Lack of understanding of the host immune response has limited progress in developing a vaccine to prevent trichomoniasis (51). Research with protein antigens is promising. There is an effective vaccine against hepatitis B, although it needs to be offered more frequently to at-risk populations, such as individuals diagnosed with other STIs and inmates in correctional facilities (52). A quadrivalent vaccine against HPV 6, 11, 16, 18 is now available for women age 11–26 to significantly reduce the risk of many squamous cell cancers of the genital track, as well as genital warts. Vaccines for HSV-2 and CMV are under development. The original vaccine developed for HSV-2 was found to be effective only in HSV-1 and HSV-2 negative women (53). Clinical trials immunizing unexposed adolescent women are currently underway. Another promising avenue of prevention is seen in the development of microbicides, which are topical substances applied vaginally or rectally to reduce the risk of STI transmission and which may also have spermicidal activity. In contrast to male condoms, these agents are used by the recipient, who may be at risk. More than 60 such compounds have been studied to date (54).

Organizationally, there is a road map to follow to win the upper hand in the battle against STIs. Instead of focusing exclusively on secondary prevention (limitation of morbidity once the disease is present), investment in primary prevention (including personal protection against STDs) is needed (55). There have been localized attempts within the military to educate about safer sex practices, but the modern model for the broader population comes from the HIV program, which has done both population-oriented HIV risk reduction and case identification. Large managed care organizations are in a unique position to partner with the public health departments to provide effective primary prevention services (education) as well as secondary prevention services (detection) (56).

Integrating the reproductive health service programs may be necessary. Initiating contraception (especially emergency contraceptive pills and condoms) in the STI clinics reduces both unintended pregnancy and STI transmission in the short run. Condom use has been shown to reduce transmission of fluid-borne infections. More recently, condoms have also been shown to decrease HSV transmission—an infection typically spread by skin-to-skin contact (57). Experience has shown that many different prevention strategies and messages must be developed to reach different age, ethnic, literary, and cultural groups. Small-scale studies have shown success when the messages of safer sex and HIV prevention are gender-tailored, concrete, and culturally supportive (58).

It has been almost a decade since the National Commission on Adolescent Sexual Health released its report and recommended a move toward a sexual health program, which integrated family planning, HIV, and STI programs. This integration will take considerable effort, because the focus of each program is substantially different (59). STI clinics tend to operate in a reactive mode— generally after a person has become infected. The intervention in STI clinics is short-lived and includes diagnosis and treatment of the infected person and, hopefully, identification and treatment of his sex partner(s). Men tend to predominate as clients. Perhaps because of this orientation, one study found that in STI clinics providing contraceptive methods that were more effective than condoms, pregnancy rates were not reduced (60). In family-planning clinics, women are more likely to be the clients and the relationship is longer term and, generally, preventive. HIV clinics evolved with a third culture. The problems and risks of unprotected sex, unintended pregnancy, and STIs are linked, but the "dual protection" message against unintended pregnancy and STI/HIV may not be sufficient. A more comprehensive model of "triple protection" is needed, which includes safeguarding of fertility and avoidance of infertility caused by STIs and unsafe obstetrical practices (61).

In its landmark work on STIs, the IOM noted that these infections are "hidden from the public view because many Americans are reluctant to address sexual health issues in an open way and because of the biological and social factors associated with these diseases" (3). What will make the most difference in our ability to combat the challenges of STIs will be a profound change in our society's attitude toward human sexuality. Rather than being a shameful, taboo subject associated with profane words, we need to develop a language to discuss sexuality positively and professionally. We need to stop considering sex as a dirty act with dire consequences (the "scare them straight" approach), but instead promote an image of healthy sex as worth waiting for and worth protecting. A great step toward this goal was taken by Surgeon General David Satcher, in his Call to Arms to Promote Sexual Health and Responsible Behavior 2001 when he wrote, "Sexuality is an integral part of human life. It carries the awesome potential to create new life. It can foster intimacy and bonding as well as a shared pleasure in our relationships. It fulfills a number of personal and social needs, and we value the sexual part of our being for the pleasures and benefits it afford us. Yet when exercised irresponsibly, it can also have negative aspects such as sexually transmitted diseases including HIV/AIDS, unintended pregnancy, and coercive or violent behavior. To enjoy the important benefits of sexuality, while avoiding negative consequences, some of which may have long-term or even lifetime implications, it is necessary for individuals to be sexually healthy, to behave responsibly, and to have a supportive environment—to protect their own sexual health, as well as that of others" (62).

Satcher presents a positive vision for us to embrace as health care providers and to share with our patients. However, as Welling et al. remind us, "No general approach to sexual health promotion will work everywhere, and no single-component intervention will work anywhere. We need to know not only whether interventions work, but why and how they do so in particular social contexts. Comprehensive behavioral interventions are needed that take account of the social context, attempt to modify social norms to support uptake and mainte- nance of behavioral change, and tackle the structural factors that contribute to risky sexual behavior" *(62a)*.

RESOURCES

- American Social Health Association
  This organization is dedicated to stopping STIs and their harmful consequences to individuals, families, and communities and provides updated telephone numbers for other resources.
  P.O. Box 13827
  Research Triangle Park, NC 27709
  Phone: 800-227-8922
  Web site: http://www.ashastd.org
- CDC National STD/AIDS Hotline
  This hotline provides anonymous, confidential information on STIs and how to prevent them. It also provides referrals to clinical and other services. Service is available in English 24 hours a day, 7 days a week; in Spanish 8 AM until 2 am, Eastern time, 7 days a week; and via TTY for the deaf and hard of hearing 10 AM until 10 PM, Eastern time, Monday through Friday.
  Phone: 800-342-AIDS (English)
           800-344-7432 (Spanish)
  TTY: 800-243-7889
- CDC National Prevention Information Network
  This is the US reference, referral, and distribution service for information on HIV/AIDS, STIs, and tuberculosis (in English and Spanish). 9 AM until 8 PM Eastern time, Monday through Friday.
  PO Box 6003
  Rockville, MD 20849-6003
  Phone: 800-458-5231; International: 919-361-4892
  TTY: 800-243-7012; International: 919-361-4884
  Web site: http://www.cdcnpin.org
- The Henry J. Kaiser Family Foundation
  This foundation is an independent philanthropy focusing on the major health care issues facing the nation. The Foundation is an independent voice and source of facts and analysis for policymakers, the media, the health care community, and the public. It publishes fact sheets, issue updates, and research.
  2400 Sand Hill Road
  Menlo Park, CA 94025
  Phone: 650-854-9400
  Web site: http://www.kff.org

- Sexuality Information and Education Council of the US (SIECUS)
  SIECUS' mission is to affirm that sexuality is a natural and healthy part of living; to develop, collect, and disseminate information; to promote comprehensive education about sexuality; and to advocate the right of individuals to make responsible sexual choices.
  130 West 42nd Street, Suite 350
  New York, NY 10036-7802
  Phone: 212-819-9770
  Web site: http://www.siecus.org

REFERENCES

1. World Health Organization. Guidelines for the management of sexually transmitted infec tions. Geneva: World Health Organization, 2003. Available from: http://www.who.int/repro-ductive-health/publications/rhr_01_10_mngt_stis/index.html. Accessed Nov. 24, 2006.
2. Centers for Disease Control and Prevention. Sexually transmitted diseases treatment guide-lines, 2006. MMWR Recomm Rep 2006; 55(RR-11):1–11. Available from: http://www.cdc.gov/std/treatment/. Accessed Nov. 24, 2006.
3. Eng TR, Butler WE, eds; Committee on Prevention and Control of Sexually Transmitted Diseases, Institute of Medicine. The Hidden Epidemic: Confronting Sexually Transmitted Diseases. Washington, DC: National Academy Press, 1997.
4. American Social Health Association. Sexually Transmitted Diseases in America: How Many Cases and at What Cost? Menlo Park, CA: Kaiser Family Foundation, 1998. Available from: http://www.ashastd.org/pdfs/std_rep.pdf. Accessed Nov. 24, 2006.
5. Nance B. Review of the book: Arrizabalaga J, Henerson J, French R. *The Great Pox: The French Disease in Renaissance Europe*. New Haven and London: Yale University Press, 1997. J Social History 1998; Summer. Available from: http://www.findarticles.com/p/articles/mi_m2005/is_n4_v31/ai_20870428. Accessed Nov. 24, 2006.
6. McNeill WH. Confluence of the civilized disease pools of Eurasia. *Plagues and People*. New York, NY: Doubleday, 1977, pp. 157–160.
7. Benson PM. Sexually transmitted diseases. In: *Military Dermatology*. Falls Church, VA: Department of the Army, Office of The Surgeon General, Borden Institute, 1994, p. 498.
8. Golden MR, Marra CM, Holmes KK. Update on syphilis: resurgence of an old problem. JAMA 2003; 290:1510–1514.
9. Barrett TJ, Silbar JD, McGinley JP. Genital warts—a venereal disease. JAMA 1954; 154: 333–334.
10. Meisels A, Morin C. Human papillomavirus and cancer of the uterine cervix. Gynecol Oncol 1981; 12:S111–S123.
11. Swarns RL. An AIDS skeptic in South Africa feeds simmering doubts. New York Times, March 31, 2002; Section 1:4–6.
12. World Health Organization. Global prevalence and incidence of selected curable sexually transmitted infections: overview and estimates. Geneva: World Health Organization, 2001. Available from: http://www.who.int/hiv/pub/sti/who_hiv_aids_2001.02.pdf. Accessed Nov. 24, 2006.
13. Roush S, Birkhead G, Koo D, Cobb A, Fleming D. Mandatory reporting of diseases and conditions by health care professionals and laboratories. JAMA 1999; 282:164–170.
14. World Health Organization. Global summary of the AIDS epidemic, December 2006. In the AIDS epidemic update, December 2006 Geneva: World Health Organization, 2006, pp. 1–2.

Available from: http://www.who.int/hiv/mediacentre/news62/en/index.html. Accessed Nov. 24, 2006.
15. Centers for Disease Control and Prevention. HIV and AIDS—United States, 1981–2000. MMWR Morb Mortal Wkly Rep 2001; 50:430–434. Available from: http://www.cdc.gov/mmwr/preview/mmwrhtml/mm5021a2.htm. Accessed May 6, 2005.
16. Centers for Disease Control and Prevention. Twenty-five years of HIV/AIDS—United States, 1981–2006. MMWR Morb Mortal Wkly Rep 2006; 55:585–589.
17. Centers for Disease Control and Prevention. HIV prevention in the third decade: Activities of CDC's divisions in HIV/AIDS prevention. Atlanta, GA: U. S. Department of Health and Human Services, 2005. Available from: http://www.cdc.gov/hiv/reports/hiv3rddecade/index.htm. Accessed Nov. 24, 2006.
18. Centers for Disease Control and Prevention. HIV/AIDS surveillance report: Cases of HIV infection and AIDS in the United States, 2004. Vol. 16. Atlanta, GA: U. S. Department of Health and Human Services, 2005. Available from:http://www.cdc.gov/hiv/topics/surveillance/resources/reports/2004report/default.htm. Accessed Nov. 24, 2006.
19. Corey L, Handsfield HH. Genital herpes and public health: addressing a global problem. JAMA 2000; 283:791–794.
20. Brown Z. Preventing herpes simplex virus transmission to the neonate. Herpes 2004; 11:175A–186A.
21. Centers for Disease Control and Prevention. Trends of Reportable Sexually Transmitted Diseases in the United States, 2004: National Surveillance Data for Chlamydia, Gonorrhea, and Syphilis. Atlanta, GA: U. S. Centers for Disease Control and Prevention, 2005. Available from:http://www.cdc.gov/std/stats. Accessed Nov. 24, 2006.
22. Weinstock H, Berman S, Cates W Jr. Sexually transmitted diseases among American youth: incidence and prevalence estimates, 2000. Perspect Sex Reprod Health 2004; 36:6–10.
23. Miller WC, Ford CA, Morris M, et al. Prevalence of chlamydial and gonococcal infections among young adults in the United States. JAMA 2004; 291:2229–2236.
24. Dupont J. Every six seconds. Sexually transmitted diseases on the increase. IDRC Rep 1984; 13:18–19.
25. World Bank. World Development Report 1993: Investing in Health. New York, NY: Oxford University Press, 1993. Available from: http://www-wds.worldbank.org/servlet/WDS_IBank_Servlet?pcont=details&eid=000009265_3970716142319. Accessed Nov. 24, 2006.
26. The Henry J. Kaiser Family Foundation and Seventeen Magazine. Sexually Transmitted Disease: A Series of National Surveys of Teens About Sex. Menlo Park, CA: The Henry J. Kaiser Family Foundation, 2001. Available from: http://www.kff.org/entpartnerships/seventeen_surveys.cfm. Accessed Nov. 24, 2006.
27. Kaul R, Kimani J, Nagelkerke NJ, et al. Monthly antibiotic chemoprophylaxis and incidence of sexually transmitted infections and HIV-1 infection in Kenyan sex workers: a randomized controlled trial. JAMA 2004; 291:2555–2562.
28. Reuters Health. Survey shows need for STD knowledge. SIECUS Report. 2001; 30:13.
29. Katz MH, Schwarcz SK, Kellogg TA, et al. Impact of highly active antiretroviral treatment on HIV seroincidence among men who have sex with men: San Francisco. Am J Public Health 2002; 92:388–394.
30. Centers for Disease Control and Prevention (CDC). Trends in primary and secondary syphilis and HIV infections in men who have sex with men—San Francisco and Los Angeles, California, 1998–2002. MMWR Morb Mortal Wkly Rep 2004; 53:575–578.
31. Fikree FF, Pasha O. Role of gender in health disparity: the South Asian context. BMJ 2004; 328:823–826.
32. Longfield K, Glick A, Waithaka M, Berman J. Relationships between older men and younger women: implications for STIs/HIV in Kenya. Stud Fam Plann 2004; 35:125–134.

33. Upchurch DM, Kusunoki Y. Associations between forced sex, sexual and protective practices, and sexually transmitted diseases among a national sample of adolescent girls. Womens Health Issues 2004; 14:75–84.
34. Shrier LA, Dean D, Klein E, Harter K, Rice PA. Limitations of screening tests for the detection of Chlamydia trachomatis in asymptomatic adolescent and young adult women. Am J Obstet Gynecol 2004; 190:654–662.
35. Landers DV, Wiesenfeld HC, Heine RP, Krohn MA, Hillier SL. Predictive value of the clinical diagnosis of lower genital tract infection in women. Am J Obstet Gynecol 2004; 190:1004–1010.
36. Ledger WJ, Monif GR. A growing concern: inability to diagnose vulvovaginal infections correctly. Obstet Gynecol. 2004; 103:782–784.
37. Centers for Disease Control and Prevention (CDC). Voluntary HIV testing as part of routine medical care—Massachusetts, 2002. MMWR Morb Mortal Wkly Rep 2004; 53: 523–526.
38. Ferris DG, Dekle C, Litaker MS. Women's use of over-the-counter antifungal medications for gynecologic symptoms. J Fam Pract 1996; 42:595–600.
39. Augenbraun M, Bachmann L, Wallace T, Dubouchet L, McCormack W, Hook EW III. Compliance with doxycycline therapy in sexually transmitted diseases clinics. Sex Transm Dis 1998; 25:1–4.
40. Bernstein KT, Curriero FC, Jennings JM, Olthoff G, Erbelding EJ, Zenilman J. Defining core gonorrhea transmission utilizing spatial data. Am J Epidemiol 2004; 160:51–58.
41. Bajos N, Warszawski J, Gremy I, Ducot B. AIDS and contraception. Unanticipated effects of AIDS prevention campaigns. Eur J Public Health 2001; 11:257–259.
42. Cagampang HH, Barth RP, Korpi M, Kirby D. Education Now and Babies Later (ENABL): life history of a campaign to Postpone Sexual Involvement. Fam Plann Perspect 1997; 29: 109–114.
43. Bruckner H, Bearman P. After the promise: the STD consequences of adolescent virginity pledges. J Adolesc Health 2005; 36:271–278.
43a. Reynolds HW, Janowitz B, Homan R, Johnson L. The value of contraception to prevent perinatal HIV transmission. Sex Transm Dis 2006; 33:350–356.
44. Blake DR, Woods ER. The future is here: noninvasive diagnosis of STDs in teens. Contemp OB/GYN 2001; Mar:103,104,106,109,113,116,121.
45. Myziuk L, Romanowski B, Johnson SC. BVBlue test for diagnosis of bacterial vaginosis. J Clin Microbiol 2003; 41:1925–1928.
46. Bulterys M, Jamieson DJ, O'Sullivan MJ, et al. Rapid HIV-1 testing during labor: a multicenter study. JAMA 2004; 292:219–223.
47. California Department of Health Services. Patient-delivered therapy of antibiotics for chlamydia trachomatis: guidance for medical providers in California. Berkeley, CA: California Department of Health Services STD Control Branch, 2001. Available from: http://www.dhs.ca.gov/ps/dcdc/STD/docs/PDT_GUIDELINES_19.pdf. Accessed June 5, 2005.
48. Gunter J. Genital and perianal warts: new treatment opportunities for human papillomavirus infection. Am J Obstet Gynecol 2003; 189:S3–S11.
49. Gulmezoglu AM, Garner P. Trichomoniasis treatment in women: a systematic review. Trop Med Int Health 1998; 3:553–558.
50. Fletcher MA. Vaccine candidates in STD. Int J STD AIDS 2002; 13:38–41.
51. Petrin D, Delgaty K, Bhatt R, Garber G. Clinical and microbiological aspects of Trichomonas vaginalis. Clin Microbiol Rev 1998; 11:300–317.
52. Neff MJ, CDC. CDC updates guidelines for prevention and control of infections with hepatitis viruses in correctional settings. Am Fam Physician 2003; 67:2620, 2622, 2625.

53. Stanberry LR, Spruance SL, Cunningham AL, et al. Glycoprotein-D-adjuvant vaccine to prevent genital herpes. N Engl J Med 2002; 347:1652–1661.
54. Alliance for Microbicide Development. Available from http://www.microbicide.org/. Accessed Nov. 24, 2006.
55. Stone KM, Grimes DA, Magder LS. Personal protection against sexually transmitted diseases. Am J Obstet Gynecol 1986; 155:180–188.
56. Gunn RA, Rolfs RT, Greenspan JR, Seidman RL, Wasserheit JN. The changing paradigm of sexually transmitted disease control in the era of managed health care. JAMA 1998; 279: 680–684.
57. Wald A, Langenberg AG, Link K, et al. Effect of condoms on reducing the transmission of herpes simplex virus type 2 from men to women. JAMA 2001; 285:3100–3106.
58. DiClemente RJ, Wingood GM, Harrington KF, et al. Efficacy of an HIV prevention intervention for African American adolescent girls: a randomized controlled trial. JAMA 2004; 292:171–179.
59. Kempner ME. True Integration of Prevention Programs Required Broad Focus on Sexual Health. SIECUS Rep. 2003; 31:5–7.
60. Shlay JC, Mayhugh B, Foster M, Maravi ME, Baron AE, Douglas JM Jr. Initiating contraception in sexually transmitted disease clinic setting: a randomized trial. Am J Obstet Gynecol 2003; 189:473–481.
61. Brady M. Preventing sexually transmitted infections and unintended pregnancy, and safeguarding fertility: triple protection needs of young women. Reprod Health Matters 2003; 11:134–141.
62. Office of the Surgeon General. The Surgeon General's call to action to promote sexual health and responsible sexual behavior. Rockville, MD:2001. Available from: http://www.surgeongeneral.gov/library/sexualhealth/default.htm. Accessed Nov. 24, 2006.
62a. Wellings K, Collumbien M, Slaymaker E, et al. Sexual behavior in context: a global perspective. Lancet 2006; 368:1706–1728.

2

Human Papillomavirus and Genital Warts

Linda Goldman

INTRODUCTION

Unknown until the second half of the 20th century, human papillomavirus (HPV) is now recognized as being one of the most common sexually transmitted infections (STI) in the United States, accounting for more than one-third of the new cases of STIs each year *(1)*. HPV is a group of more than 120 viruses, at least 30 types of which can infect the anogenital areas. Most HPV infections cause no symptoms, other types can cause genital warts, and still others cause invasive squamous cell anogenital carcinoma. The total health care costs for HPV related disease in 1998 were estimated to be $3.4 billion, two-thirds of which were spent on prevention and screening *(2)*. This chapter provides an overview of HPV infection—its transmissibility and epidemiology. It focuses on genital warts in its discussion of the clinical consequences of HPV infection. The contribution HPV infection makes to various genital cancers is mentioned, but the screening, diagnosis, and treatments of these conditions are outside the scope of this book.

FAST FACTS

- HPV is one of the most common STI in United States.
- About 70% of sexually active people acquire the infection at sometime during one's lives.
- Most people infected with HPV clear the infection spontaneously within 3 years.
- HPV can infect the genital skin and epithelium of the vagina, cervix, rectum, and urethra. Nongenital infections are also possible.
- Genital warts can result from initial, recurrent, or persistent HPV infection.
- Virtually all squamous cell cancer of the cervix results from persistent HPV infection, with high-risk HPV types.

From: *Current Clinical Practice: Sexually Transmitted Diseases:*
A Practical Guide for Primary Care
Edited by: A. L. Nelson and J. A. Woodward © Humana Press, Totowa, NJ

PREVALENCE/INCIDENCE

Precise estimates of the incidence of HPV infection are not available for several reasons. First, HPV is not a reportable disease. Additionally, most infections are subclinical. Of the patients who develop findings with HPV infection, most have only indirect indication of infections, such as abnormal cervical cytology. In patients who have more obvious manifestations of infection, such as external genital warts, no formal testing is done to document the presence of HPV. Finally, HPV also causes recurrent outbreaks of lesions. Because most first infections are asymptomatic, it may be difficult to recognize new cases from recurrent infections, which must be done to calculate incidence.

Prevalence of HPV infection is also difficult to estimate. The usual technique used to estimate the number of people infected with HPV is to measure serum antibodies. However, most people who acquire the viral infection, clear that infection within 1–2 years; others may harbor the infection for years without outbreaks; others will have obvious recurrences. Some people in these groups will have positive antibody titers, so that antibodies may overstate the number of people who are currently infected (prevalence) (3). Confusing the situation even further is the fact that only 50% of individuals infected with HPV will develop detectable antibody titers to the virus, which could underestimate prevalence.

Despite these limitations, several studies performed over the past 20 years have demonstrated a steady rise in the number of new cases of genital HPV. The number of office visits for genital HPV disease has increased over the last 30 years. It has been estimated that about 15% (20–24 million) of adults in the United States are currently infected with this virus; 9.2 million of them are between the ages of 15–24 years (3–6). The prevalence of HPV infection among sexually active college women over a 3-year period has been reported to be over 40%; the greatest prevalence is among women with 3 or more lifetime partners or partners with 2 or more lifetime sexual partners (7–9). Approximately 80% of all women will have acquired this infection with at least one subtype of HPV by age 50 (5,10).

Studies that have used sensitive polymerase chain reaction (PCR) to detect latent HPV DNA in healthy men have found that penile HPV infection rates in sexually active men are at least as high as cervical HPV infection rates are in women (11). Among men seen in one sexually transmitted disease (STD) clinic, the prevalence of HPVrates was 28.2%; oncognic HPV was found in 12%. Interestingly, HPV positivity was not associated with age, as it is in women (11). In a second study, HPV DNA was found on the cotton swab of only 1.3% of healthy male volunteers but was found in of 18.5% of men who had urethritis but no penile lesions (12).

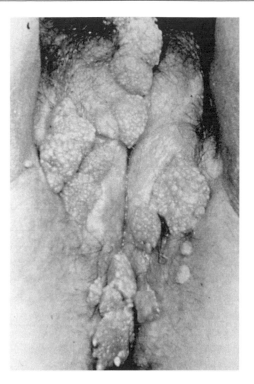

Female labia with extensive vulvar condylomata accuminata.

Investigators have found that between 5.5 and 6.2 million Americans become newly infected each year, with 4.6 million of these being young adults between the ages of 15–24. Most (70%) of women acquire HPV with onset of coital activity *(13)*. The rate of new HPV infection was 2.9% per month among women age 18–35 years of age seen for routine gynecological care in a family-planning clinic *(14)*.

It is estimated that 500,000–1 million new cases of genital warts occur each year. The prevalence of genital warts is higher; they can be found in almost 17% of the population or 1.4 million people *(15)*. This infection prompts at least 600,000 outpatient visits each year *(16)*. Women are more likely to seek care for genital warts than men are; over two-thirds of condyloma-related visits are for women *(17)*.

The Center for Disease Control and Prevention (CDC) is currently conducting a US population study and clinic-based studies to determine the epidemiology of genital HPV infection more accurately. The results of these studies are expected to yield much-needed information on actual incidence and prevalence of HPV *(3)*.

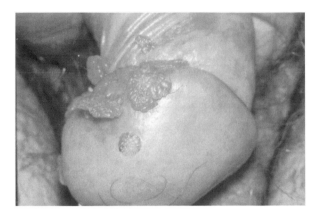

Penile genital warts.

RISK FACTORS

Acquisition of HPV is clearly related to coital activity. The highest risk groups for new infection are sexually active adolescents under the age of 19, followed by adults aged 19–30 *(18)*. The risk of HPV infection increases with number of lifetime sex partners. In one study, patients with 10 or more partners were found to have 58% current infection rates compared with an 8% rate in those with zero or one partner *(19)*. Risk factors for HPV acquisition are similar to those for other STIs, and include multiple recent sex partners and changing sex partners in the last year. Co-infection with other STDs and early age at first intercourse increase the risk of HPV infection. Expression of the virus and clearance of viral infection are related to immunocompetence of the host. Human immunodeficiency virus (HIV) infection increases the risk of HPV infection and the risk of developing HPV-related disease. All of the factors that predispose to persistent infection (those infections that do not clear) have not been elucidated. Persistent infections are associated with recurrent wart outbreaks and increased the risk of HPV-related malignancy.

INFECTIVITY AND TRANSMISSION

HPV is most commonly transmitted during sexual activity, which involves skin-to-skin contact; microabrasions in the area of contact permit the virus to be transmitted from one sexual partner to another. Transmission can occur whether or not any visible lesions exist. Even in the absence of visible lesions, such as a genital wart, the microabrasions expose the HPV-infected cells in the basal epithelium of the host and increase viral shedding. More importantly, microabrasions in the recipient expose vulnerable basal epithelial cells to the virus. About 60–66% of sex partners of HPV-infected people will develop

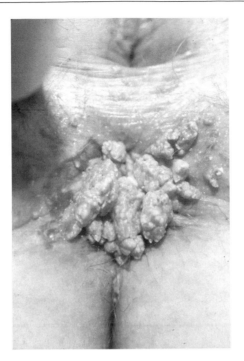

Perianal genital warts.

detectable HPV lesions, although they may be very subtle appearing or may be located in areas that escape normal detection *(20)*. About 50–55% of men whose partners have cervical HPV disease have HPV-associated penile lesions *(21)*. HPV can also be transmitted from one woman to another *(22)*.

Oral-genital contact can transmit infection. Early studies suggested that about 4% of women with external genital warts also had buccal lesions. High-risk HPV has been found in about 25% of oral cancers, supporting hypothesis there is some transmission via that route *(23)*.

Perianal infection is quite common. Transmission is possible in men and women who have anal receptive sex with men. However, the presence of genital warts around the anus does not necessarily indicate a history of receptive anal intercourse. In one study, only 10% of women who shed HPV from the anal area admitted to having anal intercourse, and 83% of those with anal virus had it in the cervix, vulva, and vaginal samples too *(24)*. The virus is found in all tissue around the genitalia; the warm, moist environment of the perianal region may be a favorable environment for growth *(25)*.

The virus can also be transmitted by fomites. Transmission of the virus to the anogenital area has been reported in tanning beds and saunas. Other nondirect

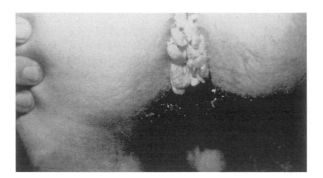

Perianal genital warts.

transmission may be possible via sex toys, exam tables, door knobs, and contamination of exam lights adjusted by examining hands *(26)*.

Vertical transmission from mother to her newborn is possible during delivery through an infected birth canal. The most serious infection that occurs is respiratory/laryngeal papillomatosis. Genital warts and facial lesions in the infant can also result from exposure during delivery.

ETIOLOGY

Papillomaviruses infect many animal species including cotton-tail rabbits, cattle, and humans. They are named and classified by their natural host. More than 120 different types of *human* papillomaviruses have been identified, but some have only been partially sequenced. HPV types are assigned new numbers when there is more than a 10% difference in gene sequences in particular regions of the viral DNA (regimens E6, E7, and L1). The types are numbered in their order of discovery.

All known HPV share a similar structure and genomic organization. They are small, nonenveloped virions with a double-stranded, circular DNA of 7800–7900 base pairs encased in an icosahedral protein capsid. They demonstrate great specificity in the anatomical locations they infect and the types of lesions they produce. At least 30 different types of HPV infect the human anogenital tract. Concurrent infection with more than one type of HPV is common.

The usual reservoirs of genital HPV infection are the moist mucosa and adjacent squamous epithelia of the male and female genitalia, the cervix, and the anus. Microabrasions that develop during sexual activity enable the infected partner to shed virus and the uninfected partner to become more susceptible to infection. Repeated trauma in the area increases infectivity as wound healing stimulates cell division, increasing episomal viral replication *(27)*. The virus enters the basal epithelial cells in areas such as the inner labia minora in woman and the prepuce and frenulum in men. Anal epithelium is also traumatized easily during sex, permitting HPV infection. The virus also preferentially infects the rapidly dividing cells within the transitional zone of the cervix.

After introduction of the virus into the host basal epithelial cells, the virus sheds its protein capsule and co-exists within the host cell as a circular episome. Infected host cells often have a characteristic microscopic appearance called *koilocytosis* after the Greek word for hollow. The nucleus of the infected cell is distorted and pushed aside by the vacuole in the cytoplasm in which the viral episome resides.

After initial infection, virus enters into a latent incubation period of 1–8 months, during which time there are no visible manifestations of the infection. The active growth phase starts when the first lesion develops. It is not known what induces the transition from latent to infective stage, but many host, viral, and environmental factors are involved. During the active infection phase, the HPV replicates independent of host cell division and induces the host cells to proliferate, creating a myriad of lesions from flat to papillary warts. Viral counts are highest in the superficial layers of the epithelium, increasing infectivity. During this phase, patients generally seek therapy. Approximately 3 months later, the host immune system mounts a response. The innate immune system is recruited and interferons slow HPV replication and trigger the cell-mediated immune response. An immunocompetent cell-mediated immune system and cytokine (interferons α, β, and γ and interleukins) production are needed for HPV clearance, but there are still challenges to viral clearance in immunocompetent hosts. HPV has some protection from the host response because the virus is intracellarly located. In addition, the epithelial cells in the perineum do not present antigens well to the host, so the HPV may not be recognized by the immune system *(28)*. HPV blocks the host response by depleting local intraepithelial lymphocytes, Langerhan's cells, and CD4+ cells and down regulating cytokine production *(27)*. However, lysis of the infected cells exposes the HPV to the host and triggers more intense defense.

About 80–90% of people will clear the infection so that the virus can no longer be detected. Only 10–20% of individuals will have persistent infection that can express itself either as a latent infection, which may be periodically reactivated, or as a persistent (and more difficult to treat) infection. Recurrences are more likely when host immune system is compromised by chemotherapy, corticosteroid therapy, or HIV infection.

HPV DNA testing now permits identification of classes of viral types in clinical practice *(29)*. In general, genital HPV types have been classified into two groups based on the oncogenic potential—low- and intermediate/high-risk groups (*see* Table 1). The low-risk types (mainly 6 and 11) are responsible for almost half of the external genital warts. However, mixed viral types may be involved in the wart formation. The low-risk viral types have also been isolated from the lesions involved in laryngeal papillomatosis/respiratory papillomatosis

Table 1
Low-Risk vs High-Risk HPV Types

Low-risk HPV types: *Possess little to no oncogenic potential*	High-risk HPV types: *Possess oncogenic potential*
HPV 6, 11, 40, 42, 43, 44, 54, 61, 70, 72, 81, and CP6108	HPV 16, 18, 31, 33, 35, 39, 45, 51, 52, 56, 58, 59, 68, 73, 82, and probably 26, 53, 66
Most commonly found on the external genitalia	Most commonly found as flat warts
Primarily responsible for external genital warts	Primarily responsible for intraepithelial neoplasias of the cervix, anus
Also responsible for juvenile respiratory papillomatosis	Also responsible for penile and anal carcinoma

(Adapted from ref. *32a*.)
HPV, human papilloma virus.

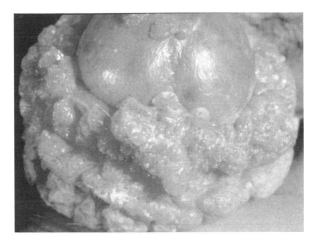

Penile genital warts.

in the tracheobronchial trees of children *(30,31)*. The high-risk HPV types are primarily involved in the development of squamous cell cancerous lesions of the uterine cervix, anus, vulva, and penis *(20,25,32)*, but also contribute to external genital warts. Four HPV types (6, 11, 16, and 18) account for 90% of genital warts. Only 1 in 1000 unscreened women with HPV infection will develop invasive cervical cancer.

CLINICAL MANIFESTATIONS

Genital warts can be found on the external genitalia, the vagina, cervix, anus, mouth, and larynx. Most patients with genital warts are asymptomatic. In a study of university women, neither acute nor persistent HPV infection (documented by viral shedding) was associated with discharge, itching, burning, soreness, or fissure *(24)*. Even women with genital warts had none of the associated symptoms. Patients with external genital warts may complain of a bump or mass they palpate or see on inspection. Infected or large lesions may be tender or associated with spotting, odor, or tenderness. Larger internal warts may produce dyspareunia or postcoital spotting. Urethral lesions may impair flow of urine or ejaculate. Condyloma acuminata are the classical external genital warts. They are raised, acuminate, exophytic lesions, which on keratinized skin are white, gray, or flesh-colored warty lesions. On mucosal surfaces, low-risk HPV tends to have finger-like projections and blend in color with surrounding tissue.

Another presentation of HPV in the genital area are papillomas. Papillomas are raised, possibly pigmented lesions, which are slow-growing and sometimes pedunculated. They are often mistaken for skin tags or moles and are most commonly found on keratinized skin.

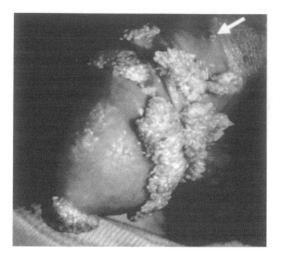

Condylomata accuminata.

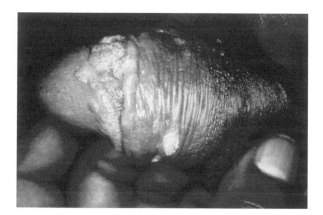

Penile genital warts.

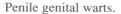

The high-risk HPV usually causes flat genital warts. They may be hyperpig-mented, white or red, depending on the impact HPV has on local melanocytes.

In men, genital warts are the only STD to be associated with penile HPV infection. However, only 46% of men with genital warts tested positive for HPV from the urethra, coronal sulcus, and glans penis (but not necessarily from the lesion) *(11)*.

In women, external warts may present anywhere on the vulva, perineum, and perianal area. External genital warts in men may involve the squamous epidermis of the penis, foreskin, scrotum, perineum, and perianal area. Internal warts affect

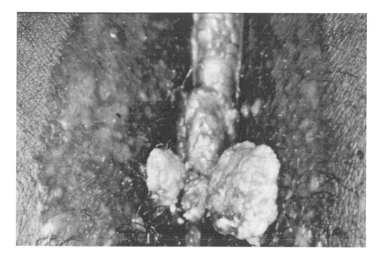

Condylomata lata.

the mucous membranes of the urethra, anus, vagina, and oral cavity. Squamous cells on the cervix can also be involved as can the transitional epithelium of the urethra. Warts are most commonly located over areas that receive friction during coitus and therefore are found near the posterior fourchette of the vulva in women and around the corona of the penis in men. Oral HPV lesions are not common, but can be found in women with external genital warts.

The differential diagnosis for genital warts in women includes vestibular papillomatosis or micropapillomatosis labialis. These are congenital papillations that fill the vestibule with symmetric, smooth-contoured projections. One single projection arises from a base. In contrast, condyloma acuminata have multiple projections from one base and vary in size and distribution. The projections with vestibular papillomatosis may turn white after the application of acetic acid, but that observation does not confirm HPV infection, because there are many other causes of acetowhitening, including acute candidal infection, contact dermatosis, etc. In men, pearly penile papules that are found circumferentially around the tip of the penis may be misdiagnosed as HPV-related external genital warts. These normal papules are symmetrical and are located just under the corona and either side of the adjacent frenulum.

Other lesions that are in the different diagnosis for the lesions caused by HPV include sebaceous cysts, molluscum contagiosum (especially in HIV-infected patients), and rudimentary hair shafts on the penis. For flat lesions, the differential diagnosis includes vulvar epithelial neoplasia, vaginal intraepithelial neoplasia, and cervical intraepithelial neoplasia depending on location. Condyloma lata, other dermopathies, and invasive carcinoma must also be considered.

Bright light and magnification with hand-held lenses are often quite helpful in diagnosing the lesion and ruling out malignancies; however, in some situations colposcopy or anoscopy may be needed to evaluate vascular changes within the lesion.

High-risk HPV types have been found in nearly 99% of all invasive squamous cell cervical carcinoma and the metastatic lesions. The high-risk HPV viruses have also been identified with squamous cell carcinomas in other genital sites, including the vagina (50–80%), the vulva (50%), and nearly all penile and anal cancers *(23)*.

TESTING FOR HPV

Testing for HPV is not useful in either the clinical diagnosis or the management of external genital warts. For cervical lesions, only tests for high-risk HPV types are useful. Currently, three types of laboratory tests are available to detect the DNA of the human papillomavirus: solution hybridization methods, PCR methods, and *in situ* hybridization methods. For clinical practice, only the Hybrid Capture II® HPV DNA assay (Digene Corporation, Gaithersburg, MD) has been approved by the Food and Drug Administration to identify HPV DNA *(33)*. The PCR and *in situ* hybridization methods for HPV detection/identification are currently used only for research and clinical laboratory applications.

DIAGNOSIS

Genital warts are commonly diagnosed by clinical examination. They may appear as typical peaked, cauliflower-like lesions; smooth papules; papules with a rough, horny layer; or as flat lesions.

Biopsy of a suspicious lesion should be performed and sent for pathological analysis. Lesions are considered suspicious when they are surrounded by thickened skin, pigmentation, or unexplained ulcerations; raised, bleeding, red, or pigmented; indurated, fixed, or large (>2 cm); unresponsive to targeted therapy; and whenever a suspicion for malignancy exists. Warts in hosts who are immunocompromised (HIV-infected) and/or who are at risk for HPV-related malignancy (chronic warts, heaving smoking) should also be biopsied. Biopsy is also indicated if the diagnosis is uncertain. Examination of other areas susceptible to infection is also necessary.

TREATMENT OF GENITAL WARTS

As the natural history of HPV infection has been better elucidated, changes have been made in the screening and management protocols for HPV-related infections. It is now recognized that the majority of women become infected with HPV with sexual debut. Estimates are that about 75% of Americans between the ages of 15–49 have been infected with genital HPV in their lifetimes. However, most of the women with new HPV infection will spontaneously clear the virus in reasonably short order. In one study, 70% of subjects were no longer infected 12 months after initial HPV infection and 81% were free of virus by 24 months. Median time to clearance was 8 months *(7)*. In another study of female university students, 42.7% developed cervical dysplasia within 3 years but virtually all resolved spontaneously. Interestingly the rates of clearance differed for the high- and low-risk types, with higher risk HPV types requiring more time for clearance *(34)*. Therefore, testing and treatment especially of cervical infections are not currently recommended until 3 years after sexual debut or age 21 (whichever comes first) *(35)*.

In one study of female university students who acquired HPV-6 or HPV-11 infections and who were followed for a mean duration of 38.8 months, 64.2% developed a clinically evident genital wart at the time of initial infection. Patients of either gender may develop genital warts. In the study of university students 64.2% developed clinically recognized genital warts *(34)*. Because the warts are disfiguring and prone to superinfection, treatment is generally recommended. However, it must be recognized that about 20–30% of patients with genital warts will spontaneously clear. In another 60% of individuals, localized destruction of the wart will recruit host defenses and clear the HPV infection.

The goal of treatment is clearance of visible warts. Some studies show that treatment may reduce infectivity, but there is no evidence that treatment of warts reduces the risk for cancer or eliminates the virus *(36)*. Therapies can be used alone or in combination. Mechanical and chemical therapies can debulk large lesions and expose the virus to the immune system and prompt host response. Therapies that directly stimulate the local immune system are also available. An important part of all therapies is the patient education and counseling. HPV infection raises all the relevant questions generally associated with STIs, but adds concerns about potential long-term risks for cancer.

The CDC treatment guidelines separate the treatments for genital warts into two general categories: treatments that are patient-applied and those that are provider-administered *(see* Table 2). The CDC treatment guidelines specify factors that may influence selection of treatment including wart size, wart number, anatomic site of wart, wart morphology, patient preference, cost of treatment, convenience, adverse effects, and provider experience *(36)*. Figure 1 shows a treatment algorithm that considers some of the variables discussed.

When deciding whether to use a patient- or provider-applied treatment regimen, it is important to consider several patient factors including patient preferences, comfort, cost, and length of time to clearance of warts. The two available patient-applied treatments (imiquimod and podofilox) have the advantage of eliminating frequent visits to a health care provider. Direct patient costs, such as insurance copayments for insured individuals, coupled with time lost from work are other factors to consider when computing the total cost of treatment *(37–40)*.

Table 2
Genital Warts—CDC STD Treatment Guidelines 2006

External genital warts—patient applied

Recommended regimens— select one of the following:	Sites	Alternative regimens— select one of the following:	Sites
Podofilox[a] 0.5% solution or gel	EGW	Patients should apply podofilox solution with a cotton swab, or podofilox gel with a finger, to visible genital warts twice a day for 3 days, followed by 4 days of no therapy. This cycle may be repeated for up to four cycles as necessary. The total wart area treated should not exceed 10 cm^2 and the total volume of podofilox should be limited to 0.5 mL per day. If possible, the health care provider should apply the initial treatment to demonstrate the proper application technique and identify which warts should be treated. The safety of podofilox during pregnancy has not been established.	
Imiquimod[a] 5% cream	EGW	Patients should apply imiquimod cream once daily at bedtime, three times a week for up to 16 weeks. The treatment area should be washed with soap and water 6–10 hours after the application. The safety of imiquimod during pregnancy has not been established.	

External genital warts—provider administered

Recommended regimens— select one of the following:	Sites	Alternative regimens— select one of the following:	Sites
Cryotherapy with liquid nitrogen	EGW, Anal, Urethral, Vaginal	Repeat applications every 1–2 weeks.	
		Intralesional interferon.	EGW
		Laser surgery	EGW

Cryotherapy with liquid cryoprobe	EGW	Repeat applications every 1–2 weeks.
Podophyllin resin[b] 10–25% compound tincture of benzoin	EGW, Urethral meatus	A small amount should be applied to each wart and allowed to air-dry. The treatment can be repeated weekly, if necessary. To avoid the possibility of complications associated with systemic absorption and toxicity, some specialists recommend that application be limited to <0.5 mL of podophyllin or an area of <10 cm^2 of warts per session. Some specialists suggest that the preparation should be thoroughly washed off 1–4 hours after application to reduce local irritation. The safety of podophyllin during pregnancy has not been established.
Trichloroacetic acid (TCA) or bichloracetic acid (BCA) 80–90%	EGW, Anal, Vaginal	A small amount should be applied only to warts and allowed to dry, at which time a white "frosting" develops. If an excess amount of acid is applied, the treated area should be powdered with talc, sodium bicarbonate (i.e., baking soda), or liquid soap preparations to remove unreacted acid. This treatment can be repeated weekly, if necessary.
Surgical removal	EGW, Anal	Either by tangential scissor excision, tangential shave excision, curettage, or electrosurgery.

Source: From ref. 36.

[a] Not recommended for pregnant and lactating women unless medical benefits outweigh the risks. (pregnancy category C).

[b] Podophyllin is not recommended for use during pregnancy.

EGW, external genital wart.

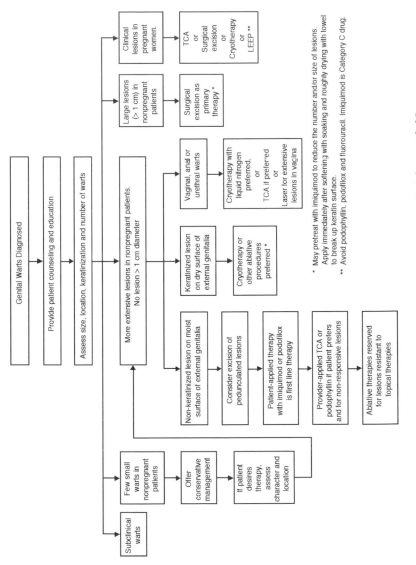

Fig. 1. Selection of therapy for genital warts. Modified from ref. 38.

Genital Warts Diagnosed

Provide patient counseling and education

Assess size, location, keratinization and number of warts

Subclinical warts

Few small warts in nonpregnant patients

Offer conservative management

If patient desires therapy, assess character and location

More extensive lesions in nonpregnant patients. No lesion > 1 cm diameter

Non-keratinized lesion on moist surface of external genitalia

Consider excision of pedunculated lesions

Patient-applied therapy with imiquimod or podofilox is first line therapy

Provider-applied TCA or podophyllin if patient prefers and for non-responsive lesions

Ablative therapies reserved for lesions resistant to topical therapies

Keratinized lesion on dry surface of external genitalia

Cryotherapy or other ablative procedures preferred *

Vaginal, anal or urethral warts

Cryotherapy with liquid nitrogen preferred, or TCA if preferred or Laser for extensive lesions in vagina

Large lesions (> 1 cm) in nonpregnant patients

Surgical excision as primary therapy *

Clinical lesions in pregnant women.

TCA or Surgical excision or Cryotherapy or LEEP **

* May pretreat with imiquimod to reduce the number and/or size of lesions. Apply immediately after softening with soaking and roughly drying with towel to break up keratin surface.

** Avoid podophyllin, podofilox and fluorouracil. Imiquimod is Category C drug.

It should be noted that warts on moist skin surfaces or intertriginous folds will usually respond to all treatments better than warts found on dry, keratinized skin *(36)*. Selection of a treatment modality should recognize that warts found on the keratinized skin of the circumcised penis or labia majora will probably require more treatment sessions than those found under the foreskin of the penis or on the inner folds of the labia minora.

Patient-Applied Therapies

IMIQUIMOD 5% CREAM

Imiquimod is a topical cell-mediated immune response modifier that is provided in single-dose foil packages. Imiquimod is recommended for the treatment of external genital warts. The patient is instructed to apply a thin layer of cream to visible genital warts three times (alternating nights) per week at bedtime. It should be washed off 6–10 hours after application *(36)*. Imiquimod is provided in monthly treatments that can be repeated for up to 4 months as long as continued improvement is noted. The individual foil package is intended for a single use but many patients report that when a small, pin-size hole is made in the foil package and the exposed edge is folded over, the cream maintains its moisture. However, there are insufficient data to recommend this practice at this time. The cream should be well-massaged into the lesion. For well-keratinized lesions, softening the surface of the wart by bathing and then disrupting it with vigorous drying with a towel has been suggested just before application. Imiquimod has a petroleum base and theoretically can weaken latex condoms or diaphragms. At any rate, sexual contact is not recommended when the cream is on the skin. Virtually all patients using the cream will develop localized erythema; however, only a small minority (10–15%) has accompanying pain. The people who do experience pain can be advised to take brief holidays from the drug.

Imiquimod acts as a local immune modulator. It induces local interferon and cytokine release, which triggers both the innate and cell-mediated immune response systems *(41,42)*. Complete clearance of warts occurs in 72–84% of women with use of imiquidmod but complete clearance rates in men are only half those seen in women *(43)*. However, many patients who do not completely clear all their lesions will have a substantial reduction in the numbers and size of remaining lesions. In clinical trials, 81% of subjects had at least a 50% reduction in wart area *(43)*. HPV recurrence rates after treatment with Imiquimod appear to be lower (5–19%) than with other self-administered treatments *(27)*. Imiquimod is in the FDA pregnancy category C.

PODOFILOX 0.5% SOLUTION OR GEL

Podofilox contains purified extract of podophyllin and is recommended for the treatment of external genital warts not involving mucosal epithelium. The solution should be applied to the lesion with a cotton swab; the gel should be applied with a finger. To avoid irritation, the patient should allow the medication to dry after application before ambulating. Podofilox is applied to visible warts two times per day for 3 consecutive days, followed by 4 days of no therapy. This cycle may be repeated up to four cycles, as needed to clear warts. The total wart area treated at any application should not exceed 10 cm^2 and the total volume of podofilox applied should be limited to 0.5 mL per day. The mechanism of action of podofilox is to disrupt cell division. It arrests the formation of the mitotic spindle in metaphase and prevents cell duplication. It may also induce damage in local blood vessels and induce immune response by releasing interleukins. The safety of podophyllin during pregnancy has not been established *(36)*. Podofilox is currently listed as pregnancy category C.

Provider-Applied Therapies

TRICHLOROACETIC ACID (TCA) 80–90% OR BICHLORACETIC ACID (BCA) 80–90%

These acids coagulate the proteins within the wart and act as chemical cautery. They can be used for the treatment of warts on keratinized and mucosal epithelia. TCA or BCA is recommended for the treatment of external genital warts, vaginal warts, and anal warts. A small amount of TCA or BCA is applied directly to visible warts and is allowed to dry. With treatment, the wart will immediately develop a white "frosting" color. Over the ensuing days to weeks, if successful, the wart will detach and leave an ulcer behind. This may be painful and must be monitored for infection. These complications limit the number of warts treated at a single session.

To ensure accurate placement of the acid on the wart, the blunt end of a wooden cotton-tipped applicator or a urethral swab can be used. If a very small area is to be treated, the wooden stick of a cotton-tipped applicator can be broken to reveal a pointed end. Building a moat of lidocaine ointment around the lesion prevents seepage into the surrounding area and provides some comfort. Other health care providers suggest that applying a small amount of lubricating jelly to the treated warts after treatment with TCA or BCA may contribute to patient comfort.

Care must be taken to avoid contamination of the clean bottle of TCA or BCA by using a new applicator stick each time, therefore an adequate supply of applicators of choice should be readily available. If excessive acid is applied to the patient, the health care provider can use either some talc, sodium bicarbonate (i.e., baking soda), or liquid soap to remove excessive acid *(36)*. This must be applied immediately because the acid will cause burns in a matter of seconds. Therefore, access to these basic substances should be readily available.

In addition, because TCA and BCA are highly caustic agents they must be stored in an area away from children's reach. Containers of TCA and BCA must also be properly labeled, and all staff working with this substance must be properly educated to avoid confusing these highly caustic agents with acetic acid (vinegar).

Clearance rates of up to 80% can be expected, but multiple applications at weekly intervals may be made. TCA and BCA are not absorbed into systemic circulation and are safe to use during pregnancy.

PODOPHYLLIN RESIN 10–25% SODIUM

This chemical is compounded in a tincture of benzoin that is cytotoxic and antimitotic and induces tissue necrosis. Podophyllin is recommended for the treatment of external genital warts and urethral meatus warts. A small amount of the solution is applied to each wart on the external genital and allowed to air-dry to prevent irritation. Treatment can be repeated weekly as needed. Podophyllin is neurotropic; it should not be applied to mucosal surfaces from which it might be systemically absorbed. Moreover, application must be limited to less than 0.5 mL or an area of less than 10 cm^2 of warts per session (36). Some specialists recommend it be washed off 1–6 hours after application to reduce the chance of a local irritation and inflammation. Podophyllin should not be applied to the cervix, vagina, oral cavity, or anal canal. The safety of podophyllin during pregnancy has not been established.

CRYOTHERAPY

Cryotherapy freezes the water within the mitochondria of the cell and causes thermally induced cytolysis. Clinicians can use liquid nitrogen (applied by cotton-tip applicator or spray) or nitrous oxide applied by cryoprobes. Regardless of the device used to deliver the cryotherapy to the lesion, application to the wart should continue until the ice ball has extended approximately 2 mm from the edge of the wart. The lesion is then allowed to thaw. Many providers have found that a second freeze session improves efficacy. It has been shown that the tissue destruction occurs during the thawing portion of this process, so adequate time must be given between the freeze–thaw sessions (38). Cryotherapy is safe to use during pregnancy.

Liquid nitrogen is recommended for the treatment of external genital warts, vaginal warts, urethral meatal warts, anal warts, and oral warts. If the liquid nitrogen is obtained from a large metal tank, it evaporates quickly; a large portion of the expense comes from frequent refilling of this large tank. A metal ladle is supplied, which is used to fill either the sealed spray canister or Styrofoam cup. Care must be taken when ladling the liquid nitrogen and protective hand coverings should be worn at all times to protect the exposed skin of the health care provider. A Styrofoam cup is used because of its excellent insulation properties; other materials are not as reliable. Regular cotton-tipped applicator sticks are used to apply the liquid nitrogen to the genital wart. Depending on the size of the lesion, it may be useful to form the cotton tip into a point before dipping it into the nitrogen.

When the nitrogen spray canister is used, it is important that the health care provider have excellent hand–eye coordination so that a steady stream of liquid nitrogen is directed at the lesion only, sparing unaffected surrounding tissue. This will take practice to become proficient, especially when treating small warts.

Nitrogen also comes as compressed gas form (nitrous oxide), which is attached to a cryoprobe with a tip that matches the size and shape of the wart. This is the same hand-held cryoprobe used to treat cervical dysplasia. Gaseous nitrogen is recommended for the treatment of external genital warts. A small amount of lubricating jelly may be applied to the cryoprobe or to the genital wart to help transfer the cold to the lesion. The trigger is pulled back, allowing the refrigerant to enter the gun, which freezes the tip and the jelly covering the wart. Because the freezing is more intense and less controlled with the cryoprobe, it is not recommended for use in cryotherapy of lesions on their mucosal surfaces such as the urethra or vagina.

Overall, clearance rates with cryotherapy are up to 90%, recurrence rates approach 40% *(23,44)*.

SURGICAL THERAPIES

In general, this therapy is reserved for large or medium lesions and those that are unresponsive to medical therapies. The warts are removed at the dermal–epidermal junction. Various techniques that can be used in different settings include scissor excision, shave excision, curettage, LEEP, electrocautery, and laser. Treatment may lead to scarring and vulvodynia if too deep a removal is performed, especially with LEEP. Often surgical excision is done under local anesthesia and requires specialist training.

However, surgical excision can be easily performed in the office to remove a wart that is pedunculated on a slender (1–2 mm) stalk. This type of wart is quite commonly seen in perianal area. After cleaning the area, lift the wart, visualize the separation line between the epidermis and the wart and cut across the base of the lesion along that line. Hemostasis is generally easily obtained by pressure and the use of Monsel solution.

Carbon dioxide laser therapy may be useful for extensive vulvar warts and anal warts, especially if other therapies have failed. It is also the preferred treatment for immunocompromised, non-pregnant patients with large lesions. All the lesions may be destroyed in one treatment, although healing may be uncomfortable. Laser therapy has been associated long-term with vulvodynia, particularly if the deeper tissue layers are burned. Recurrence rates are low in the immediate posttreatment period.

COMBINATION THERAPIES

The CDC treatment guidelines state, "Because of the shortcomings of all available treatments, some clinics employ combination therapy (i.e., the simultaneous use of two or more modalities on the same wart at the same time).

However, some specialists believe that combining modalities may increase complications without improving efficacy" *(36)*. Clinicians may want to use different treatment modalities sequentially. For example, a clinician may start therapy with TCA and have the patient return later for cryotherapy to remove persistent lesions. In another approach, at least one study has demonstrated the efficacy of up to 16 weeks of treatment with imiquimod followed by surgical removal of any remaining genital warts; recurrence rates were also reduced *(45)*.

PATIENT EDUCATION AND COUNSELING

The psychological impact of diagnosis of HPV infection may be even more profound than that of other STIs. In addition to issues of relationship fidelity, there is the issue of oncogenic potential, which requires additional counseling *(46)*.

College-aged women are at particularly high risk for acquiring HPV infection. The diagnosis can cause confusion and distress for women; they may need psychological support and information from their health care provider. Patients with HPV on pap smears report that the diagnosis created a negative effect on their sexual contact and on their relationship with their partner *(47,48)*. One large study of patients with HPV found that a majority rated their provider as fair or poor in counseling them *(49)*. Patients were most disturbed by the lack of advice about emotional issues. Survey of clinicians in college-based clinics recognized the patient's need for information but 46% spent less than 10 minutes providing education and counseling to newly diagnosed patients *(46)*.

It is not unusual for a patient to ask how long the infection has been there and when and where was the infection acquired. It is not possible for the clinician to answer these questions accurately. It has been documented that HPV infection may be subclinical (without visible lesions) for many months or years. A period of decreased immunity (as seen in pregnancy) or increased stress may trigger the growth of warts. It is important for the patient to understand three other points:

- Genital HPV infection is common among sexually active adults.
- Genital HPV infection is usually sexually transmitted, but the sex partner probably is not aware that he is affected.
- HPV testing is not warranted for the patient or the partner.

FOLLOW-UP

Follow-up at 3 months can be offered to patients who have cleared anogenital warts. This will provide an opportunity to evaluate for recurrent warts and to continue to provide patient education. Female patients who have had a history of anogenital warts should be advised to receive annual pap smears to evaluate for cervical abnormalities. Self-examination for external genital warts may be encouraged.

PARTNER NOTIFICATION
AND REPORTING REQUIREMENTS

There is no legal requirement to notify sexual contacts. It is known that most sex partners of individuals infected with HPV are themselves infected. There is no documented evidence that professional examination of sex partners is necessary. Treatment of the partner has not been shown to reduce the patient's risk for recurrence. Recurrence of anogenital warts can result from reactivation of a latent infection. For these reasons, the CDC treatment guidelines do not mandate partner notification or treatment in the absence of grossly visible lesions. However, it should be noted that a visit to a health care provider affords an excellent opportunity to provide education and to screen for other STIs in all patients. Female partners of men with external genital warts should be encouraged to receive routine pap smears (36).

PREGNANCY-RELATED ISSUES

During pregnancy, HPV tends be expressed or reactivated. It is thought that this is owing to suppression of the pregnant woman's immune system. The expression of the wart virus does not necessarily mean a recent inoculation/infection with HPV, but probably represents a latent infection or a reactivation of an old infection. The incidence of laryngeal papillomatosis is extremely rare (less than 1 in 25,000). Despite the possibility of vertical transmission, vaginal delivery is the preferred method of delivery for women with genital warts. However, occasionally, a cesarean section will be recommended for maternal indications when extensive lesions obstruct the outlet of the birth canal or they create a concern that laceration/episiotomy repair would not be possible. Treatment of external genital warts during pregnancy is generally advocated because the lesions tend to grow in the immunocompromised state and may become superinfected. However, tiny lesions may not warrant treatment, if they are asymptomatic, because they will often regress spontaneously after delivery.

POTENTIAL FOR VACCINES
AND OTHER PREVENTIVE MEASURES

A quadrivalent vaccine against HPV types 6, 11,16, and 18 is available for women ages 11–26. Vaccinated women not previously exposed to these HPV types are expected to have a 90% reduction in genital warts from those HPV types (see Chapter 16; 50–53).

Avoiding skin-to-skin contact with an infected partner is the most effective approach to prevent HPV infection. A comprehensive review of the literature confirmed that there is insufficient evidence to demonstrate that condom use decreases HPV infection, but evidence exists to demonstrate that correct and consistent condom use does clearly reduce the HPV-related diseases, such as genital warts in men and cervical dysplasia in women. A recent clinical trial of uninfected young adults found that young women whose partners used male condoms with every sexual encounter had an incidence of less than 50% of the HPV-related genital infection rates of women whose partners used condoms infrequently (*see* Chapter 15; *54,55*).

CASE STUDY

Belinda, age 30, noticed a bump on her left labia that appears to be growing. She is accompanied by her female partner of 12 years, who thinks it may be a genital wart and wants to know how this happened. Belinda's last pap smear was more than 6 months ago. On exam, Belinda has a 0.3-cm exophytic wart on a broad base on her labia majora near the perineum. Belinda is worried that it might be contagious and that it could become cancerous.

Questions

1. Does she need a biopsy?
2. Does she need viral typing?
3. Does she need a pap smear?
4. What do you tell her and her partner?
5. How would you treat her genital wart?

Answers

1. Biopsy is needed only for large (>1 cm) lesions, those that do not respond to therapy, and those that look suspicious or questionable. Belinda's wart is very characteristic in its appearance and is still small. It does not require biopsy now.
2. Viral typing is not appropriate. It does not provide information that will help in the treatment of the wart or the patient.
3. She does not need another pap smear now. She recently had one that was normal 6 months ago. The most common HPV types involved in genital warts are HPV-6 and HPV-11, which do not have oncogenic potential. However, because there can be co-infection with other HPV types, routine pap smear screening is still advised at her next annual exam.
4. The counseling messages are important for couples. HPV is a sexually transmitted infection, but the development of a wart at any one time does not necessarily mean a new infection. People carry the virus with them for years and may express (or share) it at any point. This wart, by itself, does not mean there has been any lack of monogamy. It is important to realize that HPV can be transmitted by an array of sexual practices and other sites of potential contact be checked, such as the mouth and vagina. Belinda's partner should come for examination if she notes any lesions on herself.
5. Belinda's wart is small enough to be easily treated with either patient-applied treatments (imiquimod or podofilox) or provider-provided treatments (TCA, BCA, or podophyllin). If the lesion were thickly keratinized, TCA might be more appropriate. Cryotherapy, LEEP, or laser are not needed at this time.

REFERENCES

1. The Henry J. Kaiser Family Foundation. Fact Sheet: Sexually Transmitted Diseases in the U.S. Available from: http://www.kff.org/womenshealth/1447-std_fs.cfm. Accessed Nov. 24, 2006.
2. Insinga RP, Glass AG, Rush BB. The health care costs of cervical human papillomavirus-related disease. Am J Obstet Gynecol 2004; 191:114–120.
3. Gerberding JL. Report to Congress: prevention of genital human papillomavirus infection. Centers for Disease Control and Prevention, Department of Health and Human Services; 2004.
4. Cates W Jr. Estimates of the incidence and prevalence of sexually transmitted diseases in the United States. American Social Health Association Panel. Sex Transm Dis 1999; 26:S2–S7.
5. Myers ER, McCrory DC, Nanda K, Bastian L, Matchar DB. Mathematical model for the natural history of human papillomavirus infection and cervical carcinogenesis. Am J Epidemiol 2000; 151:1158–1171.
6. Weinstock H, Berman S, Cates W Jr. Sexually transmitted diseases among American youth: incidence and prevalence estimates, 2000. Perspect Sex Reprod Health 2004; 36:6–10.
7. Ho GY, Bierman R, Beardsley L, Chang CJ, Burk RD. Natural history of cervicovaginal papillomavirus infection in young women. N Engl J Med 1998; 338:423–428.
8. Silins I, Kallings I, Dillner J. Correlates of the spread of human papillomavirus infection. Cancer Epidemiol Biomarkers Prev 2000; 9:953–959.
9. Sellors JW, Mahony JB, Kaczorowski J, et al. Prevalence and predictors of human papillomavirus infection in women in Ontario, Canada. Survey of HPV in Ontario Women (SHOW) Group. CMAJ 2000; 163:503–508.
10. Centers for Disease Control and Prevention. CDC fact sheet: genital HPV infection. Available from: http://www.cdc.gov/std/HPV/STDFact-HPV.htm#common. Accessed Nov. 24, 2006.
11. Baldwin SB, Wallace DR, Papenfuss MR, et al. Human papillomavirus infection in men attending a sexually transmitted disease clinic. J Infect Dis 2003; 187:1064–1070.
12. Takahashi S, Shimizu T, Takeyama K, et al. Detection of human papillomavirus DNA on the external genitalia of healthy men and male patients with urethritis. Sex Transm Dis 2003; 30:629–633.
13. Conley LJ, Ellerbrock TV, Bush TJ, Chiasson MA, Sawo D, Wright TC. HIV-1 infection and risk of vulvovaginal and perianal condylomata acuminata and intraepithelial neoplasia: a prospective cohort study. Lancet 2002; 359:108–113.
14. Giuliano AR, Harris R, Sedjo RL, et al. Incidence, prevalence, and clearance of type-specific human papillomavirus infections: the Young Women's Health study. J Infect Dis 2002; 186: 462–469.
15. Koutsky L. Epidemiology of genital human papillomavirus infection. Am J Med 1997; 102: 3–8.
16. Gunter J. Genital and perianal warts: new treatment opportunities for human papillomavirus infection. Am J Obstet Gynecol 2003; 189:S3–S11.
17. Fleischer AB Jr, Parrish CA, Glenn R, Feldman SR. Condylomata acuminata (genital warts): patient demographics and treating physicians. Sex Transm Dis 2001; 28:643–647.
18. Sellors JW, Karwalajtys TL, Kaczorowski J, et al. Incidence, clearance and predictors of human papillomavirus infection in women. CMAJ 2003; 168:421–425.
19. Bauer HM, Hildesheim A, Schiffman MH, et al. Determinants of genital human papillomavirus infection in low-risk women in Portland, Oregon. Sex Transm Dis 1993; 20:274–278.
20. Munoz N, Bosch FX, de Sanjose S, et al. Epidemiologic classification of human papillomavirus types associated with cervical cancer. N Engl J Med 2003; 348:518–527.

21. Bleeker MC, Hogewoning CJ, Voorhorst FJ, et al. Condom use promotes regression of human papillomavirus-associated penile lesions in male sexual partners of women with cervical intraepithelial neoplasia. Int J Cancer 2003; 107:804–810.

22. Marrazzo JM, Koutsky LA, Stine KL, et al. Genital human papillomavirus infection in women who have sex with women. J Infect Dis 1998; 178:1604–1609.

23. Cox T, Buck HW, Kinney W, Rubin MM. HPV types: natural history and epidemiology. Human papillomavirus (HPV) and cervical cancer. Clinical proceedings. Washington, DC: Association of Reproductive Health Professionals; 2001. Available from: http://ww.arhp. org/healthcareproviders/onlinepublications/clinicalproceedings/cphpv/types.cfm?ID=149. Accessed Nov. 24, 2006.

24. Mao C, Hughes JP, Kiviat N, et al. Clinical findings among young women with genital human papillomavirus infection. Am J Obstet Gynecol 2003; 188:677–684.

25. Byars RW, Poole GV, Barber WH. Anal carcinoma arising from condyloma acuminata. Am Surg 2001; 67:469–472.

26. Perniciaro C, Dicken CH. Tanning bed warts. J Am Acad Dermatol 1988; 18:586–587.

27. Gunter J. Genital and perianal warts: new treatment opportunities for human papillomavirus infection. Am J Obstet Gynecol 2003; 189:S3 S11.

28. Arany I, Evans T, Tyring SK. Tissue specific HPV expression and downregulation of local immune responses in condylomas from HIV seropositive individuals. Sex Transm Infect 1998; 74:349–353.

29. Stubenrauch F, Laimins LA. Human papillomavirus life cycle: active and latent phases. Semin Cancer Biol 1999; 9:379–386.

30. Blackledge FA, Anand VK. Tracheobronchial extension of recurrent respiratory papillomatosis. Ann Otol Rhinol Laryngol 2000; 109:812–818.

31. Silverberg MJ, Thorsen P, Lindeberg H, Grant LA, Shah KV. Condyloma in pregnancy is strongly predictive of juvenile-onset recurrent respiratory papillomatosis. Obstet Gynecol 2003; 101:645–652.

32. Rubin MA, Kleter B, Zhou M, et al. Detection and typing of human papillomavirus DNA in penile carcinoma: evidence for multiple independent pathways of penile carcinogenesis. Am J Pathol 2001; 159:1211–1218.

32a. Munoz N, Bosch FX, de Sanjose S, et al. International Agency for Research on Cancer Multicenter Cervical Cancer Study Group. Epidemiologic classification of human papillomavirus types associated with cervical cancer. N Engl J Med. 2003 Feb 6;348(6):518–527.

33. Wright TC, Cox JT. Clinical Uses of Human Papilloma Virus (HPV) DNA Testing. Hagerstown, MD: American Society for Colposcopy and Cervical Pathology; 2004.

34. Winer RL, Kiviat NB, Hughes JP, et al. Development and duration of human papillomavirus lesions, after initial infection. J Infect Dis 2005; 191:731–738.

35. Saslow D, Runowicz CD, Solomon D, et al. American Cancer Society guideline for the early detection of cervical neoplasia and cancer. CA Cancer J Clin 2002; 52:342–362.

36. Centers for Disease Control and Prevention. Sexually transmitted diseases treatment guidelines 2006. MMWR Recomm Rep. 2006; 55(RR-11):62–67. Available from: http://www.cdc. gov/std/treatment. Accessed Nov. 24, 2006.

37. Langley PC, Richwald GA, Smith MH. Modeling the impact of treatment options in genital warts: patient-applied versus physician-administered therapies. Clin Ther 1999; 21:2143–2155.

38. Kodner CM, Nasraty S. Management of genital warts. Am Fam Physician 2004; 70:2335–2342.

39. Lacey CJ, Goodall RL, Tennvall GR, et al. Randomised controlled trial and economic evaluation of podophyllotoxin solution, podophyllotoxin cream, and podophyllin in the treatment of genital warts. Sex Transm Infect 2003; 79:270–275.

40. Alam M, Stiller M. Direct medical costs for surgical and medical treatment of condylomata acuminata. Arch Dermatol 2001; 137:337–341.
41. Dahl MV. Imiquimod: an immune response modifier. J Am Acad Dermatol 2000; 43:S1–S5.
42. Tyring SK, Arany I, Stanley MA, et al. A randomized, controlled, molecular study of condylomata acuminata clearance during treatment with imiquimod. J Infect Dis 1998; 178: 551–555.
43. Edwards L, Ferenczy A, Eron L, et al. Self-administered topical 5% imiquimod cream for external anogenital warts. Arch Dermatol 1998; 134:25–30.
44. Maw RD. Treatment of anogenital warts. Dermatol Clin 1998; 16:829–834.
45. Carrasco D, vander Straten M, Tyring SK. Treatment of anogenital warts with imiquimod 5% cream followed by surgical excision of residual lesions. J Am Acad Dermatol 2002; 47:S212–S216.
46. Linnehan MJ, Groce NE. Psychosocial and educational services for female college students with genital human papillomavirus infection. Fam Plann Perspect 1999; 31:137–141.
47. Campion MJ, Brown JR, McCance DJ, et al. Psychosexual trauma of an abnormal cervical smear. Br J Obstet Gynaecol 1988; 95:175–181.
48. Filiberti A, Tamburini M, Stefanon B, et al. Psychological aspects of genital human papillomavirus infection: a preliminary report. J Psychosom Obstet Gynecol 1993; 14:145–152.
49. Guy H. Survey shows how we live with HPV. HPV news. 1993; 3:1,4–8.
50. Koutsky LA, Ault KA, Wheeler CM, et al. A controlled trial of a human papillomavirus type 16 vaccine. N Engl J Med 2002; 347:1645–1651.
51. Goldenthal KL, Pratt DR. FDA briefing document # 2. Preventive human papillomavirus (HPV) vaccines—background information. Bethesda, MD: Vaccines and Related Biological Products Advisory Committee; November 28–29, 2001.
52. Harper DM, Franco EL, Wheeler C, et al. Efficacy of a bivalent L1 virus-like particle vaccine in prevention of infection with human papillomavirus types 16 and 18 in young women: a randomised controlled trial. Lancet 2004; 364:1757–1765.
53. Villa LL, Costa RL, Petta CA, et al. Prophylactic quadrivalent human papillomavirus (types 6, 11, 16, and 18) L1 virus-like particle vaccine in young women: a randomised double-blind placebo-controlled multicentre phase II efficacy trial. Lancet Oncol 2005; 6:271–278.
54. National Institute of Allergy and Infectious Diseases. Workshop summary: scientific evidence on condom effectiveness for sexually transmitted disease (STD) prevention. Washington, DC: National Institutes of Health, Department of Health Services, 2001. Available from: http://www.niaid.nih.gov/dmid/stds/condomreport.pdf. Accessed Nov. 24, 2006.
55. Winer RL, Hughes JP, Feng Q, et al. Condom use and the risk of genital human papillomavirus infection in young women. N Engl J Med 2006; 354:2645–2654.

3

Genital Herpes

Gene Parks

INTRODUCTION

Herpes simplex virus (HSV) has a long and confusing history. More than 2500 years ago, Hippocrates first used the word "herpes," derived from the Greek word "to creep," to describe how the lesions of this contagious ulcerative disease seemed to creep or crawl along the skin *(1)*. Galen first noted that recurrences develop at the same anatomic site. However, over time, the word herpes was used to describe many skin conditions from lupus to zoster. The definition of herpes (particularly oral lesions) became more rigorous in the 17th century. In the 1830s, recurrent genital herpes was described and 60 years later was identified as a "vocational disease"—a sexually transmitted infection (STI). The virus itself was not identified until the 1950s. In 1971, it was proposed that two different types of HSV caused infection. HSV-1 commonly causes labial or pharyngeal infection, and transmission is primary by nongenital contact. HSV-2 typically affects the genital area and is transmitted by intimate sexual contact. However, both viruses are capable of causing either genital or oral-pharyngeal infections that appear identical on examination. In the United States, HSV infection is one of the most common STIs and is the leading cause of genital ulcers.

FAST FACTS

- Genital herpes is one of the most prevalent STIs in the United States. About 50 million Americans have genital HSV infection.
- HSV is the leading cause of genital ulcers. HSV-2 infections at least doubles the risk of sexual acquisition of human immunodeficiency virus (HIV) and also increases transmission.
- Herpes is a chronic, life-long infection; patients can shed virus, not only during outbreaks but also during asymptomatic periods.
- Intrapartum transmission of HSV-2 can cause neonatal death or permanent neurological damage.

From: *Current Clinical Practice: Sexually Transmitted Diseases:*
A Practical Guide for Primary Care
Edited by: A. L. Nelson and J. A. Woodward © Humana Press, Totowa, NJ

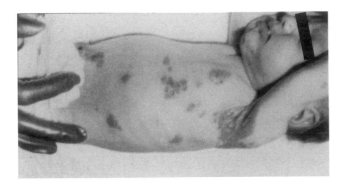

Neonatal herpes simplex virus type 2.

- Testing for HSV-2 antibodies is not recommended for general population screening.

PREVALENCE AND INCIDENCE

The full extent of the HSV epidemic in the United States is not known because (1) HSV infection is not a reportable disease in most states, (2) most people carrying the virus are not aware that they are infected, and (3) it is not possible in many cases for people to distinguish between an initial outbreak (incidence) and a recurrence (prevalence).

Serology studies suggest that 50 million people in the United States have genital HSV infection. In Europe, HSV-2 is found in 8–15% of the general population. In Africa, the prevalence rates are 40–50% in 20-year-olds. Between the two most recent iterations of National Health and Nutritional Examination Surveys (NHANES)—NHANES in 1988–1994 and NHANES in 1999–2004—the seroprevalence of HSV-2 among civilian, noninstitutionalized people aged 14–49 in the United States decreased by 19% from 21 to 17% *(2)*. By contrast, 57.7% of the same group were seropositive for HSV-1 in 1999–2004, which represents a 6.9% decline. Seroprevalence for HSV-2 increases with age, being virtually nonexistent in children under age 12, and stabilizing after age 30; this pattern is consistent with the virus being an STI. By contrast, HSV-1 seroprevalence in children under 5 is 20% and rises in a linear fashion until age 20. This pattern is not characteristic of an STI. More than 85% of the world's adult population is seropositive for HSV-1 (23.1%).

The NHANES surveys found that women (23.1%) are more likely to be seropositive than men (11.2%). Seropositivity is highest among blacks (40.3%), followed by whites (13.7%) and Mexican Americans (11.9%). Lifetime numbers of sex partners influenced seropositivity, varying from 2.6% of patients with no sex partners to 39.9%, for people with at least 50 partners *(2)*.

Patient history is very unreliable for obtaining information about this infection. Of the 50 million Americans who are HSV seropositive, only 9% is aware of having had a previous infection *(3)*. Even when seropositive individuals are asked specific questions, only 25–33% admit having had symptoms consistent with genital herpes. Approximately 75% of source partners discover their own infection only when their newly infected partner is diagnosed *(4)*.

It is estimated that there are 1.6 million new cases of genital HSV infections in the United States each year *(5)*, and 10 million recurrences annually *(6)*. Worldwide, 20 million new people are infected each year *(7)*.

Herpes infections are troubling enough by themselves, but they also represent a risk factor for acquiring and spreading other STIs. Herpes is one of the most common infections found in HIV-infected adults; 90% of HIV patients are also infected with HSV *(see* Chapter 5). Several studies have established a causative relationship between HSV genital ulcerations and HIV acquisition, transmission, and progression *(8)*. High titers of HIV are found in genital herpes ulcerations *(9)*. In addition, HIV infection reactivation is accompanied by an increase in plasma HIV viral load *(10)*. A meta-analysis of studies that documented HSV-2 infection before HIV acquisition found that the HSV more than doubled the risk; the relative risk was 2.1 (95%, C1: 1.4–3.2). About 52% of HIV infection is attributable to HSV-2 coinfection. The population attributable risk percentage varied with HSV-2 prevalence and ranged from 19 to 47% *(11)*.

RISK FACTORS

HSV-2 infects all economic classes, race, ages, and ethnic groups. However, there are identifiable risk factors for HSV-2 infection, which reflect biological and behavioral influences. Major risk factors for seropositivity include female gender, ethnicity (African-American or Hispanic), history of STIs, increasing number of sex partners, sexual contact with commercial sex workers, cocaine use, and low socioeconomic status or level of education. In addition, older age and young age at sexual debut are important factors *(12)*. Each additional sex act per week increases the risk of acquiring genital herpes *(13)*. In a study of discordant monogamous couples, risk factors for HSV acquisition were female gender and the absence of HSV-1 antibodies *(4)*. Other risk factors that have been shown to be independent predictors of HSV-2 infection in women include cigarette smoking, douching, history of having intercourse with an uncircumcised male partner, the presence of vaginal group B streptococcus, and abnormal vaginal flora *(14)*.

INFECTIVITY AND TRANSMISSION

Herpes is highly contagious. Seventy-five percent of sexual partners of HSV-2-infected people contract the disease. In a study of seronegative sexually active individuals, the annual rates of infection were 1.6% for HSV-1 and 5.1% for HSV-2 *(15)*; the primary route of transmission of HSV-2 infection is genital-to-genital skin contact with an infected partner who is shedding virus symptomatically or asymptomatically. HSV-2 is responsible for about 80% of genital herpes infections, even though there are as many initial cases with HSV-1 infection, which is usually acquired through oral–genital contact, HSV-2 is more likely to cause recurrent episodes. HSV-1 genital infections are higher in men who have sex with men (MSM) *(16)*.

Asymptomatic shedding is responsible for most of the transmission of HSV *(4,17)*. HSV DNA has been detected by polymerase chain reaction (PCR) from genital samples of HSV-2-infected women on 28% of days *(18)*. In discordant couples, 69% of transmission occurred when the infected partner was asymptomatic *(4)*. Transmission of HSV between discordant sexual partners occurs at a rate of about 10% per year *(19)*. Asymptomatic shedding is more common with HSV-2 than with HSV-1 infection *(20)*.

Although transmission of HSV infections generally results from intimate skin-to-skin contact with an infected individual, it can also result from exposure to infected saliva, semen, vaginal secretions, or fluid from active herpetic lesions. Drying and room temperature quickly inactivate the virus. Therefore, HSV transmission is not believed to occur often through exposure to fomites *(21)*.

ETIOLOGY

HSV belongs to the Herpesviridae family, which also includes the cytomegalovirus, Epstein-Barr virus, and varicella-zoster virus. HSV-1 and HSV-2 are two of the eight human herpesviruses; neither is found in other animal species. HSV is an enveloped, double-stranded DNA virus. HSV-1 and HSV-2 are distinguished by antigenic differences in their envelope proteins *(4)*. However, the genomes of the two viruses are 50% homologous. There are multiple specific strains of HSV-1 and HSV-2.

After contact with abraded skin or mucosal surfaces, the virus replicates and initiates infection in the epidermal cells of the target area. Following this initial infection, the virus travels in a retrograde fashion within axons of sensory nerves to the dorsal nerve root ganglion where it continues to replicate to establish lifelong latency *(3)*. HSV-2 usually migrates to the sacral nerve roots (S_2, S_3, and S_4). Recurrent outbreaks localized to the dermatomes innervated by the infected nerve are quite common, especially with HSV-2. In patients with an initial primary episode of genital herpes, the risk of having at least one recurrence during the first year is nearly 90% *(22)*. Although some HSV-2-infected patients may not experience symptomatic recurrences, virtually all will have repeated episodes of asymptomatic viral shedding from their genital secretions. This shedding places their sexual contacts at risk for acquiring the infection.

Table 1
Definition of Genital Herpes Syndromes

Initial primary infection
Initial infection with either herpes type 1 or herpes type 2 in a patient who
has had no prior exposure to either HSV-1 or HSV-2 (seronegative for HSV-
1 and HSV-2).

Initial non-primary infection
First clinical infection with either HSV-1 or HSV-2 in a patient who has had
prior exposure to the other HSV.

Recurrent infection
A recurrence, not a re-infection. The infection results from reactivation of a
latent virus.

Source: Modified from ref. *26*, p. 102.
HSV, herpes simplex virus.

CLINICAL MANIFESTATIONS

There are three types of HSV genital infections: primary infection, nonprimary
initial infection, and recurrent infection (*see* Table 1). A primary infection is the
first HSV infection that occurs in a patient without prior exposure to HSV, as
demonstrated by the fact that the patient has no antibodies to HSV. An initial,
nonprimary infection is defined as a first HSV infection with one HSV type in
a patient who is already infected with another type of HSV (e.g., a new HSV-2
infection in a patient with prior HSV-1 infection). Because HSV-1 is so prevalent, most initial genital infections (usually with HSV-2) are initial, nonprimary
infections. Recurrent infections are outbreaks owing to reactivation of a previously acquired HSV infection (not a reinfection).

The incubation period after genital exposure to HSV-1 or HSV-2 is approximately 4 days (range 2–12 days) *(23)*. Almost half of first-episode genital herpes
is caused by HSV-1. The local and systemic symptoms with primary genital infections are generally the same intensity and duration for both HSV-1 and HSV-2 *(24)*.

The classical clinical presentation of genital herpes starts with widespread
multiple painful macules and papules, which then mature into clusters of clear,
fluid-filled vesicles and pustules. The vesicles rupture and form ulcers. Skin
ulcers crust, whereas lesions on mucous membranes heal without crusting *(23)*.
Scarring does not usually occur after re-epithelization. Secondary bacterial
infections may produce ulcers that extend into the dermis or that cause cellulitis.
In women, the ulcers occur at the introitus, labia, perineum, or perianal area.
Patients complain of dysuria, vulvar pain, dyspareunia, and increased vaginal
discharge and bleeding. Patients may volitionally retain urine because the pain
with urination is so severe. On average, initial primary infections last 12 days,
but viral shedding continues for 20–21 days *(25)*. The infection may be spread

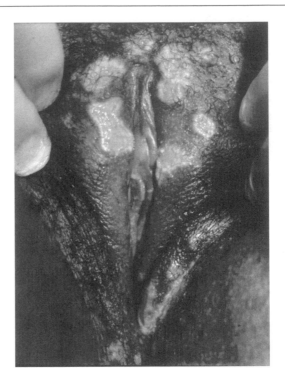

Vulvar herpes.

by autoinoculation to other areas of the genitalia as well as to the buttocks and thighs and to distant sites, such as the conjunctivae. Urethral involvement is common; 82% of patients with initial infection have urethritis with positive urethral cultures. Cervical infection, which is found in 80% of women, causes increased vaginal discharge and postcoital spotting and bleeding. Men usually develop lesions on the penile shaft or glands. The patient usually develops tender inguinal adenopathy. Perianal infections are also common in MSM. Pharyngitis may develop with oral exposure.

Initial primary infection is associated with a higher rate of systemic involvement and greater severity of local disease than is seen with initial nonprimary genital herpes infection. With primary infections, 66% of women and 40% of men develop constitutional symptoms such as fever, malaise, nausea, headache, myalgia, hepatitis, meningitis, and autonomic nervous system dysfunction as a result of viremia (23). Approximately 30% of women and 10% of men have headache, stiff neck, and photophobia with or without fever (23); 4% of individuals will develop viral meningitis (26). The meningitis is transient and requires no treatment; it resolves without any sequelae. Infection in the sacral plexus may affect sensation in the pelvis as well as detrusor function; 10–15% of women with

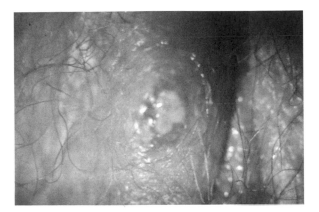

Penile genital herpes.

initial disease will develop urinary retention that requires catheterization. This nerve dysfunction may last 6–7 weeks *(3)*. HIV-infected individuals are at higher risk of developing the more serious clinical manifestations, including dissemination, encephalitis, and meningoencephalitis *(26a)*.

Most initial genital herpes infections are not "classical" in their presentation. The majority of initial infections are asymptomatic or atypical; patients note nonspecific symptoms of discharge, dysuria, pain, erythema, back pain, pruritus, soreness, fissure, and folliculitis and think they have a rash, allergy, yeast infection, cystitis, zipper trauma, jock itch, or bike seat irritation *(27)*. Clinicians often fail to diagnose HSV infection and attribute the signs and symptoms to other diagnoses, particularly when there are only small blisters or ulcers, vaginal lesions, urethritis or cervicitis without external lesions, excoriation, fissures, or nonspecific erythema *(28)*. About 1 in 7 men who present with sores, blisters, ulcers, crusting, or small cuts/slits had HSV and about 1 in 9 women with redness, irritation, or rash have HSV *(28a)*. The relative mildness of the symptoms and subtlety of the physical findings may occur because most initial infections with HSV-2 occur in people who carry antibodies to HSV-1. There are generally fewer lesions with these nonprimary initial infections. Systemic symptoms develop in only 16% of people with initial nonprimary infections. The duration of infection in this situation is shorter (9 days) and viral shedding lasts only 1 week *(29)*. Thus, genital herpes infection should be considered routinely in any patient with genital lesions. This would include patients with genital erythema, rash, skin fissuring, pain, burning, or genital itch.

Recurrent infections are more common and occur more frequently with HSV-2 than with HSV-1 infection. Within 1 year of diagnosis of initial primary HSV-2 genital infections, 90% of people will have at least one recurrence, whereas only 55% of HSV-1-infected people have repeat outbreaks. In one study, nearly 40% of

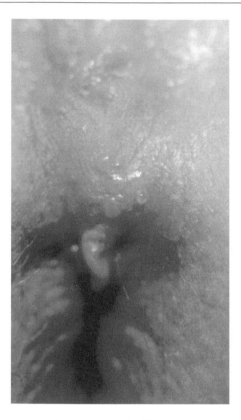

Recurrent genital herpes.

the HSV-2-infected subjects had six or more recurrences *(22)*. Median time to recurrence with HSV-2 was 49 days, whereas median time to recurrence of HSV-1 was 310 days. Most recurrences are asymptomatic. About half of patients who recognize recurrences report prodromal symptoms, such as localized tingling, pruritus, or pain 30 minutes to 48 hours before eruption. Some patients experience more painful and prolonged prodromes including shooting pain in the buttocks, hips, or legs for up to 5 days *(23)*. Recurrent herpes outbreaks are usually less severe than primary outbreaks. The numbers of lesions are generally fewer. The lesions may appear the same as in primary outbreaks but heal in half the time or they may present as fissures or vulvar erythema rather than typical ulcers. About 10–15% patients with recurrent genital herpes will have co-existing cervical disease. Systemic manifestations do not occur with recurrences in immunocompetent patients. Over time, recurrence rates decrease *(30)*.

Frequently, women who have HSV-related ulcers become superinfected with Candida. Prompt attention to treating that infection can decrease the patient's discomfort.

Factors other than HSV type that have been associated with frequency of recurrent outbreaks include fatigue, menstruation, intercourse, and trauma. The most common cause of recurrence of HSV in HIV-infected patients is the degree of immunosuppression. Although it is commonly believed that acute episodes of stress are associated with onset of recurrent herpes, studies have concluded that only persistent stress lasting longer than 1 week and depression arc psychological stressors that are associated with onset of recurrent outbreaks *(3)*.

TESTING TECHNIQUES

Until recently, viral isolation in cell culture and determination of the type of HSV with fluorescent staining has been the mainstay of herpes testing in patients presenting with characteristic genital lesions. The cytopathic cell changes induced by the herpes virus in tissue culture usually occurs within 3 days of inoculation but the cell culture is not considered negative for herpes until a final negative reading on day 15 *(31)*. The rate of recovery of the virus depends on the stage of the clinical disease being tested. There is a 90% chance of obtaining a positive culture when the specimen is obtained from the base of a freshly unroofed vesicle or pustule, but that sensitivity decreases to 70% when the specimen is obtained from an existing herpes ulcer and drops to only 27% when a crusted lesion is used as a specimen source *(31)*. The probability of recovery of the virus from a patient with recurrent herpes, which has a much shorter duration of viral shedding and a lower viral load, is only 30%. Direct Fluorescent Antibody (DFA) staining of vesicle scrapings is as specific as viral culture but not as sensitive *(31)*.

The Tzanck preparation is a histological examination of lesions that identifies the presence of a DNA virus with multinucleated giant cells typical of HSV. Although the test is rapid, it is not specific for HSV. Similar changes can be found in sites infected with the varicella virus. Similarly, cytological detection of HSV infection (e.g., from pap smear) is not only insensitive, it is nonspecific and has a low positive predictive rate. It should not be used for diagnosis.

PCR assay for HSV DNA has been shown to be more sensitive than viral culture and has a specificity that exceeds 99.9%. The PCR test is the standard of care test for the diagnosis of herpes central nervous system infection. Although the PCR is highly accurate and faster than tissue culture, its use in clinical practice for other diagnoses is currently limited, because there is no FDA clearance for testing genital specimens. In addition, the cost of the test and the requirement for experienced, trained technical staff to perform the testing *(21)* restrict its use. Enzyme-Linked Virus Inducible System® is a relatively new viral detection system that is as sensitive as viral culture, but can provide rapid results *(32)*.

Commercially available blood tests that can identify prior exposure by testing for HSV-specific glycoproteins G_2 (HSV-2) and G_1 (HSV-1) immunoglobulin

Table 2
Guidelines for Type-Specific HSV Serological Tests

- Diagnosis of genital lesions/symptoms: type-specific serology tests should be available for diagnostic purposes in conjunction with virological tests at clinical settings that provide care for patients with STDs or those at risk at risk for STDs. Serology tests may be useful in the following situations:
    - A culture-negative recurrent lesion.
    - A history suggestive of herpes/atypical herpes with no lesions to culture.
    - The first presentation of genital symptoms when culture or antigen detection is negative or not available.
    - Screening for HIV-positive patients should be generally offered.
    - Patients in partnerships or considering partnerships with HSV-2 infected people (especially if it would change behavior).
- HIV-infected people may benefit from testing during their first evaluation.
- Universal screening in pregnancy should not be generally offered.
- Screening in general population should not be generally offered.
- Herpes education and prevention counseling is necessary for all people being screened for HSV-2.

HSV, herpes simplex virus; STD, sexually transmitted disease; HIV, human immunodeficiency virus.

(Ig)G antibodies. These two Food and Drug Administration (FDA)-approved tests for laboratory use are HerpeSelect™-1 enzyme-linked immunosorbent assay (ELISA) IgG, and HerpeSelect 1 and 2 Immunoblot IgG (for HSV-1 and HSV-2) (Focus Diagnostics, Herndon, VA). They have a sensitivity of detecting HSV-2 of 98% and a specificity of 97–100% because of their ability to detect glyco-protein G-2 for HSV-2 and glycoproteins G-1 and C-1 for HSV-1. Two point-of-care tests are also available: Biokit HSV-2 and SureVac HSV-2. Unfortu-nately, many commercial laboratories are still providing older assays that are inaccurate because there are high rates of cross-reactivity between HSV-1 and HSV-2. The older tests should never be ordered to determine a specific type of herpes. Seroconversion of an initial primary herpes attack will usually occur 6 weeks after the outbreak, but may take up to 6 months. Therefore, HSV-2 sero-logical testing cannot detect a primary infection; it can be used only to rule out recurrent infections.

The CDC list of appropriate use of serologic testing is summarized in Table 2. Screening in the general population should generally not be offered. More detail of situations in which testing might be appropriate is provided here.

1. Diagnosis of HSV-2:
   a. Patients who present with a 3-month or greater history of recurrent genital lesions suggestive of recurrent genital herpes but have no lesions on exam or have recent negative viral culture for herpes. A negative HSV-1 and HSV-2 serological test would rule out genital herpes as the cause of the lesions, whereas a positive HSV-2 serology would support the diagnosis of recurrent genital herpes. Interpretation of a positive HSV-1 test would be more difficult. However, it must be recognized that the recurrent symptoms may be owing to an unrelated lesion.
   b. Patients who have first presentation of genital symptoms when culture or antigen detection is negative or not available. Note: testing would have to be delayed by 6 weeks to allow for antibody formulation.
2. HIV-infected patients. Because of to the high co-infection rate with HSV, all HIV-infected patients should be offered type-specific HSV serological testing.
3. Partner consideration. The evaluation of patient who is in a partnership or is considering partnership with a person with documented genital herpes and is concerned about the possible transmission. If the asymptomatic person is HSV-2-seropositive, then the couple can be reassured that further transmission between them cannot take place. If the asymptomatic person is seronegative, then the couple should be counseled regarding preventive measures (condom use) to reduce the chance of transmission.
4. Screening can be selectively offered to those patients as part of a comprehensive evaluation of individuals with a STI and those who are at risk for STIs.
5. Pregnancy applications. The CDC recommends against universal screening in pregnancy. However, screening should be offered to asymptomatic pregnant women whose partners have genital herpes, as well as prenatal patients who are HIV-infected. Discordant couples with an infected man should be counseled regarding the risk of acquiring and transmitting herpes and advised about preventive measures (e.g., abstinence during the third trimester) to avoid an initial primary infection. If the women is seropositive, she should be counseled regarding the signs and symptoms of genital herpes near term and counseling on plans for route of delivery (*see* "Pregnancy-Related Issues").
6. Other authors have suggested a broader utilization of serological testing in clinically apparent initial infections, although these applications have not been endorsed or found to be cost effective. These authors have suggested that an HSV-2 titer could be used to counsel women on the likelihood of recurrence (HSV-2 is more likely to occur than HSV-1 infection). Others have recommended routine serological testing for both HSV-1 and HSV-2 antibodies to establish if the clinical outbreak is a primary, nonprimary, or a recurrent lesion. The rationale is that if the patient has an HSV infection and if the serology is HSV-1- and HSV-2-negative, then the patient has an initial primary outbreak with exposure during the 14 days before the onset of symptoms. On the other hand, if the serology is HSV-1-positive but HSV-2-negative, then this is an initial nonprimary outbreak;

in such settings, one could probably come to that conclusion because 80% of genital herpes is HSV-2. However, the patient would require a repeat testing for HSV-2 in 3 months to confirm this diagnostic impression. If the serology is HSV-2-positive, then the patient has an initial nonprimary clinical outbreak of recurrent genital herpes with exposure sometime more 14 days prior.

DIAGNOSIS

The clinical diagnosis of genital herpes can be difficult. This is because the infection presents with "nonclassical" or atypical characteristics or with no symptoms at all. Although the most common cause of genital ulceration is an HSV infection, other etiologies should be considered, including chancroid, traumatic ulceration, primary syphilis, Behçet's syndrome, recurrent aphthous ulcers, fixed drug reaction, Crohn's disease, contact dermatitis, Reiter's syndrome, psoriasis, erythema multiforme, and lichen planus (23). The clinical diagnosis of genital herpes should always have laboratory confirmation, if possible.

For the last 20 years, the gold standard for diagnosis has been a positive viral culture. Viral culture results can be available in 48–72 hours and have a false-negative rate of 5–30%. Patients who present with new onset of genital herpes should also be tested for HIV infection. Testing for other STDs depends on the clinical presentation. Cultures are more likely to detect the virus if they are obtained from the freshly exposed base of a newly ruptured vesicle than if they come from an ulcerated or crusted lesion. Primary infections are more likely to produce positive result than are recurrent infections. Because of the transient nature of viral shedding, a negative culture does not exclude genital herpes. In the patient who has recurrent infections in which isolation of the virus has been difficult, one option is to have the patient return for viral cultures 1 or 2 days into the next outbreak. Another option is to order serological testing for type-specific HSV antibodies to rule out recurrent infections as described earlier.

TREATMENT

The CDC recommended therapies for initial infections and episodic and suppressive therapies for recurrent infection are displayed in Table 3.

Treatment Recommendation for Initial Herpes Genitalis

All patients with initial clinical episodes of symptomatic genital herpes should be treated with an antiviral agent for 7–10 days or until the lesions clear. Local measures, such as saline irrigation, sitz baths, topical anesthesia, use of electric blow dryer on cool setting, and warm compresses are helpful to prevent secondary infection of the lesions and to offer comfort. Careful attention must be paid to limit the spread of infection by autoinoculation. Because the effectiveness of antiviral therapy is dependent on initiation of therapy as early in the clinical stage

Table 3
Herpes Simplex Virus—CDC STD Treatment Guidelines 2006

Recommended regimens

First clinical episode of genital herpes

Acyclovir[a]	400	mg orally three times a day for 7–10 days	OR
Acyclovir[a]	200	mg orally five times a day for 7–10 days	OR
Famciclovir[a]	250	mg orally three times a day for 7–10 days	OR
Valacyclovir[a]	1	g orally twice a day for 7–10 days	

Note: Treatment may be extended if healing is incomplete after 10 days of therapy.

Episodic therapy for recurrent genital herpes

Acyclovir[a]	400	mg orally three times a day for 5 days	OR
Acyclovir[a]	800	mg orally twice a day for 5 days	OR
Acyclovir[a]	800	mg orally three a day for 2 days	OR
Famciclovir[a]	125	mg orally twice a day for 5 days	OR
Famciclovir[a]	1000	mg orally twice daily for 1 day	OR
Valacyclovir[a]	500	mg orally twice a day for 3 days	OR
Valacyclovir[a]	1.0	g orally once a day for 5 days	

Note: Treatment may be extended if healing is incomplete after initial days of therapy.

Suppressive therapy for recurrent genital herpes

Acyclovir[a]	400	mg orally twice a day	OR
Famciclovir[a]	250	mg orally twice a day	OR
Valacyclovir[a]	500	mg orally once a day[b]	OR
Valacyclovir[a]	1.0	g orally once a day	

Severe disease

Acyclovir[a]	5–10	mg/kg body weight intravenously every 8 hours for 2–7 days or until clinical improvement is observed, followed by oral antiviral therapy to complete at least 10 days total therapy

Episodic genital herpes infection in persons infected with HIV

Acyclovir[a]	400	mg orally three times a day for 5–10 days	OR
Famciclovir[a]	500	mg orally twice daily for 3 days	OR
Valacyclovir[a]	1.0	g orally once a day for 5 days	

Suppressive therapy for genital herpes infections in persons infected with HIV

Acyclovir[a]	400–800	mg orally two to three times a day	OR
Famciclovir[a,b]	500	mg orally twice a day	OR
Valacyclovir[a]	500	mg orally twice a day	

[a] The safety of systemic acyclovir, famciclovir, and valacyclovir therapy in pregnant women has not been established. Available data do not indicate an increase for major birth defects.

[b] Valacyclovir 500 mg once a day might be less effective than other valacyclovir or acyclovir dosing regimens in patients who have very frequent recurrences (i.e., ≥10 episodes per year).

CDC, Center for Disease Control and Prevention; STD, sexually transmitted disease; HIV, human immunodeficiency virus.

of disease as possible, treatment with antivirals should be started based on presumptive clinical diagnosis alone, before culture results are available.

The CDC lists three different drugs in four different treatment options for initial clinical episodes of genital herpes (*see* Table 3) *(33)*. Acyclovir (Zovirax™) was the first drug approved for the treatment of genital herpes. Acyclovir is a purine nucleoside analog that is a competitive inhibitor of viral DNA polymerase. Acyclovir completely inactivates the viral DNA polymerase and terminates viral DNA chain elongation. If given early in the initial stage of HSV infection, acyclovir will reduce the duration of symptoms by an average of 2 days, the time to heal the ulcers by 4 days, and viral shedding by 7 days compared to placebo *(4)*. In contrast to valacyclovir and famciclovir, acyclovir has poor oral bioavailability and a relatively short intracellular half-life, which means that acyclovir requires a three-times-a-day oral dosing schedule. For severe herpes infection requiring hospitalization, an intravenous formulation of acyclovir is available. The advantage of oral acyclovir therapy over other oral agents is lower cost, small tablets, and the availability of a liquid formulation. The disadvantages of oral acyclovir are the three-times-a-day dosing frequency and the development of resistant isolates.

Valacyclovir (Valtrex™) is a prodrug of acyclovir that is converted to acyclovir in the liver. The oral bioavailability of valacyclovir is much better than acyclovir and approaches the level of intravenous acyclovir. The advantage of valacyclovir is a twice-daily dosing schedule. The disadvantage of valacyclovir is higher cost and unavailability of nonoral formulations.

Famciclovir (Famvir™) is the oral form of penciclovir, a nucleoside analog with properties similar to acyclovir with an improved oral bioavailability *(34)*. Famciclovir is more expensive than acyclovir.

All oral antiviral agents have been shown to be equally effective *(3)*. Acyclovir, valacyclovir, and famciclovir have excellent safety profiles with few adverse side effects. It is estimated that more than 80 million people have taken either acyclovir or valacyclovir without significant complications *(35)*. HSV infections that are resistant to any of the recommended antiviral therapies are rare and generally restricted to immunocompromised patients. If resistance to acyclovir/valacyclovir/famciclovir develops, foscarnet 40 mg/kg body weight intravenously every 8 hours is frequently effective. Compounded topical cidofovir gel 1% applied to lesions once daily for 5 days also might be effective. Acyclovir has been used daily by patients for more than 10 years without any significant adverse effects.

After initiation of therapy, a follow-up visit with the patient should be scheduled in 7–10 days. Test results are usually available by that time, which will provide the caregiver the opportunity to provide more extensive counseling. If examination reveals new lesions or a failure of lesions to reach the crusting phase, then an additional course of antiviral agents should be prescribed.

The use of topical 5% acyclovir ointment is no longer an FDA-approved as treatment during the initial outbreak because the oral medication is more effective and the use of ointment increases the risk of autoinoculation. Other treatments that should be discouraged owing to documented lack of treatment efficacy include L-lysine, goldenseal, and garlic. Lithium has been noted to decrease frequency of recurrent herpes but has not been proven effective in the treatment of the initial infection *(36)*.

Treatment of Recurrent Genital Herpes

If started at the first prodromal symptoms or sign of a recurrence, antiviral treatment of episodic outbreaks will not only reduce the severity and duration of lesions, but may also completely abort the clinical attack, stopping the lesions from progressing beyond the papule stage. The episodic dosing schedules recommended by the CDC for acyclovir (Zovirax) vary by dose and duration of treatment. The episodic recommended dose for valacyclovir and famciclovir are also specified in the CDC recommendation.

The antiviral dosage schedule for suppressive therapy may be different for patients with more frequent (>10) outbreaks annually. All three antivirals appear to be equally effective in preventing outbreaks of genital herpes and reduce asymptomatic viral shedding by 80–90%.

In serodiscordant couples, suppressive daily antiviral therapy should be strongly considered to reduce further transmission of the infection during the first year when the incidence of asymptomatic viral shedding is highest. However, it should be noted that many couples who are discordant for genital herpes by patient history are found to be concordant by serological testing.

Immunocompromised patients are more likely to have prolonged or severe episodes of herpetic outbreak. Higher dose therapy is recommended for episodic therapy for HIV-infected persons, e.g., acyclovir 400 mg orally three times daily for 5–10 days; famciclovir 500 mg orally twice daily for 5–10 days; or valacyclovir 1.0 g orally twice a day for 5–10 days. For daily suppressive therapies, acyclovir 400–800 mg is recommended orally twice to three times a day or 500-mg doses of famciclovir or valacyclovir orally twice a day.

COUNSELING

The patient diagnosed with genital herpes may have more difficulty dealing with the psychological impact of the infection than with the physical discomfort. Studies have documented that patients frequently report anger, guilt, decreased self-esteem, loss of interest in intimacy or sex, fear of transmission to their sexual partner, and difficulty with personal relationships because of their diagnosis *(37)*. Mental and physical health scores in patients diagnosed with genital herpes were lower than the general population *(25)*. Although it is not currently possible, patients want reassurance that their genital herpes will never recur. Most patients will eventually accept their diagnosis and learn to cope with this chronic condition. The goals of counseling are patient education, partner notification (in order to break the chain of transmission), education on recognizing outbreak episodes, availability of treatment for viral transmission, as well as risk-reduction maneuvers.

The 2006 CDC Guidelines also provide guidance about patient counseling (*see* Table 4). In general, counseling of patients with recurrent herpes should emphasize that there is no known therapy to prevent establishment of latency of the herpes virus in the sensory ganglia of the sacral plexus or to prevent recurrent disease. In other words, there is no cure for herpes. The patient with recurrent disease should avoid intercourse during outbreaks beginning at the onset of prodromal symptoms until crusting over of the lesions several days later. Another option is to use latex condoms at all times, but particularly during genital outbreaks. Information about local self-help and support groups can be helpful.

The major concern of patients with genital herpes remains the fear of transmission to their sexual partners. In serodiscordant couples the transmission is most likely to occur in the first 3–6 months. It is estimated to occur at a rate less than 10% per year thereafter owing to decreased incidence of viral shedding and clinical outbreaks *(19)*.

Patients should also be advised about the risks of neonatal herpes and the strategies that should be taken to prevent vertical transmission.

PREGNANCY-RELATED ISSUES

About 22% of pregnant women are infected with HSV-2 and 2% will acquire HSV during pregnancy *(38)*. Initial HSV infection is particularly severe if it develops during pregnancy; pregnancy does not appear to increase the rate of recurrence of maternal outbreaks.

The most serious consequences of maternal infection are adverse fetal impacts and newborn infection. An initial maternal genital herpes outbreak in the first trimester of pregnancy has been associated with fetal chorioretinitis, microcephaly, and skin lesions but not spontaneous abortion or fetal death *(39)*. Neonatal HSV infection occurs in about 1500 cases each year *(40,40a)*. Neonatal HSV infection has three clinical presentations: disseminated disease involving multiple organs, such as the liver, lungs, and the central nervous system (25% of cases); disease localized to the skin, eyes, and mouth (40% of cases); and localized central nervous system disease (35% of cases). Up to 30% of infected neonates will die and up to 40% of survivors will have neurological damage, despite antiviral therapy *(40a)*.

Infection can be transmitted from the mother to her fetus/newborn in three ways: transplacentally (5–8%), intrapartum exposure (85%), or postpartum

Table 4
2006 CDC Counseling Guidelines for Patients With Herpes Genitalis

1. Information about the natural history of the disease, with emphasis on the potential for recurrent episodes, asymptomatic viral shedding, and attendant risks of sexual transmission.

2. Information about episodic or suppressive treatment with antiviral medication to shorten the duration of or prevent symptoms.

3. All patients with genital HSV infection should be encouraged to inform their current sex partners that they have genital herpes and to inform future partners before initiating a sexual relationship.

4. Persons with genital herpes should be informed that sexual transmission of HSV can occur during asymptomatic periods. Asymptomatic viral shedding is more frequent in genital HSV-2 infection than in genital HSV-1 infection and is most common in the first 12 months following acquisition of HSV-2, but may persist for years, less frequently, in some individuals.

5. Patients should be advised to abstain from sexual activity when lesions or prodromal are present.

6. The risk of HSV sexual transmission can be decreased by the daily use of antiviral agents by the infected person.

7. Latex condoms, when used consistently and correctly, can reduce the risk of genital herpes when the infected areas are covered or protected by the condom.

8. Sex partners of infected persons should be advised that they might themselves be infected even if they have no symptoms. Type-specific serological testing of asymptomatic partners of persons with genital herpes can determine whether risk for HSV acquisition exists.

9. The risk of neonatal infection should be explained to all patients, including men. Pregnant women and women of childbearing age who have genital herpes should inform their providers who care for them during pregnancy, as well as those who will care for their newborns infants. Pregnant women who are not infected with HSV-2 should be advised to avoid intercourse during the third trimester with men who have genital herpes. Similarly, pregnant women who are not infected with HSV-1 should be counseled to avoid genital exposure to HSV-1 (e.g., oral sex with a partner with oral herpes and vaginal intercourse with a partner with genital HSV-1 infection) during the third trimester.

10. Asymptomatic persons diagnosed with HSV-2 infection by type-specific serological testing should receive the same counseling messages as persons with symptomatic infection. In addition, such persons should be taught about the clinical manifestations of genital herpes.

HSV, herpes simplex virus; HIV, human immunodeficiency virus.

exposure (8–10%) *(40)*. The likelihood and severity of neonatal infection is influenced by the mother's antibody status. If a woman develops initial primary infection during pregnancy, there is a 5% chance of transplacental transmission to the baby.

Most neonatal infections result from fetal exposure during delivery. The remaining confirmed cases of neonatal herpes may have been acquired postnatally, either from the mother, a relative, or hospital worker as a result of oral contact or contact with an infected finger (whitlow) *(41)*.

Neonatal herpes infections develop in 30–50% of exposed infants whose mothers have an initial primary infection near time of delivery *(10)*. The risk of neonatal herpes from an asymptomatic mother with a history of recurrent HSV at term or who acquire HSV in the first-half of pregnancy is much lower (<1%). Only infants delivered to women who are actively shedding from recurrent infections at the time of delivery will acquire infection. It has been estimated by PCR techniques that 6–10% of HSV-2-seropositive women shed virus in labor *(42)*. However, because of the ubiquitous nature of this infection, more neonatal infections result from recurrent infections than from initial maternal infections. Infrequently, the infant may be infected by a caregiver with oral herpetic lesion or herpes whitlow, which involves the distal fingers.

The role of testing for HSV infection in pregnancy is under debate. The cost-effectiveness of routine HSV screening in pregnancy is controversial *(43,44)*. It has been suggested that type-specific HSV-2 serology testing be performed on women who have no personal history of HSV but whose partners are known to be infected. Women who tested negative could be advised to avoid sexual contact, at least during the third trimester and encouraged to use condoms (or abstinence) throughout the rest of pregnancy. The effectiveness of antiviral therapy for the partner to decrease the risk of HSV transmission to pregnant women has not been studied.

Women who develop primary HSV infection during pregnancy should be treated with acyclovir *(40,45)*. Acyclovir, valacyclovir, and famciclovir are classified as pregnancy category B drugs by the FDA. More than 1200 pregnancy outcomes have been followed in infants exposed *in utero* at all stages of fetal development to acyclovir. No significant differences in rates of birth defects or adverse pregnancy outcomes have been reported *(35)*. Experience with valacyclovir and famciclovir is too limited in the CDC estimation to provide information about the safety of its use in pregnancy.

For women who are known to have frequent recurrent outbreaks of genital lesions, suppressive therapy with antiviral agents starting at 36 weeks gestational age has also been shown to reduce the rate of symptomatic outbreaks and asymptomatic shedding and the need for cesarean section *(46)*. The concern that suppressive therapy might mask asymptomatic shedding can be addressed by culturing the women in labor who are candidates for vaginal delivery. No data support the treatment of seropositive women who have no history of lesions. The use of scalp monitors in labor should be discouraged in women who are known to shed HSV, but the American College of Obstetricians and Gynecologists says the use is not contraindicated if needed to assess fetal condition adequately in women with a history of HSV but without symptoms or lesions *(47)*.

Cesarean delivery is recommended for women who have active genital lesions or prodromal symptoms at the time of rupture of membranes or labor. Operative delivery has been shown to reduce the risk of transmission significantly in initial infection. Vaginal delivery is recommended for women who do not have lesions or symptoms at the time of delivery. Some experts recommend culturing the cervix and the area of recurrent outbreaks at the time of labor to learn postpartum if the woman was asymptomatically shedding, in which case the newborn will need antiviral therapy. C-section is not needed if the patient has lesions in extragenital areas, such as the buttocks or legs. The lesions can be covered and the patients can be allowed to deliver vaginally.

The pediatrician should always be informed of the maternal/patient history of herpes and the status of the mother at the time of delivery. Many experts recommended newborn surveillance cultures. Acyclovir may be recommended if the mother acquired the infection during pregnancy (especially third trimester) pending the results of the maternal and/or newborn culture.

Breastfeeding is not contraindicated except in mothers who have active HSV infections on the nipple or other sites on their breasts. Mothers should use caution when handling newborns and may take antiviral therapies when breastfeeding to diminish shedding.

PARTNER NOTIFICATION AND REPORTING REQUIREMENTS

HSV is not a reportable disease in most states. Patients should be advised to talk with their sex partners about their diagnosis. If the partner is infected with the same HSV type, no precautions need to be taken. Patients should understand most infected partners are not aware that they carry the virus. All new sex partners should be informed of the potential for infection and that safer sex practices may reduce, but do not eliminate, the possibility of transmission.

PREVENTION

Latex condoms are impermeable to passage of the 160 nm HSV-2. In 2002, an National Institutes of Health expert panel reviewed the literature and found that there was not sufficient data to allow it to form any conclusions about the effectiveness/ineffectiveness of correct and consistent condom usage in reducing the risk of genital herpes infection (6). However, a subsequent study of discordant couples found that when condoms were used more than 25% of the time, the risk of transmission to an uninfected woman was reduced by more than 90% (see Chapter 15) (12). More recently, analysis of data collected as part of a clinical trial of an ineffective candidate vaccine for HSV-2 revealed that those who reported more frequent condom use were at lower risk for acquiring HSV-2 than those who used condoms less frequently (48). Counseling for consistent condom use is needed because, despite the fact that there is a risk of transmission from asymptomatic shedding, couples are less likely to use condoms when active lesions are absent (49).

A recent trial of a glycoprotein D adjuvant vaccine was found to be 75% effective in preventing HSV-2 infection in women who were seronegative for HSV-1 and HSV-2. The vaccine was not effective in women who were seropositive for HSV-1 or in men. These findings demonstrate that early vaccination will be necessary if this vaccine is to be utilized *(47)*. Updated vaccine trial results are pending (*see* Chapter 16).

CASE STUDY

Jessica, age 51, has been a widow for 2 years. She is thinking about starting a new relationship and is worried about what she should do. Twenty years ago, Jessica had to have a cesarean section because she was suffering a painful genital infection that was diagnosed as herpes. Her daughter was not infected. Because she assumed that she had acquired the infection from her husband, she never worried about having to protect her partner. She has never had any recurrent outbreaks to the best of her knowledge. Recently, she saw ads warning that she may be contagious even if she has no symptoms. She is concerned because of her pending new romance and because she has been told that herpes increases her risk of getting a cancer. She wants to learn if she has to take medicine for the rest of her life. Her physical exam reveals no visible lesions.

Questions

1. What other questions would you like to ask?
2. What tests would you like to order, and for whom?
3. If she has had past exposure to HSV-2, what should she ask her potential partner to do?
4. How good are condoms at reducing female-to-male transmission of HSV-2?
5. How good is daily antiviral suppression at reducing HSV transmission?
6. Is she at any increased risk for developing cancer?

Answers and Teaching Points

1. We would like to learn if she or her husband had oral outbreaks (cold sores). Did her husband ever have genital herpes outbreaks? Did her potential partner ever have genital herpes outbreaks?
2. Type-specific serology testing for HSV-2 would be appropriate for Jessica. It is unusual for someone to have an initial symptomatic HSV-2 infection with no symptomatic recurrences. That pattern is much more common with HSV-1 infection.
3. If she has antibodies to HSV-2, testing of her potential new partner would be prudent if he has no prior history of genital herpes. Given the prevalence of HSV-2, there is a good chance he has already been exposed, even in the absence of any symptoms.
4. If there is discordance between them, condoms would be most appropriate if she were the vulnerable partner. There are no studies demonstrating that condom use protects men.

5. The role of suppressive antiviral therapy is questionable. Most recurrences occur within the first 1–3 years. Asymptomatic shedding continues, but at an extremely reduced rate. Jessica's original infection was more than 20 years ago.

6. She is not at any increased risk for developing cancer unless HSV is a marker of other infections, such as HPV.

SELECTED RESOURCES

- American Social Health Association

  A comprehensive resource for patients, their partners, and care givers. Offers herpes prevention, screening, and disease management information.

  Home of the National Herpes Resource Center
  Web site: http://www.ashastd.org/
  Phone: 800-783-9877 for a free catalog

- Herpes Web

  A comprehensive up-to-date information on herpes for patients. Includes interactive online questionnaires, discussion, and comments.

  Web site: http://www.herpesweb.net/general/menupage/general_info.htm

- The International Herpes Management Forum

  Wide range of herpes issues for both physicians and patients.

  Web site: http://www.ihmf.org/Patient/PatientResources.asp

- Fact Sheet on Genital Herpes

  From the CDC National Center for HIV, STD, and TB Prevention in the Division of Sexually Transmitted Diseases.

  Web site: http://www.cdc.gov/std/Herpes/STDFact-Herpes.htm

- National STD Hotline

  Health information hotline dedicated to providing accurate, basic information, referrals, and educational materials on a wide variety of STDs. Hotline specialists answer basic questions about STDs and refer callers to public health clinics and other local resources.

  Phone: 800-227-8922
  (8 AM–11 PM Eastern Standard Time, Monday through Friday).

- National Herpes Hotline

  Operated by American Social Health Association (ASHA) as part of the National Herpes Resource Center. Free counseling on herpes as well as referrals. A list of local support groups is available at: http://www.ashastd.org/hrc/help grp1.html

  Phone: 919-361-8488
  (9 AM–6 PM Eastern Standard Time, Monday through Friday)
  Web site: herpesnet@ashastd.org

- Planned Parenthood:

    Offers educational programs about diagnosis and treatment of genital herpes and living with the disease.

    Web site: http://www.plannedparenthood.org

    Phone: 800-230-PLAN

    24-hour information line: 800-549-0000 ext. 5326

REFERENCES

1. Roizman B, Whitley RJ. The nine ages of herpes simplex virus. Herpes 2001; 8:23–27.
2. Xu F, Sternberg MR, Kottiri BJ, et al. Trends in herpes simplex virus type 1 and type 2 seroprevalence in the United States. JAMA 2006; 296(8):964–973.
3. Yeung-Yue KA, Brentjens MH, Lee PC, Tyring SK. Herpes simplex viruses 1 and 2. Dermatol Clin 2002; 20:249–266.
4. Mertz GJ, Benedetti J, Ashley R, Selke SA, Corey L. Risk factors for the sexual transmission of genital herpes. Ann Intern Med 1992; 116:197–202.
5. Corey L, Wald A, Patel R, et al. Once-daily valacyclovir to reduce the risk of transmission of genital herpes. N Engl J Med 2004; 350:11–20.
6. National Institute of Allergy and Infectious Diseases. Workshop summary: scientific evidence on condom effectiveness for sexually transmitted disease (STD) prevention. Washington, DC: National Institutes of Health, Department of Health Services; 2001. Available from: http://www.niaid.nih.gov/dmid/stds/condomreport.pdf. Accessed June 4, 2005.
7. World Health Organization. Global prevalence and incidence of selected curable sexually transmitted infections: overview and estimates. Geneva: World Health Organization; 2001. Available from: http://www.who.int/emc-documents/STIs/whocdscsredc200110c.html. Accessed July 10, 2005.
8. Schacker T. The role of HSV in the transmission and progression of HIV. Herpes 2001; 8: 46–49.
9. Schacker T, Ryncarz AJ, Goddard J, Diem K, Shaughnessy M, Corey L. Frequent recovery of HIV-1 from genital herpes simplex virus lesions in HIV-1-infected men. JAMA 1998; 280:61–66.
10. Mole L, Ripich S, Margolis D, Holodniy M. The impact of active herpes simplex virus infection on human immunodeficiency virus load. J Infect Dis 1997; 176:766–770.
11. Wald A, Link K. Risk of human immunodeficiency virus infection in herpes simplex virus type 2-seropositive persons: a meta-analysis. J Infect Dis 2002; 185:45–52.
12. Wald A. Herpes simplex virus type 2 transmission: risk factors and virus shedding. Herpes 2004; 11:130A–137A.
13. Wald A, Langenberg AG, Link K, et al. Effect of condoms on reducing the transmission of herpes simplex virus type 2 from men to women. JAMA 2001; 285:3100–3106.
14. Cherpes TL, Meyn LA, Krohn MA, Hillier SL. Risk factors for infection with herpes simplex virus type 2: role of smoking, douching, uncircumcised males, and vaginal flora. Sex Transm Dis 2003; 30:405–10.
15. Langenberg AG, Corey L, Ashley RL, Leong WP, Straus SE. A prospective study of new infections with herpes simplex virus type 1 and type 2. Chiron HSV Vaccine Study Group. N Engl J Med 1999; 341:1432–1438.
16. Lafferty WE, Downey L, Celum C, Wald A. Herpes simplex virus type 1 as a cause of genital herpes: impact on surveillance and prevention. J Infect Dis 2000; 181:1454–1457.
17. Wald A, Zeh J, Selke S, et al. Reactivation of genital herpes simplex virus type 2 infection in asymptomatic seropositive persons. N Engl J Med 2000; 342:844–850.

18. Wald A, Corey L, Cone R, Hobson A, Davis G, Zeh J. Frequent genital herpes simplex virus 2 shedding in immunocompetent women. Effect of acyclovir treatment. J Clin Invest 1997; 99:1092–1097.

19. Bryson Y, Dillon M, Bernstein DI, Radolf J, Zakowski P, Garratty E. Risk of acquisition of genital herpes simplex virus type 2 in sex partners of persons with genital herpes: a prospective couple study. J Infect Dis 1993; 167:942–946.

20. Koelle DM, Benedetti J, Langenberg A, Corey L. Asymptomatic reactivation of herpes simplex virus in women after the first episode of genital herpes. Ann Intern Med 1992; 116: 433–437.

21. Scoular A. Using the evidence base on genital herpes: optimising the use of diagnostic tests and information provision. Sex Transm Infect 2002; 78:160–165.

22. Benedetti J, Corey L, Ashley R. Recurrence rates in genital herpes after symptomatic first-episode infection. Ann Intern Med 1994; 121:847–854.

23. Kimberlin DW, Rouse DJ. Clinical practice. Genital herpes. N Engl J Med 2004; 350:1970–1977.

24. Corey L, Adams HG, Brown ZA, Holmes KK. Genital herpes simplex virus infections: clinical manifestations, course, and complications. Ann Intern Med 1983; 98:958–972.

25. Patel R, Boselli F, Cairo I, Barnett G, Price M, Wulf HC. Patients' perspectives on the burden of recurrent genital herpes. Int J STD AIDS 2001; 12:640–645.

26. Sweet RL, Gibbs RS. Herpes simplex virus infection. In: *Infectious Diseases of the Female Genital Tract*, 4th Ed. Philadelphia, PA: Lippincott, Williams & Wilkins, 2002; pp. 101–117.

27. Kessler HA, Baker DA, Brown ZA, Leone PA. Herpesvirus management: special considerations for the female patient. A monograph based on a symposium held May 6, 2002. New York, NY: New World Health; 2002.

28. Ebel C, Wald A. *Managing Herpes: How to Live and Love with a Chronic STD*, 3rd Ed. Research Park Triangle, NC: American Social Health Association; 2002.

28a. Schacker T. The role of HSV in the transmission and progression of HIV. Herpes 2001; 8(2):46–49.

29. Kaufman RH, Gardner HL, Rawls WE, Dixon RE, Young RL. Clinical features of herpes genitalis. Cancer Res 1973; 33:1446–1451.

30. Benedetti JK, Zeh J, Corey L. Clinical reactivation of genital herpes simplex virus infection decreases in frequency over time. Ann Intern Med 1999; 131:14–20.

30a. Fleming DT, Leone P, Esposito D. Herpes virus infection and genital symptoms in primary care patients. Sex Transm Inf 2006; 33(7):416–421.

31. Waggoner-Fountain LA, Grossman LB. Herpes simplex virus. Pediatr Rev 2004; 25:86–93.

32. Crist GA, Langer JM, Woods GL, Procter M, Hillyard DR. Evaluation of the ELVIS plate method for the detection and typing of herpes simplex virus in clinical specimens. Diagn Microbiol Infect Dis 2004; 49:173–177.

33. Centers for Disease Control and Prevention. Sexually transmitted diseases treatment guidelines 2002. MMWR Recomm Rep 2002; 51:1–78.

34. Diaz-Mitoma F, Sibbald RG, Shafran SD, Boon R, Saltzman RL. Oral famciclovir for the suppression of recurrent genital herpes: a randomized controlled trial. Collaborative Famciclovir Genital Herpes Research Group. JAMA 1998; 280:887–892.

35. Tyring SK, Baker D, Snowden W. Valacyclovir for herpes simplex virus infection: long-term safety and sustained efficacy after 20 years experience with acyclovir. J Infect Dis 2002; 186:S40–46.

36. Parks DG, Greenway FL, Pack AT. Prevention of recurrent herpes simplex type II infection with lithium carbonate. Med Sci Research 1988; 16:971–972.

37. Alexander L, Naisbett B. Patient and physician partnerships in managing genital herpes. J Infect Dis 2002; 186:S57–S65.

38. Brown ZA, Gardella C, Wald A, Morrow RA, Corey L. Genital herpes complicating pregnancy. Obstet Gynecol 2005; 106(4):845–856.
39. Eskild A, Jeansson S, Stray-Pedersen B, Jenum PA. Herpes simplex virus type-2 infection in pregnancy: no risk of fetal death: results from a nested case-control study within 35,940 women. BJOG 2002; 109:1030–1035.
40. Brown Z. Preventing herpes simplex virus transmission to the neonate. Herpes 2004; 11: 175A–186A.
40a. Kimberlin DW. Neonatal herpes simplex infection. Clin Microbiol Rev 2004; 17(1):1–13.
41. Smith JR, Cowan FM, Munday P. The management of herpes simplex virus infection in pregnancy. Br J Obstet Gynaecol 1998; 105:255–260.
42. Watts DH, Brown ZA, Money D, et al. A double-blind, randomized, placebo-controlled trial of acyclovir in late pregnancy for the reduction of herpes simplex virus shedding and cesarean delivery. Am J Obstet Gynecol 2003; 188:836–843.
43. Thung SF, Grobman WA. The cost-effectiveness of routine antenatal screening for maternal herpes simplex virus-1 and -2 antibodies. Am J Obstet Gynecol 2005; 192:483–488.
44. Baker D, Brown Z, Hollier LM, et al. Cost-effectiveness of herpes simplex virus type 2 serologic testing and antiviral therapy in pregnancy. Am J Obstet Gynecol 2004; 191:2074–2084.
45. American College of Obstetricians and Gynecologists. ACOG practice bulletin. Management of herpes in pregnancy. Number 8 October 1999. Clinical management guidelines for obstetrician-gynecologists. Int J Gynaecol Obstet 2000; 68:165–173.
46. Sheffield JS, Hollier LM, Hill JB, Stuart GS, Wendel GD. Acyclovir prophylaxis to prevent herpes simplex virus recurrence at delivery: a systematic review. Obstet Gynecol 2003; 102: 1396–1403.
47. Stanberry LR, Spruance SL, Cunningham AL, et al. Glycoprotein-D-adjuvant vaccine to prevent genital herpes. N Engl J Med 2002; 347:1652–1661.
48. Wald A, Langenberg AG, Krantz E, et al. The relationship between condom use and herpes simplex virus acquisition. Ann Intern Med 2005; 143(10):707–713.
49. Rana RK, Pimenta JM, Rosenberg DM, et al. Sexual behaviour and condom use among individuals with a history of symptomatic genital herpes. Sex Transm Inf 2006; 82(1):69–74.

4

Viral Hepatitis

Michelle L. Geller and Jeremy R. Herman

INTRODUCTION

Various forms of viral hepatitis have been identified as being sexually transmitted infections (STIs), whereas other forms are transmitted primarily via oral fecal routes. The most common forms of viral hepatitis are hepatitis A, B, and C. Hepatitis A virus (HAV) infection is most often a benign self-limiting disease; however, it can progress to fulminant liver failure. Fecal–oral transmission though contact with infectious sources in combination with poor hygiene or sanitation is the major route of HAV acquisition. Infection with hepatitis B virus (HBV) can be either acute and self-limited or can become chronic. HBV carriers are at increased risk of cirrhosis, hepatocellular carcinoma (HCC), and death from chronic liver disease. HBV can be transmitted perinatally, percutaneously, or across mucous membranes by sexual contact or by close person-to-person contact through open cuts and sores. Hepatitis C virus (HCV) is a blood-borne virus transmitted primarily by parenteral exposure to infected blood. The role of sexual exposure in transmission is minimal in HCV infection.

In patients who present with signs and symptoms of viral hepatitis, an acute viral hepatitis panel may be very helpful to distinguish among the various viral types. This chapter describes the epidemiology, transmission, clinical presentation, diagnostic work-up, management, and prevention methods of the most common forms of viral hepatitis.

FAST FACTS

- Immunization programs have significantly reduced the incidence of hepatitis A and B over the last decade.
- Hepatitis A is now more frequently transmitted by sexual contact than it was in the past.
- Hepatitis B virus is more contagious sexually than human immunodeficiency virus (HIV).

From: *Current Clinical Practice: Sexually Transmitted Diseases:*
A Practical Guide for Primary Care
Edited by: A. L. Nelson and J. A. Woodward © Humana Press, Totowa, NJ

- The incidence of hepatitis C infections has decreased since the blood supply has been tested, but the future treatment of individuals already infected is expected to be prohibitively expensive.
- Approximately 5–25% of chronic HBV and HCV infected people will die prematurely from cirrhosis and liver cancer.
- Effective therapies for viral hepatitis are available, but most people with chronic HCV infection are unaware of their infections (1).

HEPATITIS A

Prevalence and Incidence

HAV is the most common cause of acute infectious hepatitis worldwide. Although hepatitis A is not generally an STI except perhaps among men who have sex with men (MSM), HAV must always be included in the differential diagnosis of viral hepatitis and, therefore, is summarized in this chapter. Most often a benign self-limited disease, HAV infection can progress to fulminant liver failure in a small, well-defined subgroup of patients. The National Health and Nutrition Survey II conducted in the United States before modern immunization practices detected HAV antibody in 38% of persons (1a). Presence of HAV antibody correlates with age because of increasing opportunity for exposure; 75% of US adults over 70 years of age have serological evidence of past HAV infection. The Centers for Disease Control and Prevention (CDC) estimates that there were approximately 90,000 symptomatic and 180,000 asymptomatic new cases in the United States in 1997 (2). Since the introduction of hepatitis A vaccines in 1995, reports of HAV infection have declined by over 80% (2a). There were only 5683 cases reported in 2004 (3). In the United States, the HAV vaccine has been given to individuals at risk, including international travelers, MSM, substance abusers, and children in states with high rates of infection (4). Many of the disparities in HAV infection between ethnic groups and geographic regions have disappeared with these targeted vaccination programs (4).

Worldwide, HAV is considered highly endemic in developing countries with variable sanitation practices, such as Africa, Asia, and Central and South America. The World Health Organization estimates that approximately 80% of the global population has HAV antibodies (5). Low rates of symptomatic disease in children enable a large reservoir of disease, whereas the major burden of illness tends to occur in sporadic (e.g., travelers) and epidemic (e.g., community outbreaks) cases.

Etiology

HAV is a single-stranded nonenveloped positive-sense RNA virus. At a pH of 1.0, it is a stable, heat-resistant member of the *Picornaviridae* family, allowing infection through water, fomites, and under-cooked food sources. A well-defined enterohepatic life cycle enables fecal–oral transmission. Four genotypes are recognized and genetic heterogeneity may contribute to some of the variability of symptom penetrance observed with HAV infection *(6)*.

Transmission

Fecal–oral transmission though contact with infectious sources in combination with poor hygiene or sanitation is the major route of HAV acquisition. Parenteral exposure to contaminated blood is known to occur but documentations are rare *(6)*. Maximal source infectivity occurs from 2 weeks before to 1 week after clinical symptoms when the largest amount viral particles can be found in stool *(7)*. Thus, the infection can be spread even before the patient develops symptoms and could take measures to reduce transmission.

Person-to-person contact accounted for the most frequently reported cases (11.6% in 2002), likely attributed to household or sexual contact, whereas approximately 5% of cases occurred in children and staff attending day-care centers. Travelers from nonendemic countries, where HAV immunity levels are low, to endemic countries accounted for 9.4% of cases that year. For persons from the United States, travel to Mexico is the most commonly reported source. Most cases within the United States occur in community-wide outbreaks, which have been associated with food and water in 2–3% of cases. Those outbreaks are usually in group settings, such as restaurants, day-care centers, schools, and health care facilities. Illegal drug use accounted for 5.9% of infections. In rare cases, transmission occurs via transfusion of blood or blood products. Although likely attributed to contact with unidentified cases, the transmission mechanism is not known in approximately 50% of HAV infections *(4)*.

Sexual transmission is an increasingly important contributor to HAV infection. Infection rates have steadily increased over the last decade among MSM and accounted for 8.4% of reported cases in 2002 *(4)*. Both heterosexual and homosexual behavior likely contributes to a large amount of HAV transmission via unapparent or gross fecal contamination *(6,8)*. Certain studies have identified greater number of sexual partners, frequent oral–anal contact, penetration through anal intercourse, or evidence of other STIs as risk factors, whereas other studies found no specific associations *(9,10)*. Injection drug use is a major risk factor for HAV infection, although it is uncertain whether equipment sharing activities or poor hygiene is more significant in this viral transmission *(11)*.

Clinical Presentation

The incubation period for HAV averages 28 days, but ranges from 15 to 50 days and is inversely related to age. The risk of developing symptoms, however, is directly related to age; most children are asymptomatic but 80% of adults have identifiable symptoms. Acute viral hepatitis is characterized most commonly by a prodrome of nonspecific constitutional symptoms such as malaise, fever, anorexia, and headache, which shortly develops into abdominal pain, nausea, and vomiting. In 2002, more than 70% of reported cases had jaundice; 25% required hospitalization *(4)*. Within 1–2 weeks, the icteric phase begins with the development of dark urine and pale stools and progresses to overt jaundice. Hepatosplenomegaly and right upper quadrant tenderness may occur but are less common. The icteric phase usually lasts for 2 weeks; convalescence ensues over the next several weeks. Liver function tests (LFTs) reveal hepatocellular disease with mixed bilirubinemia peaking at 10–15 mg/dL and markedly elevated alanine transaminase (ALT) to more than 1000 IU/dL. A major clue to HAV infection lies in identification of a high-risk exposure within 10–50 days before prodromal symptoms corresponding to the viral incubation time. Symptomatic disease is common with adult infection (75–90%), whereas children are symptomatic much less often (only 5–20% of those less than 5 years of age) *(5)*.

There is no chronic infection with hepatitis A, but relapsing hepatitis occurs in 4 to 20% of symptomatic patients *(12)*; 10–15% experience a relapse within 6 months. Relapsing hepatitis A is defined by two or more bouts of acute HAV occur over 6 to 10 weeks with symptom-free intervals. Less common symptomatic variations of HAV infection are known to occur. Cholestatic hepatitis A occurs in 10% of symptomatic patients *(13)* and is associated with prolonged symptoms of fever, pruritus, and jaundice with persistently elevated bilirubin after other LFTs normalize *(14)*.

Fulminant hepatic failure requiring transplantation is rare (0.3%). It is characterized by progressive jaundice, prothrombin time prolongation and encephalopathy within the first week of disease. Patients older than 49 years of age and persons with other underlying liver disease (chronic HBV or HCV, alcoholic disease) are at increased risk for developing HAV-induced liver failure *(15,16)*. The mortality rate from HAV infection in 2002 was 0.5% *(4)*.

Testing and Diagnosis

HAV cannot be differentiated from other forms of acute hepatitis (HBV, HCV) without serological testing. Clinical evidence of acute hepatitis should prompt testing for immunoglobulin (Ig)M anti-HAV, which indicates recent infection. Antibody can be detected 5–10 days before the onset of symptoms and may persist for up to 6 months following infection *(17)*. Highly sensitive and specific kits are available and do not require reflex confirmation. Previous exposure or immunization is reflected in testing of IgG. Total anti-HAV testing does not distinguish between acute and chronic infection.

Treatment

Symptomatic HAV infection is a benign self-limiting illness in the vast majority of patients because clinical and biochemical recovery occurs within 3 months.

Most patients can be treated as outpatients, although hospitalization may be indicated in those with dehydration, food intolerance, major comorbidities, or evidence of fulminant disease. If admitted to the hospital, contact isolation is only required for diapered patients and those incontinent of stool (18). Patients at high risk for progressing to liver failure should be transferred to institutions capable of performing liver transplantation. Medications that require hepatic metabolism or that could inflict hepatic damage should be used with caution during the acute HAV infection.

Partner Notification and Reporting Requirements

Health care practitioners should report all persons that have symptoms of acute hepatitis who are IgM anti-HAV positive to state and/or local health departments (19). Cases should be investigated as soon as possible once suspected or identified to permit adequate time to implement preventative postexposure measures to potential contacts. All confirmed cases of acute hepatitis A should be interviewed to identify a potential source or risk factor for infection during the 2–6 weeks before symptom onset. Risk history may be unreliable for persons who are antibody-positive without acute symptoms, as IgM antibodies may persist up to 6 months after infection. Postexposure prophylaxis should be provided for contacts recently exposed to a person with acute hepatitis A (see "Prevention and Postexposure Prophylaxis" below).

Pregnancy-Related Issues

The incidence of maternal HAV infection in pregnancy is 1 in 1000 (20). Perinatal transmission of the HAV does not occur (21) and unlike hepatitis E virus (HEV), pregnancy is not a risk factor for progression to liver failure. The hepatitis A vaccine is likely safe in pregnancy because it is inactivated but is considered a class C drug because there is no safety or efficacy data in animals or humans. Risk of vaccination should be weighed against the risk for HAV infection, but is generally recommend for persons at high risk for HAV infection (22). Immune globulin is safe in pregnancy and should not affect indications of use (23).

Prevention and Postexposure Prophylaxis

Hepatitis A infection is one of the most frequently reported vaccine-preventable diseases (2). Prevention of disease can occur by implementing general infection precautions as well as active and passive immunization efforts. Public health practices that may diminish HAV transmission include improved personal hygiene, especially during food preparation, improved sanitation of water processing and sewage disposal techniques, avoidance of illegal drug use, and reducing contact with infected individuals. Condom use does not have a role in the prevention of sexually acquired HAV (7).

Table 1
Indications for Intramuscular Immune
Globulin to Prevent the Hepatitis A Virus

- Unvaccinated sexual partner, sharer of intravenous drugs (7) or household contact exposed to a serologically confirmed person infected with HAV in the past 2 weeks.
- Unvaccinated attendee or staff of a day care center if one or more cases of HAV are diagnosed in children or employees or two or more cases of HAV are diagnosed in households of center attendees.
- Persons in common-source exposure situations (e.g., patrons of a food establishment with an HAV-infected food handler) if risk of transmission is determined to be high.
- Food handlers if another food handler in the same establishment is diagnosed with HAV.
- Travelers to highly endemic areas (see Table 2) within 2 weeks of departure.

Adapted from refs. 2, 30, and 30a.

Current CDC immunization strategy is based on preventing disease and eliminating global burden by recommending passive and/or active immunization for persons with well-defined risks and implementation of general childhood vaccination policies in communities with high HAV prevalence. Passive immunization consists of intramuscular (IM) administration of pooled human Ig to those persons in which active vaccination will not provide timely protection (see Table 1). For persons exposed to HAV, IM administration of pooled human immunoglobulin (Ig) (0.02 mL/kg) is effective in preventing progression to clinical disease in most cases if administered within 2 weeks of exposure (24). Ig is effective in preventing HAV in more than 85% of recipients for approximately 3 months with a low-dose (0.02 mL/kg) preparation and for 5 months with a higher dose (0.06 mL/kg). Ig is generally well-tolerated; however, it is contraindicated in patients with selective IgA deficiency because of reports of anaphylaxis after repeated administrations (25). Ig may decrease immunogenicity of concomitant administration of live attenuated virus vaccinations (i.e., measles, mumps, rubella). HAV vaccine and Ig can be administered concomitantly at different anatomical sites (2).

In 1995, the Food and Drug Administration approved two formalin-inactivated cell-cultured derived HAV vaccines (HAVRIX® [SmithKline Beecham Biologicals], two doses at 6–12 months apart and VAQTA® [Merck & Co., Inc.], two doses at 6–18 months apart), for use in persons older than 12 months of age. Recently, an effective combination hepatitis A–hepatitis B (TWINRIX® [GlaxoSmithKline], three doses at 0, 1, and 6 months) vaccine was approved for persons 18 years or older (26). All vaccines are highly immunogenic in most adults and children. Of vaccinated persons, 94–97% demonstrate neutralizing

Table 2
Indications for Active Immunization With the Hepatitis A Vaccine

- Children over 2 years of age and adults living in a state, county, city, or community with more than 20 new cases per 100,000 persons per year
- Traveling to or working in high endemic areas such as those located in Central or South America, Mexico, the Caribbean, Asia (except Japan), Africa, and Eastern Europe. Administer 2 to 4 weeks before departure
- Men who have sex with men (MSM)
- Illegal drug users [a]
- Persons with occupational risks working with laboratory hepatitis A virus (HAV)- or HAV-infected primates
- Persons who are receiving treatment with clotting factor
- Persons with chronic liver disease

[a] Both injection and noninjection drugs.
Adapted from refs. 2 and 30a.

antibodies after the first dose and virtually all have them after the second dose (27–29). The CDC recommends vaccination for all children in highly prevalent communities (when prevalence exceeds twice the national average) as well as those at high risk for acquisition (see Table 2) (2). Some authors, however, have recommended routine vaccination for all children in the United States because new cases in highly prevalent communities only represent 50% of cases (23).

Routine and prevaccination screening for anti-HAV is generally not indicated. However, if population seroprevalence is high, screening of persons recommended to receive HAV vaccine with serum HAV IgG may be cost-effective; for example, the CDC suggests to consider prevaccination testing if the prevalence in the population is more than 33% (2). Examples of these populations include the elderly, adolescents and adults of specified ethnicities (e.g., Native Americans, Alaskan Natives, and Hispanics) and foreign-born persons from endemic countries (6,30).

Decreased immunogenicity to HAV vaccination occurs in infants who obtain passive maternal antibodies, supporting the rationale not to immunize persons less than 2 years of age. Additional populations with diminished immunogenicity include patients with chronic liver disease (93%) (31), immunocompromised persons (88%) (32), and transplant recipients (26%) (33). Immunity lasting up to 9 years has been observed and CDC models indicate that protection should continue for 20 years without need for booster doses (29). The most common adverse effects include local reactions, such as injection site soreness, headache, and malaise with no evidence to suggest serious adverse effects directly attributable to HAV vaccine (2).

HEPATITIS B

Prevalence and Incidence

In the United States, between 1990 and 2005, there was a 75% decline in the number of acute hepatitis B cases; the highest percent of cases is now among adults *(3)*. This decline has been associated with a multifaceted program of vaccination in which all infants and young people under age 19 are vaccinated, as well as all at-risk individuals. In addition, all pregnant women are screened for chronic infection, and newborns receive postexposure prophylaxis.

It is estimated that more than 300 million persons worldwide are HBV carriers *(35)*. The highest prevalence (10–20%) is found in Southeast Asia, China, and sub-Saharan Africa *(36,37)*. Carriers are at increased risk of cirrhosis, hepatocellular carcinoma (HCC), and death from chronic liver disease *(38)*. Worldwide, universal hepatitis B vaccination programs have demonstrated a significant reduction in HBV carrier rates and HCC, particularly in endemic countries *(39)*.

An estimated 1.25 million US residents are HBV carriers. In the United States, most cases of acute HBV infection occur in patients aged 20–39. More men than women are infected. Non-Hispanic blacks have higher infection rates than other ethnic groups. Between 15 and 25% of chronically infected patients die prematurely. Approximately 5000 Americans die each year as a result of HBV-associated chronic liver disease. However, even in the United States, some people in high-risk populations recommended for vaccination still remain unvaccinated *(40)*.

Etiology

HBV is a double-stranded DNA hepadnavirus with seven genotypes (A–G), which vary geographically. Genotypes may predict clinical course and response to therapy, although currently there is insufficient data to alter treatment recommendations based on genotype.

Infectivity and Transmission

HBV is found in the highest concentrations in the blood. It is also found in other body fluids, such as semen and vaginal secretions. The virus can be transmitted perinatally, percutaneously, or across mucous membranes by sexual contact or close person-to-person contact through open cuts and sores. It has been estimated that HBV is 20 times more sexually contagious than HIV. Percutaneous transmission can occur from a variety of sources, including injection drug use, dialysis, needle-stick injuries, acupuncture, tattooing, and body piercing. The risk of transmission from a percutaneous exposure to HBV is 6–30% *(41)*. About 25% of regular sexual contacts of HBV-infected people will become HBV-positive *(22)*. HBV can live outside the body for up to 1 week on environmental surfaces, such as toothbrushes and razor blades *(42)*. In 2002, about 25%

of new cases were caused by sexual contact and 12% were the result of intravenous drug use, whereas only 1% of cases resulted from hemodialysis or blood transfusion. In more than 50% of cases, no causation could be identified *(4)*.

Risk Factors

High-risk populations include patients born in endemic regions, including Africa, Southeast Asia (including China, Korea, Indonesia, and the Philippines), the Middle East (except Israel), South and Western Pacific Islands, the interior Amazon River basin and certain parts of the Caribbean (Haiti and the Dominican Republic). High-risk patients from nonendemic areas include MSM, injection drug users, dialysis patients, HIV-infected patients, sexual and household contacts of HBV-infected patients, health care workers, recipients of certain blood products, and people with a recent history of multiple sex partners or a sexually transmitted disease (STD) *(43)*. High-risk patients from nonendemic areas should be tested for prior infection and vaccinated if they have not previously been exposed.

Clinical Presentation

Infection with HBV can be either acute and self-limited or can become chronic. Once a person is exposed to HBV, the incubation period is from 6 weeks to 6 months, but averages 60–90 days before the onset of symptoms begin. Approximately 50% of acute infections are symptomatic and generally present with three phases. The prodromal phase includes nonspecific symptoms, such as malaise, anorexia, nausea, vomiting, right upper quadrant abdominal pain, fever, headache, myalgias, skin rashes, arthralgias, arthritis, and/or dark urine. The icteric phase can last up to 1 to 3 weeks and presents with jaundice, light stools, and hepatomegaly with tenderness. Jaundice and the need for hospitalization increase with age *(4)*. The convalescent stage is characterized by malaise and fatigue, which can last for weeks to months. Only 1% of acute infections result in acute liver failure and/or death in adults *(7)*.

Chronic HBV infection can be asymptomatic, however, nonspecific symptoms such as fatigue can develop insidiously. Physical exam can be normal or demonstrate signs of chronic liver disease, including jaundice, splenomegaly, ascites, peripheral edema, and encephalopathy if decompensated. Other extrahepatic manifestations may include polyarteritis nodosa and renal glomerular disease. There is a much higher risk of chronic infection in infants (90%) and children under 5 years (60%) compared with adults (2–6%) *(44–47)*. If chronic infection occurs, the risk of death (i.e., from cirrhosis or HCC) is 15–25% *(7)*. In all carrier states, exacerbations of hepatitis can occur, which can lead to progressive liver fibrosis. Progression to cirrhosis is more likely in patients who are older and HBeAg-positive, and have elevated ALT levels *(48–50)*. Rapid progression is more likely in those who are co-infected with HCV and more severe liver disease is seen in co-infection with HIV *(51,52)*.

Table 3
Serological Markers in Different Stages
of Hepatitis B Virus (HBV) Infection

Stage of HBV infection	HBsAg[a]	Anti-HBs[b]	IgM Anti-HBc[c]	Total[d] Anti-HB[c]
Late incubation period	+	−	−	+/−
Acute	+	−	+	+
Chronic	+	−[d] (+ rarely)	+	−
Recent (<6 months) window period	−	+/−	+	+
Distant (>6 months); resolved[e]	−	+	+	−
Immunized	−	+[f]	−	−

[a] Hepatitis B surface antigen.
[b] Antibodies to hepatitis B surface antigen.
[c] Antibodies to hepatitis B core antigen.
[d] The total anti-HBc assay detects both immunoglobulin (Ig)M and IgG antibody.
[e] Resolved indicates that the patient no longer has the disease.
[f] Anti-HBs more than 10 mIU/mL.
Adapted from ref. 7.

Testing and Diagnosis

If HBV infection is suspected, the diagnosis can be confirmed by serological testing (see Table 3). In acute infections, IgM antibodies to hepatitis B core antigen (IgM anti-HBc) are positive. Hepatitis B surface antigen (HBsAg) may also be present, but is usually absent if the patient is in the window period (<6 months). In high-risk patients being screened for asymptomatic HBV infection, testing for HBsAg and antibody to HBsAg (anti-HBs) should be performed. Chronic HBV infection or the carrier state is determined when HBsAg is present and persists for at least 6 months (53). Presence of anti-HBs alone is seen postimmunization. Anti-HBc indicates acute, resolved, or chronic infection.

Patients diagnosed with chronic HBV infection should undergo a full history, including risk factor determination, and physical exam. Other laboratory testing should include complete blood count (including platelets), liver function tests (including aspartate aminotransferase, ALT, total bilirubin, alkaline phosphatase), albumin, prothrombin time, HIV and HCV. Hepatitis D virus (HDV) should also be tested for in patients from endemic areas. When determining the need for treatment, serum HBeAg (a marker of HBV replication and infectivity), antibody to HBeAg (anti-HBe) and HBV DNA by polymerase chain reaction (PCR) assay should be obtained. Right upper quadrant ultrasound and serum α-fetoprotein (AFP) should be obtained to screen for HCC. Liver biopsy may be helpful, although histology can vary throughout the clinical course.

Treatment

Treatment of acute HBV infections is supportive. In chronic HBV infection, patients who are seropositive for HBeAg or seronegative for HBeAg and positive for HBV DNA may be eligible for antiviral therapies, although long-term efficacy is limited. For those with HBeAg positivity, successful treatment is more likely if ALT is at least twice the upper limit of normal *(54,55)*. Response to treatment is less predictable in HBeAg-negative patients. Treatment is generally not recommended in these groups without ALT elevations, HBV DNA more than 10^5 and/or histological abnormalities. In newly diagnosed patients, treatment should be delayed up to 6 months to assess for spontaneous HBeAg seroconversion *(43)*.

In chronic HBV infection, appropriate patients are generally treated with one of the three approved antiviral therapies: interferon, lamivudine, or adefovir. Treatment should be implemented by a specialist who is experienced in treatment and management chronic HBV infection. Choice of treatment, dose, and duration is dependent on age, severity of disease, immunocompetency, likelihood of response, availability of resources, and a variety of clinical criteria. Each therapy has limitations and side effects and relapse can occur. Many new therapies are emerging, including new routes of administration as well as the use of combination therapy with existing therapies.

Follow-Up

Clearance of HBeAg, either spontaneously or in response to treatment, reduces the risk of hepatic failure and is associated with increased survival *(56–58)*. Endpoints to assess treatment response include normalized ALT values, undetectable serum HBV DNA, loss of HBeAg with or without anti-HBe, and improvement in liver histology *(59)*. For patients in the inactive HBsAg carrier state, it is recommended to monitor LFTs every 6 to 12 months, because disease can become active even after many years *(43)*. The optimal screening tools and intervals for HCC are not entirely clear, but the American Association for the Study of Liver Diseases (AASLD) guidelines, based on current evidence, suggest testing AFP alone for low-risk carriers and AFP plus ultrasound for high-risk carriers at 6 month intervals *(59)*.

If not immune to HAV, patients should be vaccinated with hepatitis A vaccine, two doses 6 to 18 months apart. Patients should be advised to abstain from alcohol use. Heavy consumption of alcohol (>40g/d) has been associated with poor outcomes *(60–62)*; However, a "safe" amount of alcohol use has not been determined. Patients should also be counseled on prevention of transmission to others (*see* "Prevention and Postexposure Prophylaxis" section on p. 83).

Partner Notification and Reporting Requirements

Health care practitioners are required to report confirmed acute hepatitis B cases to state and/or local health departments *(19)*. This should be done as soon as possible to ensure adequate time to implement preventative measures and appropriate postexposure prophylaxis of contacts. A reported case is considered confirmed if it meets both clinical and serological criteria. Serological criteria include IgM anti-HBc-positive or HBsAg-positive and IgM anti-HAV-negative. All confirmed or suspected cases of acute hepatitis B should be interviewed by the provider to identify a source or risk factor(s) for infection during the 6 weeks to 6 months before illness onset *(19)*.

Contacts of persons with acute HBV infection should receive postexposure vaccination and prophylaxis with hepatitis B immune globulin (HBIG), unless they have been previously vaccinated and known to be responders. Sexual partners of known infected persons should receive these two interventions within 14 days of sexual contact. The recommended dose of HBIG is 0.06 mL/kg. If a person is diagnosed with chronic HBV infection, hepatitis B vaccine alone should be administered to sexual partners, needle-sharing partners, and household contacts. Postvaccination testing with anti-HBs should be considered for sexual partners. If they are anti-HBs-negative, they should receive a second complete series. If they continue to be antibody-negative, abstinence and other methods of protection should be emphasized *(7)*. Victims of sexual assault and people who have percutaneous exposure (needle stick or bite) or mucosal exposure to blood or body fluids who have not previously been vaccinated should receive the vaccine series but not HBIG unless the perpetrator is known to have an acute infection.

Pregnancy-Related Issues

Early prenatal testing for HBsAg is recommended by the Advisory Committee on Immunization Practices, the American College of Obstetrics and Gynecology, and the American Academy of Pediatrics. If seronegative at the first prenatal visit, high-risk women should be screened again later in the pregnancy *(63,64)*. Because of the high rate of perinatal transmission, newborns of HBsAg-positive mothers should receive both passive and active immunization with HBIG and hepatitis B vaccine within 12 hours of delivery and then complete the recommended vaccine schedule *(65)*. Variations exist for premature and low-birthweight infants *(66)*.

The CDC recommends that all pregnant women receiving STI services should be tested for HBsAg, even if testing had been done earlier in the pregnancy. Pregnancy is not a contraindication for HBV vaccine and HBsAg-negative pregnant women at risk (e.g., STI, multiple or new sex partners, women who exchange sex for money or drugs, patient or her partner uses or has used intravenous drugs, partner is bisexual) who have not been previously vaccinated should receive the HBV vaccine. Breastfeeding has not been shown to increase the risk of transmission over formula-fed infants, if the preceding recommendations regarding HBIG and vaccination are adhered to *(67)*.

Pregnancy does not increase the risk of HBV infection; acute HBV infection occurs in 1–2 per 1000 pregnancies. If the acute HBV infection occurs during the first trimester, the risk of spontaneous abortion is increased. Infection in the third trimester is associated with preterm delivery. However, the incidence of these problems is about the same as is seen in association with other febrile infections *(22)*.

Perinatal transmission in the absence of immunoprophylaxis occurs in 20–30% of chronic carriers (HBsAg-positive). In women who are seropositive for both HBsAg and HBeAg, transmission increases to 90% without intervention *(68)*. Transmission can occur transplacentally, because of intrapartum exposure or with breastfeeding. The risk of transmission is increased if acute infection develops later in pregnancy. With the use of combined immunization listed above, only 5–15% of exposed newborns will develop HBV infection *(69)*.

The possibility of hepatitis B or hepatitis C transmission because of in vitro procedures prompted the development of regulations in artificial reproductive technology to control the spread of these viruses in cryopreserved semen and embryos. The regulations include recommendations for screening for HBsAg and HCV antibodies. Samples from known infected patients and specimens from patients with unknown status should be kept in sealed vials and stored separate from known uninfected patients.

Prevention and Postexposure Prophylaxis

Hepatitis B vaccine is recommended by the CDC for use in universal immunization of infants and previously unvaccinated children, as well as vaccination of adolescents and adults at increased risk of infection. Table 4 lists the indications for vaccinations.

Hepatitis B recombinant vaccine is a safe and well-tolerated vaccine, the most common side effect being pain at injection site. Less common side effects include low-grade fever, malaise, headache, joint pain, and myalgias. Rare cases of anaphylaxis have been reported and the vaccine is contraindicated in persons with a known anaphylactic reaction to yeast. Despite reports in the past of a possible association between the hepatitis B vaccine and multiple sclerosis, several studies have failed to demonstrate a statistically significant association *(70,71)*. In the United States, screening before vaccination in the general population for past exposure is not cost-effective, unless the population being assessed has more than a 20% risk of HBV infection *(66)*. In these cases, the vaccine should be administered at the same time serological testing occurs if there is a likelihood that the patient may not return for the vaccine. Hepatitis B vaccine is given alone or, for adults over age 18, in a combination preparation with hepatitis A vaccine. Other combined preparations with childhood vaccinations are available for children and infants *(66)*. The hepatitis B vaccine is administered intramuscularly in the deltoid muscle (adults) and the recommended dose

Table 4
Hepatitis B Vaccination Indications in Adults

Medical Indications:
- Hemodialysis patients
- Recipients of clotting-factor concentrates

Occupational Indications:
- Health care and public safety workers with exposure to blood in the workplace
- Persons in training in schools of medicine, dentistry, nursing, laboratory technology and other allied health professions

Behavioral Indications:
- Injection drug users
- More than one sexual partner in the previous 6 months
- Recently acquired sexually transmitted infection
- All clients in sexually transmitted disease clinics
- Men who have sex with men

Other Indications:
- Household contacts and sex partners of persons with chronic hepatitis B virus (HBV) infection
- Clients and staff of institutions for the developmentally disabled
- International travelers to countries with high or intermediate prevalence of chronic HBV infection for more than 6 months
- Inmates of correctional facilities

Adapted from ref. *30a.*

and schedule varies by product and age of the recipient (*see* Table 5). The minimum time between the first and second dose is at least 1 month and the between the first and third dose is at least 4 months, allowing for some flexibility in dosing schedules. If a patient starts but has not completed the hepatitis B three-dose vaccine series, do not start the series again. Instead, resume vaccination until the required three doses are complete.

Because a high percentage of adolescents and adults younger than 40 develop a protective antibody response (approximately 50%) after only the first vaccine dose, hepatitis B vaccination should not be withheld if there is concern that the series may not be completed. The CDC does not recommend either periodic antibody testing to determine immunity or booster doses after completing the series in immunocompetent persons in this age group, because a protective antibody response occurs in more than 90% after the third dose. However, in adult populations at high risk, such as health care workers, hemodialysis patients, sexual partners of carriers, and MSM, postvaccination testing is recommended 1–2 months after completion of the series. A positive immune response to the vaccine

Table 5
Recommended Dose of Hepatitis B Vaccine

	Vaccine	
Group	Recombivax HB [a] (Merck) dose (mL)	Engerix-B [a] (GlaxoSmithKline) dose (mL)
Infants [b] and children and adolescents <20	5 µg (0.5) × 3	10 µg (0.5) × 3
Adolescents 11–15 years [c]	10 µg (0.5) [c] × 3	10 µg (0.5) × 3
Adults 20 years or older	10 µg (1.0) × 3	20 µg (1.0) × 3
Dialysis patients and other immuno-compromised persons >20	40 µg (1.0) [d] × 3	40 µg (2.0) [e] × 3

[a] Usual schedule: three doses at 0, 1, and 6 months.

[b] Infants whose mothers are hepatitis B surface antigen-positive should also receive hepatitis B immune globulin (HB1G) at birth.

[c] Note: adolescents age 11–15 can receive two 10 µg doses of Recombivax HB separated by 4–6 months.

[d] Special formulation for dialysis patients.

[e] Two 1.0 mL does given at one site in a four-dose schedule at 0, 1, 2, and 6 months.

Adapted from ref. 30.

is defined as anti-HBs titer at or above 10 IU/L. Receiving additional doses beyond the three dose series is not harmful. Nonresponders, more commonly seen in hemodialysis and immunocompromised patients as well as a small percentage of healthy individuals who are genetically determined nonresponders, should be revaccinated. In HIV-infected patients, it is prudent to test for anti-HBs 1–2 months after the third vaccine dose and repeat the entire series if immunity is not demonstrated. If no response is seen at this point, patients should be advised that they might remain susceptible to HBV infection and counseled on prevention methods.

Condom use should be strongly advised for all at-risk patients, and risk of transmission should be discussed. In addition to receiving vaccination, household contacts to persons with acute or chronic HBV infection should be advised to avoid activities such as sharing a toothbrush or razor blade, in which contact to blood may occur.

HEPATITIS C

Prevalence and Incidence

In the United States, HCV is the most common chronic blood-borne infection; it is the leading cause of death from liver disease, and the most common indication for liver transplantation (4,72). The World Health Organization estimates that 170 million people worldwide are chronically infected with the virus. Since the late 1980s, the incidence of HCV has decreased by more than 80% (3).

Recent data from National Health and Nutrition Examination survey III report that 3.7 million (1.8%) Americans have evidence of HCV antibodies and 2.7 million (1.3%) have chronic infection. A vast majority of infections occur within the 20- to 39-year-old age group with a 2 to 1 male predominance. Infection is slightly more prevalent in non-Hispanic blacks and American Indians/Alaskan natives, although rates in all racial and ethnic groups have substantially declined. History of intravenous drug use is by far the most recognizable risk factor for the acquisition of HCV *(73)*. The CDC estimates that 90% of injection drug users are infected after 5 years of use. Prevalence reflects risk factors. HCV is found is found in 60–90% of people with hemophilia; 50–90% of intravenous drug abusers; 10–20% of hemodialysis patients; 4–15% of persons with a history of STIs; 6% of people transfused before 1990; and 9% of people with more than 50 lifetime sex partners *(74)*. The role of sexual exposure in transmission is likely minimal, but CDC surveillance reports that 15–20% of infected patients report high-risk sexual behavior in the absence of other risk factors *(75)*.

Etiology

HCV is a single-stranded RNA virus of the family *Flaviviridae*. Six different genotypes are recognized. Genotype is highly associated with response to therapy. In the United States, the most common are genotypes 1 (75%), 2 (10%), and 3 (10%) *(76)*.

Transmission

HCV is a blood-borne virus primarily transmitted by parenteral exposure to infected blood. The most efficient mechanism of transmission consists of large, repeated, direct percutaneous exposures. Frequent small percutaneous exposures, such as those seen in patients receiving long-term hemodialysis, impart a moderate risk *(75)*. In 2002, 26% of cases were attributed to intravenous drug use, whereas transfusion and dialysis accounted for less than 1%. In 44% of cases, the cause was unknown. However, the largest burden of HCV in the United States is from a history of blood product transfusion before high specificity testing of donors was implemented in 1992. Pooled products such as IgG and clotting factors were an additional rich source of HCV before 1987, when irradiation practices that eradicate virus were implemented *(75)*.

Low-risk transmission is seen in unapparent percutaneous or mucosal exposure. Many potential sources are implicated, including occupational mucosal exposure to blood (e.g., conjunctival splashes) or needle-stick injuries, household contact (e.g., sharing razor blades, toothbrushes, and so on), and sexual transmission. No reports of HCV transmission because of military service, medical, dental, or surgical procedures, tattooing, acupuncture, foreign travel, or body piercing have been described *(7)*.

Vertical transmission is possible. The average rate of HCV infection in infants born to HCV-infected mothers is 5 to 6% *(77)*. The rates increase to approximately 14 to 17% if the mother is co-infected with HIV *(78)*. Neither vaginal (as opposed to cesarean delivery) *(79)* nor breastfeeding *(80)* appears to increase the risk of perinatal transmission.

Sexual transmission of HCV is possible but inefficient. However, given the large burden of HCV in the United States and the high frequency of sexual contact, sexual transmission was responsible for 11% of new HCV cases in 2002 *(4)*. Efforts aimed at detecting virus in semen, vaginal secretions, and saliva have had variable success. The virus is most often not detected and when it is found, very low (<10 copies/mL) numbers are present *(81,82)*. To date, no animal model or cell culture has demonstrated genital mucosal penetration or STI. Additionally, a study including MSM often at high risk for acquiring other blood-borne STIs found infection rates similar to that of heterosexuals *(83)*, calling into question the concept of sexual transmission of HCV *(7)*. In the absence of a proven biological mechanism, sexual transmission is suggested by multiple case reports of temporal sexual relationships with an HCV-infected partner that resulted in HCV infection when the possibility of nonsexual transmission has been excluded and highly concordant viral genomic sequence homology has been demonstrated. However, monogamous partners of HCV-infected persons have a minimal risk of acquiring HCV *(84)*. Current best estimates of incidence indicate that 0 to 0.6% of monogamous partners of HCV-positive persons will become infected each year *(85)*. Persons with multiple sex partners (more than one partner in 6 months) or those with high risk for STDs (e.g., female sex workers, persons with other STDs, attendees of STD clinics and, possibly, MSM) acquire HCV at a rate of 0.4 to 1.8% per year. Seroprevalence data suggest that 1.5% (0–4.4%) of monogamous partners of HCV-infected persons have HCV, whereas the values for groups at risk for STDs may be up to 4%.

Risk Factors

The most common risk factor for HCV infection is intravenous drug use. Factors that may increase the risk of sexual HCV transmission include HIV co-infection, attendance of an STI clinic, presence of other STIs, and traumatic sexual practices such as anal receptive sex. Some studies have reported independent associations with HCV infection, including exposure to an infected partner, increasing number of partners, failure to use a condom, history of STIs, heterosexual sex with a male intranvenous drug user, and traumatic sexual activities *(86)*. These associations may be surrogates for increased nonsexual risk factors in those specific populations. High HCV RNA levels, such as those observed in patients with pooled product exposure, may increase risk of sexual transmission *(87)*. Limited data appears to suggest that women may be slightly more prone to acquiring HCV from male partners than men are from women *(83,85)*.

Clinical Manifestations

The incubation period for HCV averages 6–7 weeks, but ranges between 2 and 26 weeks. Acute HCV infection goes unnoticed in 60–70% of cases. Onset of symptoms is insidious in symptomatic patients. Nonspecific symptoms such as anorexia, malaise, or abdominal pain are seen in only 10–20% of patients; jaundice is seen in 20–30% of cases *(75)*. Mortality rates from acute infections are low (0.2–0.4%). Most infected patients develop chronic hepatitis; only 15 to 25% of cases resolve spontaneously and have no detectable viral RNA. Serum anti-HCV will persist, even though the RNA clears; these persons will not develop liver disease and are not infectious. Chronic HCV infection is even more likely to be asymptomatic than acute illness, but when symptoms occur, nonspecific findings such as fatigue, vague right upper quadrant pain, and pruritus are noted *(76)*. Of all patients with chronic disease, 5–20% will develop cirrhosis after 20 years *(88)*. Approximately 60–70% of chronically infected persons will have evidence of liver disease detectable by abnormal ALT levels *(89)*. Patients with persistently abnormal ALT levels progress to cirrhosis more often than patients with normal ALT levels, who rarely develop any advanced fibrotic liver disease.

Many host-related factors and exposures have been associated with progression to cirrhosis in HCV-infected individuals. Strong associations include chronic alcohol intake of more than 50 g/day, advanced age, and co-infection with HBV or HIV. Other likely associations include male sex, obesity, diabetes mellitus type 2, nonalcoholic steatohepatitis, specific genetic factors, and tobacco use *(90)*.

Testing and Diagnosis

Initial testing for HCV should include testing for HCV antibody (anti-HCV enzyme immunoassay or chemiluminescence assay). A negative result has sufficient predictive value to determine that a person is not infected given ample time after exposure for seroconversion (4–6 months). If early detection is needed, quantitative and qualitative nucleic acid tests such as reverse transcriptase-PCR (RT-PCR) testing for HCV RNA (e.g., AMPLICOR®, Roche Molecular Systems) can be useful in detecting low levels of viral antigen 4 to 6 weeks after exposure. A positive anti-HCV has high predictive value of infection in patients with established risk factors but yields false-positive rates of approximately 35% when population prevalence is less than 10% (e.g., volunteer blood donors). For this reason, the CDC recommends reflex confirmation testing with a highly sensitive recombinant immunoblot assay (Chiron RIBA®, Chiron Corp.). RT-PCR testing may be unreliable in confirming HCV status because of the intermittent viremia associated with chronic disease. Patients may test negative for antibody before seroconversion has occurred and repeat testing at 6 months following exposure is indicated. Intermittent viremia of chronic disease or viral eradication by host clearance or therapy may cause RT-PCR tests to be negative.

Table 6
Indications for Testing for Anti-HCV

- History of at least one episode of injection drug use
- Received a blood product transfusion or organ donation before July 1992
- Received clotting factor concentrate produced before 1987
- Notification of transfusion from an hepatitis C virus (HCV)-positive donor
- Persistent ALT elevation[a]
- History of long-term hemodialysis
- Health care, emergency medical, and public safety workers after percutaneous or mucosal exposures to HCV-positive blood
- Children born to HCV-positive women
- Partners of HCV-infected persons[b]

[a] ALT, alanine aminotransferase. Persistent elevation is defined as two separate measurements at least 6 months apart, more than the upper limit of normal.
[b] Clinically useful in reassuring partners given the low level of monogamous sexual transmission.
Adapted from refs. 75 and 90 with permission.

Patients found to have risk factors for acquiring HCV should be tested, but routine screening of the general population is not indicated. This is partly because of the cost of screening, but also because of the high false-positive rates that occur in low-prevalence populations. A careful history will elicit the risks found in Table 6, which mandate serum testing. Currently, the CDC recommends that health care workers, public safety workers, pregnant women, and nonsexual household contacts not be routinely tested for HCV. Data regarding risk in patients with a history of transplanted tissues (e.g., cornea, skin) after 1992, intranasal cocaine use or other noninjection drug use, history of tattoos, and body piercing are inconclusive; most expert panels do not recommend screening in these populations. Rather than routine screening of HCV for persons at risk for STIs, the CDC recommends that the decision to test should be based on careful scrutiny for the presence of nonsexual risks for HCV acquisition (75).

Extrahepatic manifestations of HCV have been recognized and include mixed cryoglobulinemia associated with renal and skin disease, porphyria cutanea tarda, lichen planus, and seronegative arthritis (91). Recognition of these entities should prompt an evaluation for HCV infection.

Given the low likelihood of acute symptomatic hepatitis C infection, suspicion for disease is often based on detection of abnormal LFTs, clinical evidence of overt liver disease, or presence of high-risk factors. Initial testing for HCV should include testing for HCV antibody and, if positive, followed with reflex confirmation testing with a highly sensitive recombinant immunoblot assay. If serological diagnosis is confirmed, quantitative and qualitative nucleic acid tests for HCV RNA should be initiated, as well as referral to a specialist for consideration for treatment for chronic HCV infection.

Treatment

Acute HCV infections are treated with supportive care as described for HBV infections. Persons chronically infected with HCV are at risk for progression to decompensated liver disease. The American Association for the Study of Liver Diseases published practice guidelines in April 2004 detailing the recommendations for treatment *(90)*. The decision to treat persons with chronic HCV infection should be based on careful assessment of the risks and benefits of therapy done by referral to specialists. Optimal therapy consists of 6 to 12 months (based on genotype) of Pegylated Interferon in combination with Ribavirin. However, because only half of patients respond to a therapy associated with significant side effects and the majority of persons with chronic HCV do not progress to cirrhosis, targeting those with the greatest likelihood to benefit from therapy is imperative. Only patients with a high likelihood of progressing to cirrhosis or end-stage liver disease should be considered for treatment. The gold standard for defining risk of progression is demonstration of advanced fibrosis by liver biopsy. However, persistent elevations in ALT levels in the absence of a biopsy may allow for initiation of treatment. Patients with symptomatic hepatitis C or extrahepatic manifestations should also be considered for treatment. Several factors are associated with response to therapy, the most significant being viral genotype. There are several contraindications to therapy, including pregnancy and decompensated liver disease. Side effects of treatment are common and can be debilitating. The mainstay of therapy in patients with decompensated liver disease remains referral for liver transplantation *(90)*.

In order to prevent progression of liver disease, liver failure, and increased fatality, all patients with HCV infection should be immunized with standard regimens of the Hepatitis A and B vaccine if they have not had prior exposure. Patients should be immunized as early as possible, because response to vaccination is diminished in patients with advanced liver disease *(92)*. Additionally, patients should be counseled to abstain from alcohol and not take any over-the-counter medications without consulting their physician.

Follow-Up

Surveillance is also an integral part of managing patients with HCV. Patients with persistently normal ALT levels and no histological evidence of advanced fibrosis are often not treated because of lower risks of progression to advanced liver disease. Given the waxing and waning pattern of ALT in chronic HCV, serum liver function tests should be drawn every 6 to 12 months to detect the presence of progressive disease. Patients with clinical or histological evidence of cirrhosis need to be screened every 6 months with liver ultrasound or other liver imaging and serum AFP levels to detect emergence of HCC. Patients with decompensated liver disease should undergo endoscopic evaluation for varices at least every 2 years *(90)*.

Partner Notification and Reporting Requirements

Laboratory reporting of anti-HCV results is encouraged as a method to iden tify persons with HCV infection, however, most cases identified this way are chronic rather than acute infections *(19)*. Investigating these cases is not an efficient mechanism to identify acute cases unless clinical data is available. The CDC recommends that case investigations be conducted by local health departments in suspected cases of acute hepatitis C (i.e., clinical and laboratory evidence of acute infection with absence of alternative causes of acute hepatitis). Health departments should also interview all confirmed cases of acute hepatitis C to identify risk factors for infection during the 2 weeks to 6 months before illness onset. Given that hepatitis C rarely presents in the acute phase, it is difficult to identify these cases. Recently, the AASLD has recommended testing partners of HCV-infected persons in order to provide reassurance given the low risk of sexual transmission among monogamous couples *(90)*.

Pregnancy-Related Issues

The prevalence of HCV antibodies in pregnant women varies from 2.3 to 4.5% *(22)*, although among HIV-infected pregnant women, seroprevalence may be as high as 33%. Very little is know about the effect of HCV on pregnancy, but there does not seem to be an increase in adverse pregnancy outcomes in HCV-infected women. Routine screening of pregnant women is not recommended, but testing of women with risk factors listed in Table 6 is recommended.

Vertical transmission to neonates varies by maternal RNA titers and HIV co-infection status. The overall rate of HCV transmission in HIV-negative, HCV-positive women is 10%. However, the risk of transmission was 33% in women with HCV RNA titers 10^6 copies/mL or more. No woman with titers below 10^4 copies/mL transmitted virus to her newborn *(93)*. Perinatal transmission of HCV is higher in women co-infected with HIV. Most infants delivered to HCV-infected mothers progress to chronic hepatitis *(22)*. Vaginal delivery does not appear to increase the risk of perinatal infection *(79)*.

The role of breastfeeding in HCV transmission is still not clear. HCV RNA has been isolated in colostrum of HCV-infected women with detectable levels of HCV RNA. However, infection through breastfeeding has not been demonstrated *(80)*. Therefore, at the current time, breastfeeding is not contraindicated in patients with HCV unless the mother has cracked or bleeding nipples according to the American Academy of Pediatrics *(94)*.

Screening of men and women seeking infertility services may be appropriate to identify those who need therapy before conception. Because transmission through intercourse is controversial, use of condoms is not needed by couples who are trying to conceive. Infants born to HCV-infected mothers should be tested for anti-HCV no sooner than 12 months of age to allow for passively acquired maternal antibody to clear. RT-PCR, although not licensed by the Food and Drug Administration, can be used to detect HCV RNA as early as 1–2 months of age *(95)*. Ribavirin is teratogenic and is contraindicated in pregnancy.

Prevention

No vaccine is available to prevent acquisition of HCV. Therefore, education of individuals at risk for transmitting or acquiring infection remains the mainstay of primary prevention of HCV. Patients who inject illegal drugs should be counseled to stop and enter a drug rehabilitation program. If they are unable to stop, single-use unshared equipment, such as sterile syringes, needles, cookers, cottons, and water should be used every time they inject to prevent spread of disease. Persons with chronic HCV should be counseled not to donate blood, semen, body organs, or tissues. Additionally, infected persons and household contacts should be instructed not to share any products that may be contaminated with infected blood, such as razors, toothbrushes, or nail hygiene equipment. Covering open wounds is recommended. However, it is not necessary to avoid close contact with infected people or to avoid sharing meals or eating utensils. Given the very low risk of acquisition of HCV from an infected sexual partner, persons in stable monogamous sexual relationships with HCV-infected persons do not need to change their current sexual habits. Persons at risk for STIs including persons with multiple partners, female sex workers, attendees of STI clinics, and individuals infected with other STIs should be counseled on general precautions to lower their risk of acquiring blood-borne STIs (e.g., HIV, HBV, and HCV). These recommendations should include abstinence or use of a barrier method, such as a condom, and avoidance of sexual relationships with injection drug users *(7)*.

OTHER FORMS OF VIRAL HEPATITIS

Several other forms of viral hepatitis have been identified. HDV is a defective, circular, single-stranded RNA virus, which requires the presence of HBV for infection *(96)*. HDV should be considered in patients with risk factors similar to those of HBV, including intravenous drug users, MSM, as well as in patients from endemic countries such as southern Italy, North Africa, the Middle East, and the Amazon Basin. It should also be suspected in those who present with unusually severe hepatitis or in a patient with chronic hepatitis B whose condition suddenly worsens. Symptoms are usually abrupt. Mortality rates are 2–20%, but can rise to 30% with superinfection with hepatitis B. About 25% of chronic HBV carriers are co-infected or superinfected with HDV. Approximately 70–80% of patients with HDV will develop cirrhosis or portal hypertension.

Other forms of viral hepatitis have also been identified, including hepatitis E virus (HEV) and hepatitis G virus (HGV). HEV is generally spread by fecally contaminated water in endemic regions (Mexico, Asia, and Africa) and is generally self-limited. There is documented transmission of HEV from mother to infant, but sexual contact has not been identified as a risk factor for transmission. Mortality rate overall is usually 1–2%, but rises to 15–20% in pregnant women, especially if infection occurs in the third trimester *(97)*. The role of HGV in acute and chronic hepatitis remains to be fully defined, however, HGV does not appear to be an important cause of clinical liver disease *(98)*. HGV is generally transmitted by transfusion but it has been suggested in the literature that HGV may be associated with sexual transmission *(99)*. These and other potential forms of viral hepatitis and their clinical significance are currently under further investigation.

CASE STUDY

After attempting to donate blood, Samantha, age 35, is notified that she needs follow-up on abnormal hepatitis results. She has a letter from a blood donation center that indicates that she has HBsAg. She has been married for 1 year, but had two previous sex partners earlier in life. She is second-generation American, her grandmother was born in Indonesia. She denies any illicit drug use. She wants to know what she should do. She and her husband are planning a pregnancy in about 6 months. Will this make her infertile? Will it affect the baby?

Answers and Teaching Points

- Samantha is a chronic carrier of HBV, which she may have acquired through vertical transmission or from a sex partner.
- She needs to have her liver function tests checked and a full hepatitis panel done to determine if she has any other hepatitis infection, particularly HDV.
- Her husband needs to be tested for prior exposure if he has not been immunized. If he is vulnerable to infection, he should receive the HBV vaccine series.
- Samantha's fertility is not compromised by HBV infection, but her newborn will need HBIG at birth as well as HBV vaccinations.
- Longer term, chronic HBV infection increases her risk for hepatic carcinoma.

REFERENCES

1. Custer B, Sullivan SD, Hazlet TK, Iloeje U, Veenstra DL, Kowdley KV. Global epidemiology of hepatitis B virus. J Clin Gastroenterol 2004; 38(10 Suppl):S158–S168.
1a. Shapiro CN, Coleman PJ, McQuillan GM, Alter MJ, Margolis HS. Epidemiology of hepatitis A: seroepidemiology and risk groups in the USA. Vaccine 1992; 10:S59–S62.

2. Centers for Disease Control and Prevention. Prevention of hepatitis A through active or passive immunization: recommendations of the Advisory Committee on Immunization Practices (ACIP). MMWR Recomm Rep 1999; 48:1–37.

2a. Centers for Disease Control and Prevention. Hepatitis awareness month—May 2006. MMWR Morb Mortal Wkly Rep 2006; 55:505.

3. Centers for Disease Control and Prevention. Summary of notifiable diseases—United States, 2004. MMWR Morb Mortal Wkly Rep 2006; 53(53):1–79. Available from: http://www.cdc.gov/mmwr/summary.html. Accessed Nov. 24, 2006.

4. Centers for Disease Control and Prevention. Hepatitis surveillance report no. 61. Atlanta, GA: US Department of Health and Human Services, Centers for Disease Control and Prevention, 2004. Available from: http://www.cdc.gov/ncidod/diseases/hepatitis/resource/PDFs/hep_surveillance_61.pdf. Accessed Nov. 24, 2006.

5. World Health Organization. Hepatitis A. Department of communicable disease surveillance and response. Geneva: World Health Organization; 2001. Available from: http://www.who.int/csr/disease/hepatitis/whocdscsredc2007.html. Accessed Nov. 24, 2006.

6. Cuthbert JA. Hepatitis A: old and new. Clin Microbiol Rev 2001; 14:38–58.

7. Centers for Disease Control and Prevention. Sexually transmitted diseases treatment guidelines 2006. MMWR Recomm Rep 2006; 55(RR-11):69–78. Available from: http://www.cdc.gov/std/treatment/. Accessed Nov. 24, 2006.

8. Ross JDC, Ghanem M, Tariq A, Gilleran G, Winter AJ. Seroprevalence of hepatitis A immunity in male genitourinary medicine clinic attenders: a case control study of heterosexual and homosexual men. Sex Transm Infect 2002; 78:174–179.

9. Katz MH, Hsu L, Wong E, Liska S, Anderson L, Janssen RS. Seroprevalence of and risk factors for hepatitis A infection among young homosexual and bisexual men. J Infect Dis 1997; 175:1225–1229.

10. Corona R, Stroffolini T, Giglio A, et al. Lack of evidence for increased risk of hepatitis A infection in homosexual men. Epidemiol Infect 1999; 123:89–93.

11. Roy K, Howie H, Sweeney C, Parry J, Molyneaux P, Goldberg D, Taylor A. Hepatitis A virus and injecting drug misuse in Aberdeen, Scotland: a case-control study. J Viral Hepat 2004; 11:277–282.

12. Glikson M, Galun E, Oren R, Tur-Kaspa R, Shouval D. Relapsing hepatitis A. Review of 14 cases and literature survey. Medicine (Baltimore). 1992; 71:14–23.

13. Gordon SC, Reddy KR, Schiff L, Schiff ER. Prolonged intrahepatic cholestasis secondary to acute hepatitis A. Ann Intern Med 1984; 101:635–637.

14. Kemmer NM, Miskovsky EP. Hepatitis A. Infect Dis Clin North Am 2000; 14:605–615.

15. O'Grady J. Management of acute and fulminant hepatitis A. Vaccine 1992; 10:S21–S23.

16. Vento S, Garofano T, Renzini C, et al. Fulminant hepatitis associated with hepatitis A virus superinfection in patients with chronic hepatitis C. N Engl J Med 1998; 338:286–290.

17. Liaw YF, Yang CY, Chu CM, Huang MJ. Appearance and persistence of hepatitis A IgM antibody in acute clinical hepatitis A observed in an outbreak. Infection 1986; 14:156–158.

18. Garner JS. Guideline for isolation precautions in hospitals. The Hospital Infection Control Practices Advisory Committee. Infect Control Hosp Epidemiol 1996; 17:53–80 and Am J Infect Control 1996; 24:24–52.

19. Centers for Disease Control and Prevention. Guidelines for viral hepatitis surveillance and case management. Atlanta, GA; 2005. Available from: http://www.cdc.gov/ncidod/diseases/hepatitis/resource/PDFs/revised_GUIDELINES_formatted5.pdf. Accessed Nov. 24, 2006.

20. Leikin E, Lysikiewicz A, Garry D, Tejani N. Intrauterine transmission of hepatitis A virus. Obstet Gynecol. 1996; 88:690–691.

21. American College of Obstetricians and Gynecologists. ACOG educational bulletin. Viral hepatitis in pregnancy. Number 248, July 1998 (replaces No. 174, November 1992). Int J Gynaecol Obstet 1998; 63:195–202.

22. Practice Committee of the American Society for Reproductive Medicine. Hepatitis and reproduction. Fertil Steril 2004; 82:1754–1764.

23. Craig AS, Schaffner W. Prevention of hepatitis A with the hepatitis A vaccine. N Engl J Med 2004; 350:476–481.

24. Stokes J, Neefe JR. The prevention and attenuation of infectious hepatitis by gamma globulin; preliminary note. JAMA 1945; 127:144–145.

25. Ellis EF, Henney CS. Adverse reactions following administration of human gamma globulin. J Allergy 1969; 43:45–54.

26. Diaz-Mitoma F, Law B, Parsons J. A combined vaccine against hepatitis A and B in children and adolescents. Pediatr Infect Dis J 1999; 18:109–114.

27. Clemens R, Safary A, Hepburn A, Roche C, Stanbury WJ, Andre FE. Clinical experience with an inactivated hepatitis A vaccine. J Infect Dis 1995; 171:S44–S49.

28. Ashur Y, Adler R, Rowe M, Shouval D. Comparison of immunogenicity of two hepatitis A vaccines—VAQTA and HAVRIX—in young adults. Vaccine 1999; 17:2290–2296.

29. McMahon BJ, Williams J, Bulkow L, et al. Immunogenicity of an inactivated hepatitis A vaccine in Alaska Native children and Native and non-Native adults. J Infect Dis 1995; 171: 676–679.

30. Centers for Disease Control and Prevention. Hepatitis A. In: Atkinson W, Hamborsky J, Wolfe S, eds. *Epidemiology and Prevention of Vaccine-Preventable Diseases*, 8th Ed. Washington, DC: Public Health Foundation; 2004, pp. 177–189.

30a. Centers for Disease Control and Prevention. Recommended Adult Immunization Schedule, United States, October 2006–September 2007. Available from: http://www.cdc.gov/nip/recs/adult-schedule.htm. Accessed Nov. 24, 2006.

31. Keeffe EB, Iwarson S, McMahon BJ, et al. Safety and immunogenicity of hepatitis A vaccine in patients with chronic liver disease. Hepatology 1998; 27:881–886.

32. Neilsen GA, Bodsworth NJ, Watts N. Response to hepatitis A vaccination in human immuno-deficiency virus-infected and -uninfected homosexual men. J Infect Dis 1997; 176:1064–1067.

33. Arslan M, Wiesner RH, Poterucha JJ, Zein NN. Safety and efficacy of hepatitis A vaccination in liver transplantation recipients. Transplantation 2001; 72:272–276.

34. Alter MJ, Mares A, Hadler SC, Maynard JE. The effect of underreporting on the apparent incidence and epidemiology of acute viral hepatitis. Am J Epidemiol 1987; 125:133–139.

35. Lee WM. Hepatitis B virus infection. N Engl J Med 1997; 337:1733–1745.

36. Maynard JE. Hepatitis B: global importance and need for control. Vaccine 1990; 8:S18–S23.

37. Alter MJ, Hadler SC, Margolis HS, et al. The changing epidemiology of hepatitis B in the United States. Need for alternative vaccination strategies. JAMA 1990; 263:1218–1222.

38. Centers for Disease Control and Prevention (CDC). Incidence of acute hepatitis B—United States, 1990–2002. MMWR Morb Mortal Wkly Rep 2004; 52:1252–1254.

39. Chang MH, Chen CJ, Lai MS, et al. Universal hepatitis B vaccination in Taiwan and the incidence of hepatocellular carcinoma in children. Taiwan Childhood Hepatoma Study Group. N Engl J Med 1997; 336:1855–1859.

40. MacKellar DA, Valleroy LA, Secura GM, et al. Two decades after vaccine license: hepatitis B immunization and infection among young men who have sex with men. Am J Public Health 2001; 91:965–971.

41. Papaevangelou GJ, Roumeliotou-Karayannis AJ, Contoyannis PC. The risk of nosocomial hepatitis A and B virus infections from patients under care without isolation precaution. J Med Virol 1981; 7:143–148.

42. Bond WW, Favero MS, Petersen NJ, Gravelle CR, Ebert JW, Maynard JE. Survival of hepatitis B virus after drying and storage for one week. Lancet 1981; 1:550–551.
43. Lok AS, McMahon BJ; Practice Guidelines Committee, American Association for the Study of Liver Diseases (AASLD). Chronic hepatitis B: update of recommendations. Hepatology 2004; 39:857–861.
44. Stevens CE, Beasley RP, Tsui J, Lee WC. Vertical transmission of hepatitis B antigen in Taiwan. N Engl J Med 1975; 292:771–774.
45. Beasley RP, Hwang LY, Lin CC, Leu ML, Stevens CE, Szmuness W, Chen KP. Incidence of hepatitis B virus infections in preschool children in Taiwan. J Infect Dis 1982; 146:198–204.
46. Coursaget P, Yvonnet B, Chotard J, et al. Age- and sex-related study of hepatitis B virus chronic carrier state in infants from an endemic area (Senegal). J Med Virol 1987; 22:1–5.
47. Tassopoulos NC, Papaevangelou GJ, Sjogren MH, Roumeliotou-Karayannis A, Gerin JL, Purcell RH. Natural history of acute hepatitis B surface antigen-positive hepatitis in Greek adults. Gastroenterology. 1987; 92:1844–1850.
48. Yu MW, Hsu FC, Sheen IS, et al. Prospective study of hepatocellular carcinoma and liver cirrhosis in asymptomatic chronic hepatitis B virus carriers. Am J Epidemiol 1997; 145:1039–1047.
49. Liaw YF, Tai DI, Chu CM, Chen TJ. The development of cirrhosis in patients with chronic type B hepatitis: a prospective study. Hepatology 1988; 8:493–496.
50. Realdi G, Fattovich G, Hadziyannis S, et al. Survival and prognostic factors in 366 patients with compensated cirrhosis type B: a multicenter study. The Investigators of the European Concerted Action on Viral Hepatitis (EUROHEP). J Hepatol 1994; 21:656–666.
51. Roudot-Thoraval F, Bastie A, Pawlotsky JM, Dhumeaux D. Epidemiological factors affecting the severity of hepatitis C virus-related liver disease: a French survey of 6,664 patients. The Study Group for the Prevalence and the Epidemiology of Hepatitis C Virus. Hepatology 1997; 26:485–490.
52. Housset C, Pol S, Carnot F, et al. Interactions between human immunodeficiency virus-1, hepatitis delta virus and hepatitis B virus infections in 260 chronic carriers of hepatitis B virus. Hepatology. 1992; 15:578–583.
53. Lok AS, Heathcote EJ, Hoofnagle JH. Management of hepatitis B: 2000—summary of a workshop. Gastroenterology. 2001; 120:1828–1853.
54. Chien RN, Liaw YF, Atkins M. Pretherapy alanine transaminase level as a determinant for hepatitis B e antigen seroconversion during lamivudine therapy in patients with chronic hepatitis B. Asian Hepatitis Lamivudine Trial Group. Hepatology 1999; 30:770–774.
55. Perrillo RP, Lai CL, Liaw YF, et al. Predictors of HBeAg loss after lamivudine treatment for chronic hepatitis B. Hepatology 2002; 36:186–194.
56. Fattovich G, Brollo L, Giustina G, et al. Natural history and prognostic factors for chronic hepatitis type B. Gut 1991; 32:294–298.
57. de Jongh FE, Janssen HL, de Man RA, Hop WC, Schalm SW, van Blankenstein M. Survival and prognostic indicators in hepatitis B surface antigen-positive cirrhosis of the liver. Gastroenterology 1992; 103:1630–1635.
58. Lau DT, Everhart J, Kleiner DE, et al. Long-term follow-up of patients with chronic hepatitis B treated with interferon alfa. Gastroenterology 1997; 113:1660–1667.
59. Lok AS, McMahon BJ; Practice Guidelines Committee, American Association for the Study of Liver Diseases. Chronic hepatitis B. Hepatology 2001; 34:1225–1241.
60. Villa E, Rubbiani L, Barchi T, et al. Susceptibility of chronic symptomless HBsAg carriers to ethanol-induced hepatic damage. Lancet 1982; 2:1243–1244.
61. Kim YI, Heathcote J, Wanless IR. The hepatitis B carrier state—a follow-up study of 100 consecutive cases. Clin Invest Med 1987; 10:383–387.

62. Chevillotte G, Durbec JP, Gerolami A, Berthezene P, Bidart JM, Camatte R. Interaction between hepatitis B virus and alcohol consumption in liver cirrhosis. An epidemiologic study. Gastroenterology 1983; 85:141–145.

63. Gall SA. Maternal immunization. Obstet Gynecol Clin North Am 2003; 30:623–636.

64. Poland GA, Jacobson RM. Clinical practice: prevention of hepatitis B with the hepatitis B vaccine. N Engl J Med 2004; 351:2832–2838.

65. Stevens CE, Toy PT, Tong MJ, et al. Perinatal hepatitis B virus transmission in the United States. Prevention by passive-active immunization. JAMA 1985; 253:1740–1745.

66. Centers for Disease Control and Prevention. Hepatitis B. In: Atkinson W, Hamborsky J, Wolfe S, eds. *Epidemiology and Prevention of Vaccine-Preventable Diseases*, 8th Ed. Washington DC: Public Health Foundation; 2004, pp. 191–212.

67. Hill JB, Sheffield JS, Kim MJ, Alexander JM, Sercely B, Wendel GD. Risk of hepatitis B transmission in breast-fed infants of chronic hepatitis B carriers. Obstet Gynecol 2002; 99: 1049–1052.

68. Okada K, Kamiyama I, Inomata M, Imai M, Miyakawa Y. e antigen and anti-e in the serum of asymptomatic carrier mothers as indicators of positive and negative transmission of hepatitis B virus to their infants. N Engl J Med 1976; 294:746–749.

69. Hsu HM, Chen DS, Chuang CH, et al. Efficacy of a mass hepatitis B vaccination program in Taiwan. Studies on 3464 infants of hepatitis B surface antigen-carrier mothers. JAMA 1988; 260:2231–2235.

70. Ascherio A, Zhang SM, Hernan MA, et al. Hepatitis B vaccination and the risk of multiple sclerosis. N Engl J Med 2001; 344:327–332.

71. Confavreux C, Suissa S, Saddier P, Bourdes V, Vukusic S; Vaccines in Multiple Sclerosis Study Group. Vaccinations and the risk of relapse in multiple sclerosis. Vaccines in Multiple Sclerosis Study Group. N Engl J Med 2001; 344:319–326.

72. Kim WR. The burden of hepatitis C in the United States. Hepatology. 2002; 36:S30–S34.

73. Alter MJ, Kruszon-Moran D, Nainan OV, et al. The prevalence of hepatitis C virus infection in the United States, 1988 through 1994. N Engl J Med 1999; 341:556–562.

74. Rosenberg J. Hep C Action Report. Medical Board of California; 1999, pp. 2–3.

75. Centers for Disease Control and Prevention. Recommendations for prevention and control of hepatitis C virus (HCV) infection and HCV-related chronic disease. MMWR Recomm Rep 1998; 47:1–39.

76. Flamm SL. Chronic hepatitis C virus infection. JAMA 2003; 289:2413–2417.

77. Ohto H, Terazawa S, Sasaki N, et al. Transmission of hepatitis C virus from mothers to infants. The Vertical Transmission of Hepatitis C Virus Collaborative Study Group. N Engl J Med 1994; 330:744–750.

78. Thomas DL, Villano SA, Riester KA, et al. Perinatal transmission of hepatitis C virus from human immunodeficiency virus type 1-infected mothers. Women and Infants Transmission Study. J Infect Dis 1998; 177:1480–1488.

79. Zanetti AR, Tanzi E, Newell ML. Mother-to-infant transmission of hepatitis C virus. J Hepatol 1999; 31:96–100.

80. Lin HH, Kao JH, Hsu HY, et al. Absence of infection in breast-fed infants born to hepatitis C virus-infected mothers. J Pediatr 1995; 126:589–591.

81. Pekler VA, Robbins WA, Nyamathi A, Yashina TL, Leak B, Robins TA. Use of versant TMA and bDNA 3.0 assays to detect and quantify hepatitis C virus in semen. J Clin Lab Anal 2003; 17:264–270.

82. Belec L, Legoff J, Si-Mohamed A, et al. Cell-associated, non-replicating strand (+) hepatitis C virus-RNA shedding in cervicovaginal secretions from chronically HCV-infected women. J Clin Virol 2003; 27:247–251.

83. Thomas DL, Zenilman JM, Alter HJ, et al. Sexual transmission of hepatitis C virus among patients attending sexually transmitted diseases clinics in Baltimore—an analysis of 309 sex partnerships. J Infect Dis 1995; 171:768–775.

84. Vandelli C, Renzo F, Romano L, et al. Lack of evidence of sexual transmission of hepatitis C among monogamous couples: results of a 10-year prospective follow-up study. Am J Gastroenterol 2004; 99:855–859.

85. Terrault NA. Sexual activity as a risk factor for hepatitis C. Hepatology 2002; 36:S99–S105.

86. Dienstag JL. Sexual and perinatal transmission of hepatitis C. Hepatology 1997; 26:66S–70S.

87. Hisada M, O'Brien TR, Rosenberg PS, Goedert JJ. Virus load and risk of heterosexual transmission of human immunodeficiency virus and hepatitis C virus by men with hemophilia. The Multicenter Hemophilia Cohort Study. J Infect Dis 2000; 181:1475–1478.

88. Seeff LB. Natural history of chronic hepatitis C. Hepatology 2002; 36:S35–S46.

89. Alter MJ, Margolis HS, Krawczynski K, et al. The natural history of community-acquired hepatitis C in the United States. The Sentinel Counties Chronic non-A, non-B Hepatitis Study Team. N Engl J Med 1992; 327:1899–1905.

90. Strader DB, Wright T, Thomas DL, Seeff LB; American Association for the Study of Liver Diseases. Diagnosis, management, and treatment of hepatitis C. Hepatology 2004; 39:1147–1171.

91. Hoofnagle JH. Course and outcome of hepatitis C. Hepatology 2002; 36:S21–S29.

92. Koff RS. Risks associated with hepatitis A and hepatitis B in patients with hepatitis C. J Clin Gastroenterol 2001; 33:20–26.

93. Alter MJ. Epidemiology of hepatitis C in the West. Semin Liver Dis 1995; 15:5–14.

94. Gartner LM, Morton J, Lawrence RA, et al. Breastfeeding and the use of human milk. Pediatrics. 2005; 115:496–506.

95. Alter MJ, Kuhnert WL, Finelli L; Centers for Disease Control and Prevention. Guidelines for laboratory testing and result reporting of antibody to hepatitis C virus. Centers for Disease Control and Prevention. MMWR Recomm Rep 2003; 52:1–13, 15

96. Taylor J, Negro F, Rizzetto M. Hepatitis delta virus: From structure to disease expression. Rev Med Virol 1992; 2:161–167.

97. Tsega E, Krawczynski K, Hansson BG, Nordenfelt E. Hepatitis E virus infection in pregnancy in Ethiopia. Ethiop Med J 1993; 31:173–181.

98. Alter MJ, Gallagher M, Morris TT, et al. Acute non-A-E hepatitis in the United States and the role of hepatitis G virus infection. Sentinel Counties Viral Hepatitis Study Team. N Engl J Med 1997; 336:741–746.

99. Ramia S, Mokhbat J, Sibai A, Klayme S, Naman R; HIV Epidemiology Research Study Group. Exposure rates to hepatitis C and G virus infections among HIV-infected patients: evidence of efficient transmission of HGV by the sexual route. Int J STD AIDS 2004; 15:463–466.

5

HIV Infection and AIDS

Gunter Rieg

INTRODUCTION

In the summer of 1981, the Centers for Disease Control and Prevention (CDC) reported clusters of unusual infections (*Pneumocystis carinii* pneumonia, now called *Pneumocystis jiroveci*) and tumors (Kaposi sarcoma) among homosexual men in California and New York. This was the beginning of the acquired immune deficiency syndrome (AIDS) pandemic. Initially, infection with the human immunodeficiency virus (HIV) appeared to be associated with homosexual activities, which led to the initial naming of gay-related immune deficiency syndrome. However, it soon became clear that heterosexual and direct blood contact could also transmit the newly recognized pathogen. Since then, HIV infection and AIDS have been spreading rapidly around the world, affecting millions of people and resulting in millions of deaths. In his speech at the 2003 International AIDS Conference in Paris, France, President Nelson Mandela declared HIV/AIDS the "greatest health crisis in human history."

HIV infection and AIDS are not yet curable. Highly active antiretroviral therapy (HAART)—where available—prolongs survival of HIV/AIDS patients. However, prevention of HIV transmission is the key component to fight the HIV and AIDS epidemics. It is critical to understand the mechanisms of the sexual transmission of HIV and to recognize preventive interventions in clinical practice in order to counsel patients properly. On a global scale, those elements are needed not only to protect individual patients, but also to prevent future spread of the infection. This chapter focuses on risk factors and mechanisms of HIV transmission, prevention measures, diagnostic tests, and symptoms of acute HIV infection. Care of patients with established HIV infection should be reserved for an HIV specialist and is not addressed in this chapter.

FAST FACTS

- The number of HIV-infected people continues to rise in all parts of the world, including in the United States.

From: *Current Clinical Practice: Sexually Transmitted Diseases:
A Practical Guide for Primary Care*
Edited by: A. L. Nelson and J. A. Woodward © Humana Press, Totowa, NJ

- Sexual transmission of HIV is variable and influenced by multiple factors. Anal intercourse carries the highest risk of HIV transmission followed by vaginal intercourse. Oral sex has a low risk of HIV transmission.
- Correct and reliable use of barrier methods, such as latex condoms, is protective against HIV transmission. Guidelines for postexposure prophylaxis for unprotected high-risk exposure have been published by the CDC.
- Routine screening of at-risk individuals, including all prenatal women, is recommended.
- Symptoms of acute HIV infection are nonspecific and require special awareness to pursue a diagnostic work-up. Care and treatment of established HIV infection and AIDS should be reserved for a HIV-trained health care provider.

PREVALENCE AND INCIDENCE

United States

The CDC publishes an annual surveillance report of AIDS cases *(1)*. AIDS is a reportable disease in all 50 states in the United States, District of Columbia, and US dependencies and possessions. The CDC estimates that AIDS reporting is more than 85% complete. By 2003, HIV infection (not AIDS) had been reported in 41 areas; however, the 2005 CDC report included data from only 35 states and territories, from which surveillance data on HIV infection (not AIDS) had been available since at least 2000.

In the United States and its territories, 944,306 AIDS cases had been reported from the initial recognition of AIDS to the end of 2004. At that time, an estimated 462,792 people in the 35 areas were known to be living with HIV/AIDS. These 35 areas represent approximately 61% of the epidemic in the United States.

The estimated number of HIV/AIDS cases in the 35 areas decreased year by year from 2001 through 2003, but increased 1% from the end of 2003 through the end of 2004. The number of AIDS cases increased each year since 2002. Since the introduction of HAART, the number of deaths resulting from AIDS has decreased by 8% from 2000 through 2004. Because the twin pressures including an increasing number of people newly acquiring the infection each year and the increase in years of life of those already infected, it is apparent that the number of persons living with HIV and AIDS will continue to grow for the foreseeable future. In addition, it is estimated that 40,000 new HIV infections occur every year in the United States *(2)*.

Nearly three out of four adults and adolescents living with HIV/AIDS in the United States are male. The 40- to 44-year-old age group accounts for most cases of HIV/AIDS (22%). Sexual contact is responsible for 89% of all HIV/AIDS cases diagnosed in 2004. Heterosexual transmission is responsible for 78% of cases in women diagnosed with HIV/AIDS in 2004, whereas male-to-male sexual contact now accounts for 74% of cases among men. Minorities are disproportionately affected by HIV and AIDS. African-Americans and Hispanics account for the majority of all reported AIDS cases in the United States at the end of 2004. African-Americans continue to be the most commonly affected minority; they accounted for 50% of all new cases of HIV/AIDS reported in 2004. Minority women are even more disproportionately affected by HIV and AIDS. More than 75% of all female AIDS cases in the United States occur in minority women; African-American women account for more than half of these cases. In the 29 states with HIV reporting during 1999–2002, blacks had an HIV diagnosis rate of 75.6 per 100,000 in 2002, nearly 10 times the rate of whites and 2.5 times the rate of Hispanics *(3)*.

Worldwide

The picture of HIV/AIDS internationally is significantly different from that found in the United States. The Joint United Nations Program on HIV/AIDS reported that 38.6 million people worldwide were living with HIV at the end of 2005 *(4)*. Disturbingly, an estimated 4.1 million people (10.5%) became newly infected with HIV and 2.8 million lost their lives to AIDS that year alone. The AIDS epidemic continues to expand in many regions in the world, whereas in several countries the proportion of people living with HIV leveled off. Sub-Saharan Africa has the greatest number of HIV-infected persons (24.5 million), with an estimated 2.7 million new infections in 2005. HIV epidemics are also spreading rapidly in Eastern Europe and Asia. In Asia an estimated 8.3 million people are living with HIV. India has the largest number of people living with AIDS outside Africa: more than 5.5 million people are HIV infected.

The worldwide pandemic of HIV is a heterosexually transmitted infection. Women now account for 59% of all people living with HIV in sub-Saharan Africa. In South Africa, almost one in three pregnant women attending public prenatal clinics were living with HIV in 2004. Only limited resources are available in developing nations for prevention measurements and treatment of HIV. Globally, fewer than 1 in 5 people who need antiretroviral therapy have access to HIV medications. The United Nations Program on HIV/AIDS report in 2004 stated: "Despite increased funding, the AIDS epidemic continues to outpace the global response."

ETIOLOGY

HIV is the third human retrovirus to be identified. It is now believed that humans became infected with HIV in the early- to mid-20th century by nonhuman primates infected with the simian immunodeficiency virus (SIV), a closely related virus found in monkeys. HIV is classified by types 1 and 2, with HIV-1 primarily responsible for the current worldwide epidemic. HIV-1 is further divided in three groups—group M (the main group responsible for the pandemic), group

O (found primarily in Western Africa) and group N (found in some patients from Cameroon). HIV-1 group M is further divided in nine subgroups. Subgroups A, B, and C account for nearly 90% of HIV infections worldwide, and HIV-1 group M subgroup B is the predominant HIV in the United States.

In general, viruses are obligate intracellular organisms. HIV enters the human cells using the CD4 receptor and chemokine co-receptors. The major human cells infected by HIV are CD4-positive T lymphocytes and cells of the nervous system.

The initial step in sexually transmitted HIV infection is entry of the virus into the cells of activated T cells, macrophages, or dendritic cells in the genital tract or bowel. The initial cellular targets for HIV are tissue dendritic cells (Langerhans cells), which are located just below the epithelium of the genital tract. The virus binds to the CD4 molecule on the dendritic cell. However, uptake of the virus into the cell requires a co-receptor. This co-receptor varies for different strains of HIV. For the most common sexually transmitted HIV (the macrophage-tropic strains), the co-receptor that is needed is called *CCR5*. Therefore, the dendritic cells that express viral co-receptor *CCR5* are susceptible to infection. Within 18 hours, the infected dendritic cells fuse with the CD4+ T-cell lymphocytes. The infected CD4+ T lymphocytes collect in the regional lymph nodes. From these nodes, systemic dissemination follows; HIV-1 can be cultured from the blood 4–11 days after infection *(5)*. Other strains of HIV have other target cells. T-cell-tropic HIV (which can be seen in parenteral transmission) requires a different co-receptor (CCR4) on the host cells for infection to occur. Dual-tropic HIV strains can infect CCR5 and CXCR4 positive cells.

RISK FACTORS

Sexual contact is the most common route of HIV transmission. Worldwide, 75–85% of HIV-infected individuals have been infected through sexual contact. Although the risk of HIV transmission through direct, skin-penetrating blood exposure (e.g., needle-stick injuries, needle sharing, and transfusions) is well-defined, the rate of HIV transmission through sexual contact is much more variable. Sexual transmission of HIV can occur in a single sexual encounter or might not occur for years in HIV-discordant couples (one HIV-infected partner and one HIV-negative partner) that have unprotected intercourse.

Transmission of HIV via mucosal surfaces of the genital, oral, or rectal tract is influenced by multiple factors. In general, sexual transmission is dependant both on the concentration of HIV in genital secretions and on the susceptibility of the exposed partner. In infected people, HIV is present in the genital tract of both women and men as well as in rectal secretions. Although HIV can be recovered from the vagina, the glandular epithelium in the transformation zone between the columnar and squamous cells of the cervix appears to be a dominant source of HIV shedding in women. Concentrations of HIV from endocervical swabs have been found to be two to three times higher than from vaginal swabs (6,7). In men, HIV can be detected in seminal cells such as lymphocytes and monocytes as well as in seminal plasma (cell-free HIV) (8). Although HIV DNA has been detected in sperm cells and their precursors (9), sperm itself appears to play no significant role in HIV transmission. Sperm cells do not possess CD4 receptors, which are the main cell receptors for HIV. Experience from assisted reproduction clinics—using washed and isolated spermatozoa for intrauterine insemination or for in vitro fertilization—has not been associated with HIV transmission, confirming that spermatozoa alone do not play a significant role in HIV transmission (10,11). Vasectomy in men does not significantly affect HIV concentration in seminal secretion, suggesting that the majority of HIV shedding occurs distal of the vas deference (12). Interestingly, the genital tract can act as a separate compartment for HIV replication. The correlation between the HIV concentration in blood plasma and seminal secretion is only moderate (8,12,13). Antiretroviral medication can achieve an undetectable HIV viral load in blood plasma, but this does not automatically mean that there is no virus in the seminal secretions. HIV concentration in rectal secretions has been found to be significantly elevated and even higher than HIV concentration in blood plasma and seminal fluid (14).

The exposed partner's susceptibility to HIV infection is also important in transmission efficacy. The partner's susceptibility depends on the presence of cells expressing CD4 receptors and chemokine surface receptors in the genital, oral, and/or rectal tissue (15). The cells with CD4 receptors include CD4 T lymphocytes, Langerhans' cells, and other macrophages (16). HIV-receptive cells have been found in the lamina propria of oral, cervicovaginal, foreskin, urethral, and rectal epithelia in primate models (16).

Different sexual practices are associated with different rates of transmission. Anal intercourse causes the highest risk of sexual HIV transmission. In a study of male-to-female anal sex, the transmission rate was estimated to be 140 in 10,000 to 183 in 10,000 encounters, depending on the stage of HIV disease in the index case (17). Studies in men who have sex with men (MSM) and bisexual men in the United States, the risk for HIV transmission for receptive anal sex has been estimated to be between 50 in 10,000 and 300 in 10,000 encounters (18,19). The second most risky sexual practice is penile–vaginal intercourse. In women, the vagina rather than the cervix appears to be the susceptible site for acquiring HIV infection. This was shown in an animal model of hysterectomized Rhesus monkeys who were able to be infected with SIV (20). The overall sexual transmission rate appears lower than direct, skin-penetrating blood exposure, such as needle-stick injuries or needle sharing. In large cohorts of heterosexual couples with discordant HIV status, the transmission probabilities of HIV have been estimated to range from 3 per 10,000 to 14 per 10,000 encounters *(16,21–24)*. These rates are an overall estimate and should not be used as a definite number. Also, the risk of sexual transmission is not constant from one sexual contact to another. Over time, stable HIV-discordant couples have a lower risk of transmitting HIV. In a given partnership, HIV transmission appears to occur within the early sexual contacts and is considerably less likely thereafter *(25)*. Consequently, a higher rate of HIV transmission should be expected in sexual assault cases. Sexual contact with multiple partners is associated with a higher risk of HIV transmission. Higher rates have been reported in men with contact to sex workers. A study of military recruits in Thailand who had contact with female sex workers as the principal mode of HIV transmission estimated the probability of HIV transmission per sexual contact to be between 310 and 560 per 10,000 encounters, a rate that is 100 times higher than HIV-discordant couples in long-term relationships *(26,27)*. A high rate of primary HIV infection among Thai female sex workers might have further increased the rate of HIV transmission.

US and European studies demonstrated that male-to-female transmission of HIV appears to be more likely than female-to-male transmission. A European study of 563 stable HIV-discordant couples, male-to-female transmission was 1.9 times more efficient than female-to-male transmission *(28)*. Other studies of discordant couples from the United States and Europe reported an even greater difference of transmission efficacy; the male-to-female transmission rates are eight to nine times greater than female-to-male rates *(21)*. However, studies from Africa do not show any difference in transmission risk between males and females. It is not known why the rates of intergender transmission of HIV from in Africa are comparable, whereas the transmission rates are different in Europe and the United States.

Oral sex is considered to have the lowest risk of HIV transmission. At the beginning of the AIDS epidemic, transmission of HIV through oral sex was disputed. The difficulty has been to show reliably that no other risk factors are involved in a given transmission of HIV. Several case series now report transmission of HIV through oral sex *(29–31)*, although the rate of HIV transmission through oral sex appears rather low. HIV can be detected in saliva in small concentrations *(31)*. Components of saliva, however, have an inactivating effect on HIV, which further decreases the transmissibility of HIV. Any oral lesions and/or bleeding, however, will increase the concentration of HIV and the risk of HIV transmission. In a study of MSM, the risk of HIV transmission is estimated to be 4 per 10,000 encounters for receptive oral sex for partners with unknown HIV status *(19)*. In comparison to insertive oral sex, insertive vaginal sex and anal sex have 10 times higher risks of infection, and receptive vaginal and anal sex had 20 to 100 times higher risks *(see* Table 1) *(32)*. These calculations did not control for cofactors of sexual transmission of HIV.

Table 1
Per Act Relative Risk for Acquisition of HIV

Sexual act	Relative risk
Insertive oral	1
Receptive oral	2
Insertive vaginal	10
Insertive anal	13
Receptive vaginal	20
Receptive anal	100

HIV, human immunodeficiency virus.
Adapted from ref. *32*.

Other Factors Influencing Sexual Transmission of HIV

HIGH VIRAL TITERS

There is a greater efficacy of HIV transmission when the index patient has advanced HIV disease or AIDS *(23,33–37)*. A CD4 cell count of less than 200 cells/mm *(34)*, detectable p24 antigen *(36)*, or a positive HIV culture *(33)* are risk factors for enhanced HIV transmission. Acute HIV infection also increases HIV transmission *(37,38)*. Both of these stages of HIV infection (acute and advanced HIV infection/AIDS) are associated with an elevated HIV viral load. Recent studies found a strong correlation between HIV blood plasma viral load and an increased risk of HIV transmission *(24,38–43)*. In a large study of HIV-discordant couples in Uganda, HIV blood plasma viral load of the index patient was significantly higher in couples in which the initially HIV-negative partner became infected vs those who remained uninfected (mean viral load was 90,254 vs 38,029) *(38)*. There was a significant dose–response effect of HIV viral load on HIV transmission. Despite the fact that the genital tract can act as a separate compartment for HIV replication, HIV transmission did not occur when the HIV blood plasma viral load of the index patient was less than 1500 copies per milliliter. The risk of HIV transmission increased progressively with higher HIV blood plasma viral load. Also supporting this observation is the fact that HAART, which is associated with decreased HIV viral load, reduces the likelihood of HIV transmission *(44)*. Clearly, factors other than the blood plasma viral load influence the concentration of HIV in genital secretion *(16,45)*. Using a mathematical probabilistic model, the probability of HIV transmission was calculated to be 1 per 100 episodes of intercourse when semen contains 100,000 copies/mL of HIV, but was 3 per 10,000 when the seminal HIV load was 1000 copies/mL *(46)*.

Co-Infection With Other Sexually Transmitted Infections

STIs increase the vulnerability of uninfected people to acquire HIV and increase the risk of HIV-infected individuals to infect their partners. The rate of HIV infection is considerably higher in patients who present to STD clinics with genital ulcers or mucosal inflammation *(8)*. Genital infections increase the risk for HIV transmission because of several mechanisms. Genital infection disrupts the host's mucosal barriers and/or an increase in the number of HIV susceptible cells in the genital tract *(8)*. STIs also lead to an increase in HIV shedding in the genital secretions and, therefore, increase the risk of HIV transmission. Several studies have shown an increase in the HIV viral load of genital secretions in patients with a traditional STI. A large study in Malawi showed an eightfold increase in HIV concentration in the genital secretions of HIV-infected men with urethritis in comparison to HIV-infected men with no urethritis. Gonorrhea was associated with the largest increase in HIV shedding. Treatment of the urethritis reversed the increase of HIV shedding *(47)*. In women (female sex workers in Ivory Coast), HIV shedding in genital secretion (cervix) was increased with gonorrhea (odds ratio 1.9), Chlamydia (odds ratio 2.5) infection, and cervical or vaginal ulcers (odds ratio 3.9) *(48)*. Treatment of the underlying STIs lowered the frequency of HIV shedding in genital secretions from 42 to 21% *(48)*. The impact of STI therapy/intervention on the HIV incidence in populations with low prevalence rates has also been shown in a study in Tanzania. Establishment of STI clinics, training of staff to diagnose and treat STIs, regular supply of STI drugs, and supervision reduced HIV incidence by about 40% *(49)*.

Lack of Male Circumcision

Circumcised men have a lower risk of acquiring HIV. In a meta-analysis of studies from sub-Saharan Africa, 21 of 27 studies found that circumcision was protective. The overall risk was decreased by a factor of 2–4 *(50)*.

Multiple factors have been discussed to explain the increased risk of HIV infection in uncircumcised men. The foreskin possesses an abundance of Langerhans cells on the inner surface, which are susceptible to HIV and are thought to be the primary target of transmission in uncircumcised men *(16)*. Circumcision also appears to confer a decreased risk of ulcerative STI, which will further decrease the risk for HIV transmission *(50)*. Furthermore, the diagnosis of ulcerative disease may also be delayed when the foreskin is present.

Cervical Ectopy

Cervical ectopy is the residual ring of columnar cells surrounding the cervical os that have not yet undergone squamous metaplasia. These cells have thinner epithelia and are often more friable. Cervical ectopy has been associated with enhanced HIV transmission in multiple studies, such as a large cohort study of

HIV-serodiscordant couples in Nairobi, Kenya, which found that cervical ectopy was associated with HIV infection in women (OR = 4.7) *(51)*.

GENETIC FACTORS

The chemokine receptor *CCR5* is a co-receptor for the fusion and entry of macrophage-tropic variants of HIV, which are the principal types of virus involved in person-to-person transmission. Mutation in the *CCR5* gene is common in Europeans and North Americans and is estimated to occur in 8–10% in these groups *(52,53)*. The mutation contains a 32-bp deletion (δ-32) and can occur in one or both alleles of the *CCR5* gene. δ-32 mutations in both alleles (homozygotes) of the *CCR5* genes are rare. However, consistent evidence shows that people with homozygous δ-32 mutations of the *CCR5* gene are resistant to infection by macrophage-tropic HIV *(52,54)*. Paxton et al. examined 1252 MSM enrolled in the Chicago fraction of the Multicenter AIDS Cohort Study for *CCR5* mutation. None of the HIV-infected participants was homozygous for the δ-32 mutation in the *CCR5* gene; however, 3–6% of at-risk but uninfected Caucasian participants were homozygous for the mutation *(53)*. Because this mutation is rare in native Africans and East Asians, it has been discussed that the lack of this mutation supports the more rapid rate of transmission in sub-Saharan Africa and Asia *(55)*. Further studies are needed to define the role of heterozygous δ-32 mutation of *CCR5* gene in HIV transmission.

HORMONAL CONTRACEPTION

Hormonal contraceptives do not protect against HIV. The remaining question is whether any hormonal contraceptive method increases transmission. A meta-analysis of 28 observational and cross-sectional studies in 1999 was not able to demonstrate a statistically significant increase in risk of HIV acquisition with oral contraceptive (OC) use (odds ratio of 1.19; 95% confidence interval [CI]; 0.99–1.42) *(56)*. However, the odds ratio increased to 1.32 (95% CI; 1.12–1.57) when analyzing prospective studies only *(49)*. The eight "best" studies in this meta-analysis had an overall odds ratio of 1.60 (95% CI; 1.05–2.44). Different factors have been postulated to explain the increased susceptibility of women using OCs to HIV, including cervical ectopy induced by OCs, the impact of OCs on the immune system, and possible thinning of the vaginal epithelium, which possibly enhances entry of HIV *(57)*. More recent studies demonstrated an increased expression of *CCR5* chemoreceptor on CD4 T lymphocytes in women taking hormonal contraceptives *(58)*.

OCs might not only change the susceptibility of women to HIV, but might also alter their infectivity. Increased shedding of HIV in genital secretion has been found in women using OCs. Women starting to take OCs were found to have an increase in the prevalence of HIV-infected cells in their genital secretions *(57)*.

Depot medroxyprogesterone acetate (DMPA) is also being studied carefully. Some studies have demonstrated an increased risk of HIV acquisition and transmission with DMPA use. In an animal model using SIV, subcutaneous progesterone implant led to a thinning of the vaginal epithelium and a 7.7-fold increased of SIV vaginal transmission (59). In a prospective cohort study of female sex workers in Kenya, use of DMPA was associated with an increased incidence of HIV infection (Hazard ratio of 2.0; 95% CI; 1.4–3.8) (60). Users of hormonal contraceptives should be aware of the potential increased risk of HIV susceptibility and HIV shedding and should use barrier methods to reduce their STI risks.

NONOXYNOL-9 SPERMICIDE

The currently marketed detergent-type spermicide nonoxynol-9 has been studied in multiple large clinical trials. A double-blinded, randomized, placebo-controlled trial in female sex workers in Cameroon showed no protective effect of nonoxynol-9 against HIV (61). The rate of HIV transmission was identical in the group receiving nonoxynol-9 and in the placebo group (6.7 vs 6.6 cases per 100 woman-years, respectively). A study among sex workers in several African countries and Thailand comparing nonoxynol-9 gel with a placebo showed an increased risk of HIV transmission associated with nonoxynol-9 gel use (16 vs 12%). Other international studies using different concentrations of nonoxynol-9 confirmed that it is not protective against HIV transmission (62). Higher frequency of nonoxynol-9 use has been associated with a higher rate of HIV infection suggesting a disruption of the vaginal mucosal integrity allowing higher HIV transmission (62).

ALLOIMMUNIZATION

The low HIV transmission rate among long-term HIV-discordant heterosexual partners supports the theory that in some people, an immune response of the HIV-negative partner to the HIV-positive partner's HLA antigens may occur. Because HLA antigens are present on CD4 cells, T-cells, macrophages, neutrophils, immature germ cells and HIV itself, an immune response to human leukocyte antigen in genital secretions might stimulate a local immune response. This immune response can be seen as "natural vaccination" (alloimmunization). This alloimmunization will enhance an immune response against HIV and is potentially protective against HIV transmission. In one study, peripheral blood mononuclear cells (PBMCs) of monogamous heterosexual couples were significantly more stimulated by their partner's PBMC if the couple practiced unprotected sex compared with couples who used condoms. The stimulation of PBMCs led to a decrease of HIV susceptibility in vitro. Stimulation was more significant in women than in men (63). Alloimmunization could also be used in future therapeutic vaccination research.

CONTROVERSIAL RISK FACTORS

Some studies have shown that HIV viral load in women's cervices are lowest at the time of ovulation *(64,65)* and highest just before and during menses *(65, 66)*, although other studies have found no fluctuation during the menstrual cycle. Vitamin A levels have also been studied; deficiency of vitamin A was thought to increase perinatal transmission, although this has not been a consistent finding.

CLINICAL MANIFESTATIONS

Overview

The natural history of HIV infection is characterized by an initial acute HIV infection syndrome followed by an asymptomatic, chronic phase (asymptomatic chronic HIV infection) and a late stage with symptomatic HIV infection and AIDS. During the acute phase, before immune response, it has been estimated that up to 250 billion host cells could become infected *(67)*. During the asymptomatic stage, there is rapid production and turnover of HIV, but infection, cell death, and replacement are somewhat balanced. The CD8+ cell activators keep the virus in check. However, CD8+ cell function depends on CD4+ T-cell production of interleukin-2. The CD4+ cell count drops over time. The effectiveness of CD8+ protection wanes and the third phase of HIV infection—the symptomatic HIV infection and AIDS—starts.

Symptoms of Acute HIV Infection

Symptoms of acute HIV seroconversion occur during dissemination of the virus with high-grade viremia. Acute retroviral syndrome (acute HIV infection syndrome) develops in 40–90% of patients infected with HIV and starts 2–6 weeks after exposure to HIV. It lasts for days to weeks, typically 14 days, but may persist up to 10 weeks. The development of specific antibodies against HIV marks the completion of seroconversion. Often, by the time of the onset of symptoms, the patient does not correlate the acute HIV conversion symptoms with the sexual encounter.

Symptoms of an acute HIV infection are often mononucleosis-like and commonly include fever, rash, fatigue, pharyngitis, weight loss, night sweats, lymphadenopathy, myalgias, headache, nausea, and diarrhea. Mucosal ulcers (e.g., esophageal ulcers) can also be found. Neurological manifestations, such as aseptic meningitis, radiculopathy, and cranial nerve VII palsy, occur in some symptomatic patients. Routine laboratory tests characteristically show leukopenia, thrombocytopenia, and elevated transaminases. The nonspecific clinical presentation of primary HIV infection leads to a large number of undiagnosed cases. High clinical suspicion is warranted to pursue the diagnostic work-up for HIV infection.

Table 2
AIDS Case Definition for Adolescents and Adults (1993)

		Clinical categories		
CD4 cell categories		*Asymptomatic or acute HIV infection*	*Symptomatic*	*AIDS indicator conditions (see Table 2)*
>500/mm^3	(≥29%)			■
200–499/mm^3	(14–28%)			■
<200/mm^3	(<14%)	■	■	■

The shaded areas above indicate conditions representing AIDS.
AIDS, acquired immune deficiency syndrome; HIV, human immunodeficiency virus.

Clinical recovery from the acute HIV syndrome is characterized by an immune response to the virus and is accompanied by a decline of the HIV viral load. During the following latent phase of the infection, the viral load stabilizes at a "set point" that is generally lower than the acute HIV infection phase. The CD4 cells decline slowly during the latent phase. Patients in the latent phase of an HIV infection are usually asymptomatic; however, HIV-infected patients in any stage have a higher risk for particular infections, such as pneumococcal infections and tuberculosis. With further decline of the CD4 cells, other complications, such as oropharyngeal Candida infection and seborrhoic dermatitis can occur.

The late stage of HIV infection (AIDS) is typified by an increase in HIV viral load and a further decline of the CD4 cells, which allows for the development of opportunistic infections, specific tumors, wasting, and neurological complications that are the hallmarks of AIDS. AIDS is defined as severe immune suppression with a CD4 cell count less than 200 cell/mm^3 (or <14% CD4 cells) or the onset of well-defined, characteristic infections (e.g., *P. jiroveci* pneumonia) and tumors (e.g., Kaposi sarcoma), regardless of CD4 cell count in a HIV-infected patient (*see* Tables 2 and 3). If untreated, death occurs at an average of 1.3 years after the onset of an AIDS-defining complication. The average time from infection to the development of AIDS in patient without antiretroviral therapy is about 8 years.

TESTING TECHNIQUES

All HIV diagnostic tests detect one or more molecules that comprise an HIV particle or detect antibodies that the host makes against the HIV particles *(68)*. The standard HIV test detects specific antibodies against HIV. Two different methods are used to detect antibodies. An enzyme-linked immunosorbent assay (ELISA) is used to screen for HIV-specific antibodies. The ELISA is more than

Table 3
AIDS Indicator Conditions

- Candidiasis of esophagus, trachea, bronchi, or lungs
- Cervical cancer, invasive
- Coccidioidomycosis, extrapulmonary
- Cryptococcosis, extrapulmonary
- Cryptosporidiosis with diarrhea for more than 1 month
- CMV of any organ other than liver, spleen, or lymph nodes
- Encephalopathy, HIV-related
- Herpes simplex with mucocutaneous ulcer for more than 1 month or bronchitis, pneumonitis, or esophagitis
- Histoplasmosis, extrapulmonary
- Isosporosis with diarrhea for more than 1 month
- Kaposi's sarcoma
- Lymphoma, Burkitt's, immunoblastic, primary central nervous system
- Mycobacterium avium complex or *M. kansasii*, disseminated
- Mycobacterium, other or unidentified species, disseminated or extra-pulmonary
- Mycobacterium tuberculosis
- Pneumocystis jiroveci pneumonia
- Pneumonia, recurrent bacterial more than two episodes in 12 months)
- Progressive multifocal leukoencephalopathy
- Salmonella septicemia
- Toxoplasmosis of internal organ/brain
- Wasting syndrome owing to HIV

CMV, cytomegalovirus; HIV, human immunodeficiency virus.

99% sensitive and specific *(69)*. A Western blot assay, which detects HIV-specific antibodies, is used to confirm the HIV diagnosis. These two tests should be used in combination because false-negative and false-positive tests occur. Certain types of HIV, HIV-2, and some subtypes of HIV-1 (subtype O and N, which are very uncommon in the United States), will not be reliably detected with the standard ELISA and Western blot tests. Special tests through the CDC are necessary to detect these types if suspicion for HIV infection is high.

Specific antibodies against HIV have some important clinical limitations. The ELISA and Western blot tests will be negative during the initial weeks after infection ("window period"), because antibodies are not usually detectable for 6–8 weeks. The time needed to perform the tests in the laboratory is also a disadvantage, as is the requirement for blood drawing in a clinical setting.

Newer HIV tests have been developed to either shorten the time period for a test result to be available ("rapid HIV test") or to improve patient convenience (oral HIV test, urine HIV test, HIV home kit test). The rapid HIV test must be performed by a trained laboratory technician and test results are available within 30 minutes. A positive result must be confirmed with the traditional standardized Western blot test. The oral HIV test (OraSure®) samples saliva by putting a specimen collection device (special pad) between buccal mucosal and lower gum for 2 minutes. The amount of HIV immunoglobulin G sampled from the saliva is high and sufficient for detection. Results are usually available within 3 days. The oral HIV test makes specimen collection very simple, has a reduced cost, and potentially a much better acceptance by patients. The urine test provides a more convenient sampling, but it can only be administered in a physician's office. The specificity of the urine test, however, is somewhat lower. Home test kits for patients are available. Sampling of blood is necessary (use of lancet). Negative test results can be obtained through a prerecorded phone message. Callers with a positive test result receive counseling from a counselor.

Direct testing for HIV RNA/DNA or HIV antigens (p24) can be used to detect HIV shortly after exposure, before antibodies against HIV have developed. The p24 antigen test, which detects the viral p24 antigen, is approved by the Food and Drug Administration to screen during acute HIV seroconversion and to screen blood donors to reduce the length of the "window period." Sensitivity of p24 antigen tests varies with the stage of the infection and ranges from 32 to 89%. HIV RNA and DNA testing using nucleic acid amplification assays for HIV can also detect the infection early. Polymerase chain reaction-based tests have a high sensitivity (89–100%). These tests are widely used to detect the level of HIV viremia ("viral load") and have replaced the p24 antigen test in clinical practice to detect early HIV infection, although they are not approved by the Food and Drug Administration for this indication. Any test that detects HIV or parts of HIV needs to be confirmed in an appropriate time interval by standard HIV tests (ELISA and Western blot test), which will detect HIV-specific antibodies.

HIV testing should be routinely offered to adults and adolescents. It is particularly encouraged for all pregnant women. Rules regarding the need for informed consent are being modified. In many settings, HIV testing is becoming a routine test with opt-out, instead of opt-in consenting, so many of the traditional requirements for a consent are being altered. Other barriers to testing should be reduced.

TREATMENT

Once the diagnosis of HIV infection is made, management should begin in consultation with an HIV specialist, if available. There are currently four different classes of antiretroviral medications approved for the treatment of HIV infection. Since the introduction of protease inhibitor in 1996, highly active antiretroviral therapy (HAART) has been available, which can lead to suppression of HIV to below detectable levels in the plasma. A cure of HIV is still not possible.

Antiretroviral therapy is associated with toxicities ranging from hepatic and metabolic toxicities (including lactic acidosis) to neuropathy and pancreatitis. Patients on antiretroviral therapy need to be closely monitored for toxicities and emerging resistance to the virus. Resistance to available antiretroviral agents can develop very rapidly and presents a challenge in treating patients with HIV infections. Protective methods need to be used to minimize the risk of HIV transmission.

POSTEXPOSURE PROPHYLAXIS

The use of antiretroviral agents to prevent HIV infection after exposure is now common clinical practice. For years, clinical guidelines recommended antiretroviral therapy after exposure to HIV in an occupational setting (e.g., a health care worker is accidentally exposed to blood of a known HIV-infected person). The CDC has also published guidelines for postexposure prophylaxis in nonoccupational settings. Several factors justify the use of postexposure prophylaxis. Immediately after exposure to HIV, there is an infection of dendritic cells at the site of inoculum. It takes 24–48 hours before these cell migrate to regional lymph nodes. Antiretroviral therapy during the time after exposure to HIV and the involvement of regional lymph nodes could prevent the establishment HIV infection systemically.

The choice of HAART for postexposure prophylaxis is based on first-line recommendation by the Department of Health and Human Services for HIV-infected people. No evidence indicates that any specific antiretroviral medication or combination is optimal for postexposure prophylaxis. In cases in which the source patient is known and an assessment can be made that the potentially transmitted virus has mutations leading to HIV drug resistance, the antiretroviral regimen should be individually adjusted. Counseling of possible side effects and the importance of compliance with the medication regimen should be undertaken. Ancillary medication (e.g., against nausea and diarrhea) should be offered. The patient should be followed closely. Use of antiretroviral therapy is associated with toxicity; high cost and widespread unjustified use may limit the benefit.

Non-Occupational Exposure Prophylaxis

Animal studies, mainly in macaques, have suggested that postexposure prophylaxis after genital exposure is effective (70,71). In a macaque animal model, HIV-2 was inserted atraumatically into the vagina. Antiretroviral therapy was given to the animals after 12, 36, or 72 hours. Infection rates in the treated animals were compared with infection rates in animals that received no antiretroviral therapy. No transmission occurred when antiretroviral therapy was given within 12 to 36 hours; 25% of animals became HIV-infected when antiretroviral therapy was given after 72 hours. In comparison, 75% of untreated animals became HIV infected *(70)*.

Observational studies in humans of non-occupational exposures among MSM and among sexually assaulted women in Brazil demonstrated the possible benefit of postexposure prophylaxis after high-risk sexual encounters. In study of MSM, 202 participants were given antiretroviral medication to use as prophylaxis immediately after high-risk sexual exposure. HIV seroconversion occurred in 10.9% of those who did not use postexposure prophylaxis compared with only 0.9% of men given postexposure prophylaxis *(72)*. In another non-randomized study from Brazil, postexposure prophylaxis was given to victims of sexual assaults. None of the sexually assaulted women who received 28-day postexposure prophylaxis with HIV medication within 72 hours after the assault became HIV-infected, whereas four out of 145 women (2.7%) who did not receive postexposure prophylaxis became HIV-infected *(73)*.

The CDC published guidelines for the use of non-occupational HIV prophylaxis in January 2005 *(see* Fig. 1) *(74)*. Multidrug therapy for 28 days is recommended for people who present within 72 hours of a non-occupational exposure to blood, semen, vaginal secretions, rectal secretions, breast milk, or other body fluids that are contaminated with blood of a person known to be HIV-infected. The earlier the prophylaxis is initiated, the better the chance of success. A history of the exposure, timing, and frequency of exposure, HIV status of the source as well as the exposed person and the risk for transmission needs to be assessed. Frequently exposed persons requiring frequent or even continuous prophylaxis should not receive postexposure prophylaxis. If the status of the source person is not known, an attempt should be undertaken to test the source patient (if available). Prophylaxis for the exposed person can be initiated before the HIV test result of the source patient is known. If the HIV status of the source patient is unknown, a risk assessment of the source patient should be attempted (e.g., higher HIV prevalence among MSM, bisexual men, and iv drug users) and initiation of postexposure prophylaxis should be determined on a case-by-case basis. This is expected to be the situation in virtually all cases *(75)*.

Occupational Exposure Prophylaxis

A case-controlled study of health care workers with occupational, percutaneous exposure to HIV-infected blood showed that postexposure prophylaxis with AZT lowered the risk of HIV transmission significantly (odds ratio = 0.19) *(76)*. With the advancement and introduction of newer antiretroviral agents, the CDC recommends using a combination of antiretroviral agents for occupation postexposure prophylaxis *(77)*. The risk of HIV transmission after a needle-stick injury depends on the amount of blood exposed and the severity of the injury (e.g., large-bore needle containing blood from an HIV-infected patient with a high viral load with deep percutaneous penetration and injection of blood will

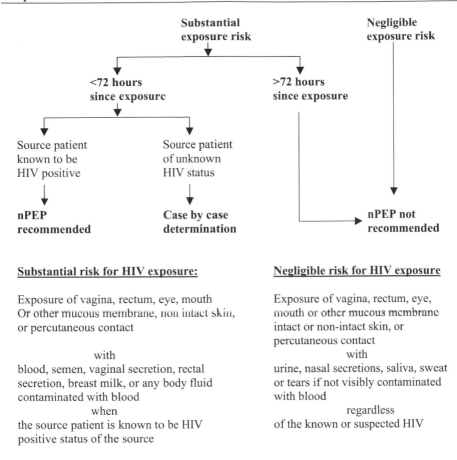

Fig. 1. Non-occupational postexposure prophylaxis.

confer highest risk). The CDC and University of California, San Francisco hotlines are available to provide guidance in individual cases. Failures of postexposure prophylaxis have been reported.

Diagnostic Tests After Postexposure Prophylaxis

HIV antibody levels of the exposed patients should be determined at baseline, 4–6 weeks, 3 months, and 6 months. In addition, testing for hepatitis B and C and other STIs should be recommended and offered. Interaction with the person seeking postexposure prophylaxis also provides an opportunity for safe sex counseling. Partner notification of the exposed person should be encouraged. If the exposed person becomes infected with HIV, partner notification is essential and required.

PARTNER NOTIFICATION AND REPORTING REQUIREMENTS

AIDS is a reportable disease in every state, and HIV infection is a reportable disease in most states. Laws and regulations covering partner notification also vary by state. In general, patients with newly diagnosed HIV infection should be encouraged to notify their prior sexual contacts and encourage them to seek testing. The newly diagnosed cases should also be counseled to advise any potential new sex partner of his/her status.

PREGNANCY-RELATED ISSUES

As heterosexual transmission rates of HIV in the United States are increasing, the risk of HIV infection during pregnancy is also increasing. Pregnancy has no impact on the clinical course or progression of asymptomatic HIV infection; elective abortion does not affect HIV infection progression. However, maternal infection may have serious adverse impacts on fetal outcome. In women with low CD4 counts, preterm birth rates have been reported to be 20%, and growth restriction has been found in 24% of newborns (78). The stillbirth rate may also be increased with maternal HIV infection (79).

Vertical transmission via early transplacental infection has been demonstrated. In general, transmission occurs at birth. Approximately 15–25% of infants born to HIV-infected mothers are HIV-infected (80). Infection is more likely in preterm births, especially if associated with prolonged rupture of membranes. In one study, preterm delivery carried a 3.7-fold increased risk of HIV infection (81). Membranes ruptured for longer than 4 hours were associated with transmission rates of 14–25% (82). Concurrent infection with syphilis increases vertical transmission. Perinatal transmission rates are most profoundly correlated with maternal viral load (HIV-1 RNA) (83). Neonatal infection occurs in about 5% of infants when maternal viral loads are less than 5000 copies/mL and more than 40% when those levels exceed 100,000 copies/mL (84,85). Transmission of HIV-1 infection with breastfeeding occurs in about 16% of cases (86). Therefore, breastfeeding is discouraged in HIV-infected women who have access to safe formula feeding. However, in underdeveloped countries where formula feeding is associated with potentially fatal diarrheal and respiratory infections, the World Health Organization and United Nations Children's Fund have recommended continued breastfeeding promotion.

Universal screening of all pregnant women is recommended at the first prenatal visit. The CDC, American College of Obstetricians and Gynecologists, and the American Academy of Pediatrics recommend that screening be offered using an opt-out approach, where a patient is notified that she will be tested for HIV as part of the routine battery of prenatal blood tests unless she declines (87). If the patient declines, her decision should be documented. She should be offered testing at every subsequent visit. Repeat testing in the third trimester is recommended routinely in areas where HIV prevalence is 0.5% or greater and when the woman has personal risk factors (history of STIs, illicit drug use, multiple sex partners, or signs or symptoms suggestive of acute HIV infection). Women who present in labor with no prenatal care or no prenatal HIV testing should be offered immediate testing with rapid HIV test technologies. Therapy should be initiated (with consent) based on the rapid test results.

Women diagnosed with HIV infection should be treated with multi-drug therapy starting at least in the second trimester to reduce viral loads and vertical transmission. Viral loads should be tested each trimester and as delivery is being planned. Women with HIV-1 RNA viral loads more than 1000 copies/mL should be delivered by a caesarian section that is planned close to 38 weeks gestational age to reduce the risk of membrane rupture *(88)*.

Intrapartum therapy with antiretroviral drugs is an important component in the prevention of vertical transmission, even for women who are acutely diagnosed in labor. Newborns should receive antiretroviral therapy for 6 weeks.

PREVENTION

Prevention of HIV infection is the key intervention in fighting HIV infection and AIDS. Despite significant advances in HIV therapy, the rate of new infection of HIV has remained unchanged over the last 10 years. Improved efforts are necessary to enhance fundamental behavior changes to prevent new HIV transmission.

Abstinence and mutual monogamy with a partner who has been tested and is known to be HIV-negative are the surest way to avoid HIV transmission. For sexually active persons with risk of HIV transmission, barrier methods (condoms) are the most efficient methods to reduce the risk for HIV transmission.

Condoms

Male condoms are widely available and are the most commonly used barrier devices. Most male condoms are commonly made out of natural latex, but other materials are also used. Polyurethane condoms are considered an alternative to latex condoms in patients with latex allergies. They appear sufficient to prevent HIV from crossing through the condom. Natural condoms do not protect against HIV transmission and are not recommended for disease prevention, because they possess natural pores that may allow HIV to cross through the condom. Overall, male latex condoms are protective against HIV transmission (*see* Chapter 15). Consistent and correct use to minimize breakage or slippage is crucial to provide protection.

The efficacy of condom use in preventing HIV transmission has been recently evaluated by Davis and Weller *(89)*. The meta-analysis included 12 cohort studies of HIV serodiscordant heterosexual couples. Condom use—when used at every encounter—was estimated to be 87% protective, which is comparable or slightly lower than its effectiveness to prevent pregnancy (89).

Data for anal intercourse are less robust. Available data confirm the protective properties of condoms during anal intercourse (36,90). Anal intercourse is perceived as being associated with a higher breakage and slippage rate because of increased friction. Some European countries recommend use of thicker/stronger condoms for anal intercourse. This recommendation has been based only on expert opinion; data to support use of thicker and stronger condoms is sparse. A few small studies report a comparable breakage rate of standard and thicker condoms during anal intercourse (91,92).

The female condom appears to be as protective as the male condom to prevent HIV transmission with correct and constant use (every time). It is less likely to break or leak when compared to the male condom (93). The United Nations program against AIDS promotes and supports female condoms in developing countries.

Other Preventive and Therapeutic Measures

MICROBICIDES

Microbicides are topical agents, which are applied to the vagina/rectum to prevent HIV transmission (see Chapter 16). So far, more than 60 microbicide candidates have been identified to have in vitro activity against HIV. Microbicides could provide potential protection against HIV transmission through several mechanisms, such as direct inactivation of HIV, preventing HIV attachment to target cells, inhibiting HIV from entering and replicating in target cells, and prevention of dissemination of HIV from target cells. Targeting HIV entry is a preferred mechanism in the more advanced microbicides designed to prevent HIV transmission.

Multiple safety and efficacy trials are ongoing using different microbicides to prevent HIV transmission. More specific microbicides are being developed to block the CCR5 co-receptor for HIV on susceptible cells in the vaginal mucosa. Animal studies appear promising (94). The development of these agents is still very preliminary (see Chapter 16 for more details).

HAART FOR INFECTED PEOPLE TO REDUCE TRANSMISSION

Since the mid-1990s, advances in HIV therapeutics led to the possibility to suppress HIV to a point where HIV is undetectable in serum. As outlined earlier, a low or undetectable HIV viral load influences the risk of HIV transmission. A very low or undetectable HIV viral load of HIV-infected person will significantly lower the risk of HIV transmission (38,44). The high cost of HAART therapy, late or delayed diagnosis of HIV infection, difficult to treat HIV infection (owing to resistant HIV) and/or non-compliance with HIV therapy are challenges.

TREATMENT OF STIs

As shown above, other STIs contribute to an increased risk of HIV transmission. HIV shedding as well as susceptibility to HIV infection are increased in patients with STIs. Aggressive treatment of other STIs has been shown to lower the risk of HIV transmission by up to 40% *(49)*.

CONCLUSION

In conclusion, HIV infection is an expanding pandemic with more than 40,000 new cases per year in the United States alone. Sexual transmission is the dominant transmission mode. HIV therapy might be able to control the virus, but a cure is not possible to date. Prevention and prophylaxis play a central role to fight the HIV epidemic. Knowledge of the risks for transmission, contributing factors, and prevention/prophylaxis methods is crucial for health care providers to counsel patients.

CASE STUDY

Marilyn, age 19, plans to enlist in the Army. She requests screening for STIs, so that she can be treated before her induction physical. She has had multiple sexual partners over the last few years, including an episode of forced sex when she was 14. She has no symptoms at this time, but she has been treated for chlamydia and genital warts in the past. She needs the test results fast. On exam, you note only a foul-smelling vaginal discharge. Microscopic examination reveals more than 20% clue cells. You send cervical specimens to test for C. trachomatis and N. gonorrhoeae. You send blood tests for syphilis and HBV surface antigen. Because she wants quick results, you test her saliva for HIV. The results are positive.

Questions

1. How do you counsel her about the test results?
2. What further tests do you perform?
3. Do you need to report her as an HIV infection?
4. Does that test result change the way you would treat any of her other infections?
5. What should she tell her partner?

Answers

1. The results of the rapid HIV test are not diagnostic, but they are suggestive. She needs to understand that she may have acquired HIV, but you will not know for certain until the blood test results are available. This two-step approach has been found to help patients adjust to their diagnosis and to plan for how they will deal with it more effectively. Because this news will have a very profound effect on her immediate plans, and because even the suggestion of HIV infec-

tion is so devastating, be prepared to offer her support and assess her response carefully to ensure that she is not suicidal (*see* Chapter 13 for more details).

2. She needs confirmatory Western blot assay. The other tests that need to assess viral load, CD4 cell count and other baseline measurements to determine her eligibility for therapy will be performed by the HIV specialist who will be managing her care after her diagnosis is confirmed.

3. You should await the results of the Western blot before reporting her infection to the local health department.

4. She can be treated with all the same drugs you would normally use to treat bacterial vaginosis and the other STIs you may detect. Be sure she has an effective contraceptive method as well as condoms.

5. At this point, she does not need to tell her partner about these test results, but she may want to talk to him if it will gain his psychological support. She should definitely avoid sex or use condoms until she learns that she is not infected.

SELECTED RESOURCES

- CDC National AIDS Hotline:
  - 800-342-AIDS [2437] English, 24 hours, 7 days a week;
  - 800-344-SIDA [7432] Spanish, 8 AM–2 AM Eastern Standard Time;
  - 800-243-7889 [TTY for hearing impaired] Monday–Friday 10 AM–10 PM Eastern Standard Time.
- University of California, San Francisco.
  - The National HIV Telephone Consultation Service (Warmline) 800-933-3413—is available from 6 AM to 5 PM (Pacific Standard Time) Monday through Friday
  - National Clinicians' Post-Exposure Prophylaxis Hotline (PEPline) 888-448-4911—is available 24 hours, 7 days a week. Both are free and confidential services.

REFERENCES

1. Centers for Disease Control and Prevention. HIV/AIDS Surveillance Report, 2005 (Vol. 16). Atlanta, GA: US Department of Health and Human Services, Centers for Disease Control and Prevention; 2005. Available from: http://www.cdc.gov/hiv/stats/hasrlink.htm. Accessed August 1, 2006.
2. Fleming PL, Byers RH, Sweeney PA, Daniels D, Karon JM, Janssen RS. HIV prevalence in the United States, 2000. In: Programs and Abstracts of the 9th Conference of Retroviruses and Opportunistic Infections. Seattle, WA: February 24–28, 2002, Abstract 11.
3. Hall HI, Ling Q, Song R, McKenna MT. Recent trends in HIV diagnosis in the United States. In: Programs and Abstracts of the 11th Conference of Retroviruses and Opportunistic Infections; San Francisco, CA: February 8–11, 2004; Abstract 86.
4. Joint United Nations Program on HIV/AIDS. Report on the global AIDS epidemic. 2006. Geneva: Joint United Nations Programme on HIV/AIDS; 2006. Available from: http://www.unaids.org. Accessed on August 1, 2006.
5. Sweet RL, Gibbs RS. HIV/AIDS. In: *Infectious Diseases of the Female Genital Tract*, 4th Ed. Philadelphia, PA: Lippincott Williams & Wilkins; 2002, pp. 238–317.

6. Clemetson DB, Moss GB, Willerford DM, et al. Detection of HIV DNA in cervical and vaginal secretions. Prevalence and correlates among women in Nairobi, Kenya. JAMA 1993; 269:2860–2864.

7. Mostad SB, Overbaugh J, DeVange DM, et al. Hormonal contraception, vitamin A deficiency, and other risk factors for shedding of HIV-1 infected cells from the cervix and vagina. Lancet 1997; 350:922–927.

8. Vernazza PL, Eron JJ, Fiscus SA, Cohen MS. Sexual transmission of HIV: infectiousness and prevention. AIDS 1999; 13:155–166.

9. Bagasra O, Farzadegan H, Seshamma T, Oakes JW, Saah A, Pomerantz RJ. Detection of HIV-1 proviral DNA in sperm from HIV-1-infected men. AIDS 1994; 8:1669–1674.

10. Bujan L, Pasquier C, Labeyrie E, Lanusse-Crousse P, Morucci M, Daudin M. Insemination with isolated and virologically tested spermatozoa is a safe way for human immunodeficiency type 1 virus-serodiscordant couples with an infected male partner to have a child. Fertil Steril 2004; 82:857–862.

11. Pasquier C, Daudin M, Righi L, et al. Sperm washing and virus nucleic acid detection to reduce HIV and hepatitis C virus transmission in serodiscordant couples wishing to have children. AIDS 2000; 14:2093–2099.

12. Krieger JN, Nirapathpongporn A, Chaiyaporn M, et al. Vasectomy and human immunodeficiency virus type 1 in semen. J Urol 1998; 159:820–826.

13. Tachet A, Dulioust E, Salmon D, et al. Detection and quantification of HIV-1 in semen: identification of a subpopulation of men at high potential risk of viral sexual transmission. AIDS 1999; 13:823–831.

14. Zuckerman RA, Whittington WL, Celum CL, et al. Higher concentration of HIV RNA in rectal mucosa secretions than in blood and seminal plasma, among men who have sex with men, independent of antiretroviral therapy. J Infect Dis 2004; 190:156–161.

15. Dragic T, Litwin V, Allaway GP, et al. HIV-1 entry into CD4+ cells is mediated by the chemokine receptor CC-CKR-5. Nature 1996; 381:667–673.

16. Royce RA, Sena A, Cates W Jr, Cohen MS. Sexual transmission of HIV. N Engl J Med 1997; 336:1072–1078.

17. Quinn TC, Wawer MJ, Sewankambo N, et al. Viral load and heterosexual transmission of human immunodeficiency virus type 1. Rakai Project Study Group. N Engl J Med 2000; 342: 921–929.

18. Leynaert B, Downs AM, de Vincenzi I. Heterosexual transmission of human immunodeficiency virus: variability of infectivity throughout the course of infection. European Study Group on Heterosexual Transmission of HIV. Am J Epidemiol 1998; 148:88–96.

19. DeGruttola V, Seage GR III, Mayer KH, Horsburgh CR Jr. Infectiousness of HIV between male homosexual partners. J Clin Epidemiol 1989; 42:849–856.

20. Mingjia L, Short R. How oestrogen or progesterone might change a woman's susceptibility to HIV-1 infection. Aust NZ J Obstet Gynaecol 2002; 42:472–475.

21. Padian NS, Shiboski SC, Glass SO, Vittinghoff E. Heterosexual transmission of human immunodeficiency virus (HIV) in northern California: results from a ten-year study. Am J Epidemiol 1997; 146:350–357.

22. Nicolosi A, Correa Leite ML, Musicco M, Arici C, Gavazzeni G, Lazzarin A. The efficiency of male-to-female and female-to-male sexual transmission of the human immunodeficiency virus: a study of 730 stable couples. Italian Study Group on HIV Heterosexual Transmission. Epidemiology 1994; 5:570–575.

23. de Vincenzi I. A longitudinal study of human immunodeficiency virus transmission by heterosexual partners. European Study Group on Heterosexual Transmission of HIV. N Engl J Med 1994; 331:341–346.

24. Gray RH, Wawer MJ, Brookmeyer R, et al. Probability of HIV-1 transmission per coital act in monogamous, heterosexual, HIV-1-discordant couples in Rakai, Uganda. Lancet 2001; 357:1149–1153.

25. Downs AM, De Vincenzi I. Probability of heterosexual transmission of HIV: relationship to the number of unprotected sexual contacts. European Study Group in Heterosexual Transmission of HIV. J Acquir Immune Defic Syndr Hum Retrovirol 1996; 11:388–395.

26. Mastro TD, Satten GA, Nopkesorn T, Sangkharomya S, Longini IM Jr. Probability of female-to-male transmission of HIV-1 in Thailand. Lancet 1994; 343:204–207.

27. Satten GA, Mastro TD, Longini IM Jr. Modelling the female-to-male per-act HIV transmission probability in an emerging epidemic in Asia. Stat Med 1994; 13:2097–2106.

28. European Study Group on Heterosexual Transmission of HIV. Comparison of female to male and male to female transmission of HIV in 563 stable couples. BMJ 1992; 304:809–813.

29. Edwards S, Carne C. Oral sex and the transmission of viral STIs. Sex Transm Infect 1998; 74:6–10.

30. Richters J, Grulich A, Ellard J, Hendry O, Kippax S. HIV transmission among gay men through oral sex and other uncommon routes: case series of HIV seroconverters, Sydney. AIDS 2003; 17:2269–2271.

31. Rothenberg RB, Scarlett M, del Rio C, Reznik D, O'Daniels C. Oral transmission of HIV. AIDS 1998; 12:2095–2105.

32. Varghese B, Maher JE, Peterman TA, Branson BM, Steketee RW. Reducing the risk of sexual HIV transmission: quantifying the per-act risk for HIV on the basis of choice of partner, sex act, and condom use. Sex Transm Dis 2002; 29:38–43.

33. Rockstroh JK, Ewig S, Bauer T, et al. Male-to-female transmission of HIV in a cohort of hemophiliacs—frequency, risk factors and effect of sexual counseling. Infection 1995; 23: 29–32.

34. Shiboski SC, Padian NS. Epidemiologic evidence for time variation in HIV infectivity. J Acquir Immune Defic Syndr Hum Retrovirol 1998; 19:527–535.

35. O'Brien TR, Busch MP, Donegan E, et al. Heterosexual transmission of human immunodeficiency virus type 1 from transfusion recipients to their sex partners. J Acquir Immune Defic Syndr 1994; 7:705–710.

36. Saracco A, Musicco M, Nicolosi A, et al. Man-to-woman sexual transmission of HIV: longitudinal study of 343 steady partners of infected men. J Acquir Immune Defic Syndr 1993; 6:497–502.

37. Seidlin M, Vogler M, Lee E, Lee YS, Dubin N. Heterosexual transmission of HIV in a cohort of couples in New York City. AIDS 1993; 7:1247–1254.

38. Vittinghoff E, Douglas J, Judson F, McKirnan D, MacQueen K, Buchbinder SP. Per-contact risk of human immunodeficiency virus transmission between male sexual partners. Am J Epidemiol 1999; 150:306–311.

39. Fiore JR, Zhang YJ, Bjorndal A, et al. Biological correlates of HIV-1 heterosexual transmission. AIDS 1997; 11:1089–1094.

40. Hisada M, O'Brien TR, Rosenberg PS, Goedert JJ. Virus load and risk of heterosexual transmission of human immunodeficiency virus and hepatitis C virus by men with hemophilia. The Multicenter Hemophilia Cohort Study. J Infect Dis 2000; 181:1475–1478.

41. Tovanabutra S, Robison V, Wongtrakul J, et al. Male viral load and heterosexual transmission of HIV-1 subtype E in northern Thailand. J Acquir Immune Defic Syndr 2002; 29:275–283.

42. Pedraza MA, del Romero J, Roldan F, et al. Heterosexual transmission of HIV-1 is associated with high plasma viral load levels and a positive viral isolation in the infected partner. J Acquir Immune Defic Syndr 1999; 21:120–125.

43. Ragni MV, Faruki H, Kingsley LA. Heterosexual HIV-1 transmission and viral load in hemophilic patients. J Acquir Immune Defic Syndr Hum Retrovirol 1998; 17:42–45.

44. Stephenson JM, Imrie J, Davis MM, et al. Is use of antiretroviral therapy among homosexual men associated with increased risk of transmission of HIV infection? Sex Transm Infect 2003; 79:7–10.

45. Coombs RW, Reichelderfer PS, Landay AL. Recent observations on HIV type-1 infection in the genital tract of men and women. AIDS 2003; 17:455–480.
46. Chakraborty H, Sen PK, Helms RW, et al. Viral burden in genital secretions determines male-to-female sexual transmission of HIV-1: a probabilistic empiric model. AIDS 2001; 15:621–627.
47. Cohen MS, Hoffman IF, Royce RA, et al. Reduction of concentration of HIV-1 in semen after treatment of urethritis: implications for prevention of sexual transmission of HIV-1. AIDSCAP Malawi Research Group. Lancet 1997; 349:1868–1873.
48. Ghys PD, Fransen K, Diallo MO, et al. The associations between cervicovaginal HIV shedding, sexually transmitted diseases and immunosuppression in female sex workers in Abidjan, Cote d'Ivoire. AIDS 1997; 11:F85–F93.
49. Grosskurth H, Mosha F, Todd J, et al. Impact of improved treatment of sexually transmitted diseases on HIV infection in rural Tanzania: randomised controlled trial. Lancet 1995; 346:530–536.
50. Weiss HA, Quigley MA, Hayes RJ. Male circumcision and risk of HIV infection in sub-Saharan Africa: a systematic review and meta-analysis. AIDS 2000; 14:2361–2370.
51. Moss GB, Clemetson D, D'Costa L, et al. Association of cervical ectopy with heterosexual transmission of human immunodeficiency virus: results of a study of couples in Nairobi, Kenya. J Infect Dis 1991; 164:588–591.
52. Hoffman TL, MacGregor RR, Burger H, Mick R, Doms RW, Collman RG. CCR5 genotypes in sexually active couples discordant for human immunodeficiency virus type 1 infection status. J Infect Dis 1997; 176:1093–1096.
53. Paxton WA, Kang S, Koup RA. The HIV type 1 coreceptor CCR5 and its role in viral transmission and disease progression. AIDS Res Hum Retroviruses 1998; 14(Suppl 1):S89–S92.
54. D'Ubaldo C, Serraino D, Peroni M, Ippolito G. Do chemokines play a role in HIV-1 heterosexual transmission? Susceptibility to HIV infection. J Biol Regul Homeost Agents 1999; 3:97–102.
55. Philpott S, Weiser B, Tarwater P, et al. CC chemokine receptor 5 genotype and susceptibility to transmission of human immunodeficiency virus type 1 in women. J Infect Dis 2003; 187:569–575.
56. Wang CC, Reilly M, Kreiss JK. Risk of HIV infection in oral contraceptive pill users: a meta-analysis. J Acquir Immune Defic Syndr 1999; 21:51–58.
57. Wang CC, McClelland RS, Overbaugh J, et al. The effect of hormonal contraception on genital tract shedding of HIV-1. AIDS 2004; 18:205–209.
58. Prakash M, Kapembwa MS, Gotch F, Patterson S. Oral contraceptive use induces upregulation of the CCR5 chemokine receptor on CD4(+) T cells in the cervical epithelium of healthy women. J Reprod Immunol 2002; 54:117–131.
59. Marx PA, Spira AI, Gettie A, et al. Progesterone implants enhance SIV vaginal transmission and early virus load. Nat Med 1996; 2:1084–1089.
60. Lavreys L, Chohan V, Overbaugh J, et al. Hormonal contraception and risk of cervical infections among HIV-1-seropositive Kenyan women. AIDS 2004; 18:2179–2184.
61. Roddy RE, Zekeng L, Ryan KA, Tamoufe U, Weir SS, Wong EL. A controlled trial of nonoxynol 9 film to reduce male-to-female transmission of sexually transmitted diseases. N Engl J Med 1998; 339:504–510.
62. Van Damme L, Ramjee G, Alary M, et al. Effectiveness of COL-1492, a nonoxynol-9 vaginal gel, on HIV-1 transmission in female sex workers: a randomised controlled trial. Lancet 2002; 360:971–977.
63. Peters B, Whittall T, Babaahmady K, Gray K, Vaughan R, Lehner T. Effect of heterosexual intercourse on mucosal alloimmunisation and resistance to HIV-1 infection. Lancet 2004; 363:518–524.

64. Money DM, Arikan YY, Remple V, et al. Genital tract and plasma human immunodeficiency virus viral load throughout the menstrual cycle in women who are infected with ovulatory human immunodeficiency virus. Am J Obstet Gynecol 2003; 188:122–128.
65. Benki S, Mostad SB, Richardson BA, Mandaliya K, Kreiss JK, Overbaugh J. Cyclic shedding of HIV-1 RNA in cervical secretions during the menstrual cycle. J Infect Dis 2004; 189:2192–2201.
66. Reichelderfer PS, Coombs RW, Wright DJ, et al. Effect of menstrual cycle on HIV-1 levels in the peripheral blood and genital tract. WHS 001 Study Team. AIDS 2000; 14:2101–2107.
67. Embretson J, Zupancic M, Ribas JL, et al. Massive covert infection of helper T lymphocytes and macrophages by HIV during the incubation period of AIDS. Nature 1993; 362:359–362.
68. Iweala OI. HIV diagnostic tests: an overview. Contraception 2004; 70:141–147.
69. Mylonakis E, Paliou M, Lally M, Flanigan TP, Rich JD. Laboratory testing for infection with the human immunodeficiency virus: established and novel approaches. Am J Med 2000; 109:568–576.
70. Otten RA, Smith DK, Adams DR, et al. Efficacy of postexposure prophylaxis after intravaginal exposure of pig-tailed macaques to a human-derived retrovirus (human immunodeficiency virus type 2). J Virol 2000; 74:9771–9775.
71. Tsai CC, Emau P, Follis KE, et al. Effectiveness of postinoculation (R)-9-(2-phosphonyl-methoxypropyl) adenine treatment for prevention of persistent simian immunodeficiency virus SIVmne infection depends critically on timing of initiation and duration of treatment. J Virol 1998; 72:4265–4273.
72. Schechter M, Largo RF, Ismerio R, et al. Acceptability, behaviorly impact, and possible efficacy of sexual exposure chemoprophylaxis (PEP) for HIV. In: Programme and Abstracts of the 9th Conference of Retroviruses and Opportunistic Infections. Seattle, WA: February 24–28, 2002.
73. Schechter M. Occupational and sexual PEP—benefit/risk? In: Programme and Abstracts of the 6th International Conference on Drug Therapy in HIV Infection. Glasgow, UK: November 17–21, 2002.
74. Smith DK, Grohskopf LA, Black RJ, et al. Antiretroviral postexposure prophylaxis after sexual, injection-drug use, or other nonoccupational exposure to HIV in the United States: recommendations from the U.S. Department of Health and Human Services. MMWR Recomm Rep 2005; 54:1–20.
75. Merchant RC, Mayer KH. Perspectives on new recommendations for nonoccupational HIV postexposure prophylaxis. JAMA 2005; 293:2407–2409.
76. Cardo DM, Culver DH, Ciesielski CA, et al. A case-control study of HIV seroconversion in health care workers after percutaneous exposure. Centers for Disease Control and Prevention Needlestick Surveillance Group. N Engl J Med 1997; 337:1485–1490.
77. US Public Health Service. Updated U.S. Public Health Service Guidelines for the Management of Occupational Exposures to HBV, HCV, and HIV and Recommendations for Postexposure Prophylaxis. MMWR Recomm Rep 2001; 50:1–52.
78. Stratton P, Tuomala RE, Abboud R, et al. Obstetric and newborn outcomes in a cohort of HIV-infected pregnant women: a report of the women and infants transmission study. J Acquir Immune Defic Syndr Hum Retrovirol 1999; 20:179–186.
79. Langston C, Lewis DE, Hammill HA, et al. Excess intrauterine fetal demise associated with maternal human immunodeficiency virus infection. J Infect Dis 1995; 172:1451–1460.
80. Centers for Disease Control and Prevention. Sexually transmitted diseases treatment guidelines 2002. MMWR 2002 51:7–11.
81. Kuhn L, Steketee RW, Weedon J, et al. Distinct risk factors for intrauterine and intrapartum human immunodeficiency virus transmission and consequences for disease progression in

infected children. Perinatal AIDS Collaborative Transmission Study. J Infect Dis 1999; 179: 52–58.

82. Landesman SH, Kalish LA, Burns DN, et al. Obstetrical factors and the transmission of human immunodeficiency virus type 1 from mother to child. The Women and Infants Transmission Study. N Engl J Med 1996; 334:1617–1623.

83. Mofenson LM, Lambert JS, Stiehm ER, et al. Risk factors for perinatal transmission of human immunodeficiency virus type 1 in women treated with zidovudine. Pediatric AIDS Clinical Trials Group Study 185 Team. N Engl J Med 1999; 341:385–393.

84. The European Collaborative Study. Maternal viral load and vertical transmission of HIV-1: an important factor but not the only one. AIDS 1999; 13:1377–1385.

85. Garcia PM, Kalish LA, Pitt J, et al. Maternal levels of plasma human immunodeficiency virus type 1 RNA and the risk of perinatal transmission. Women and Infants Transmission Study Group. N Engl J Med 1999; 341:394–402.

86. Nduati R, John G, Mbori-Ngacha D, et al. Effect of breastfeeding and formula feeding on transmission of HIV-1: a randomized clinical trial. JAMA 2000; 283:1167–1174.

87. ACOG Committee on Obstetric Practice. ACOG committee opinion number 304, November 2004. Prenatal and perinatal human immunodeficiency virus testing: expanded recommendations. Obstet Gynecol 2004; 104:1119–1124.

88. The European Mode of Delivery Collaboration. Elective caesarean-section versus vaginal delivery in prevention of vertical HIV-1 transmission: a randomised clinical trial. Lancet 1999; 353:1035–1039. Erratum in: Lancet 1999; 353:1714.

89. Davis KR, Weller SC. The effectiveness of condoms in reducing heterosexual transmission of HIV. Fam Plann Perspect 1999; 31:272–279.

90. Samuel MC, Hessol N, Shiboski S, Engel RR, Speed TP, Winkelstein W Jr. Factors associated with human immunodeficiency virus seroconversion in homosexual men in three San Francisco cohort studies, 1984–1989. J Acquir Immune Defic Syndr 1993; 6:303–312.

91. Golombok S, Sheldon J. Evaluation of a thicker condom for use as a prophylactic against HIV transmission. AIDS Educ Prev 1994; 6:454–458.

92. Golombok S, Harding R, Sheldon J. An evaluation of a thicker versus a standard condom with gay men. AIDS 2001; 15:245–250.

93. Mitchell HS, Stephens E. Contraception choice for HIV positive women. Sex Transm Infect 2004; 80:167–173.

94. Lederman MM, Veazey RS, Offord R, et al. Prevention of vaginal SHIV transmission in rhesus macaques through inhibition of CCR5. Science 2004; 306:485–487.

6

Chlamydial Infections

Albert John Phillips

INTRODUCTION

Chlamydia trachomatis is the most commonly reported infectious disease in the United States and is the most common sexually transmitted bacterial infection *(1)*. The word *chlamys* is Greek for "cloaked" or "draped," descriptive of the intracytoplasmic inclusion bodies that are "draped" around the host cell nucleus. A large reservoir of infection sustains the continued spread of *C. trachomatis* because chlamydial infections rarely cause symptoms in women, they have a long incubation period, and the infection persists for at least several months. The annual cost of short- and long-term impacts of chlamydial infections in the United States was estimated to be $2.4 billion in 1987 and has increased since that time *(2)*.

FAST FACTS

- Chlamydia is the most commonly reported bacterial infection, with an estimated 2.8 million new cases each year.
- Adolescents and young adults are most commonly infected with *C. trachomatis*.
- By age 30, 50% of US women carry antibodies, indicating prior exposure.
- The majority of infections with *C. trachomatis* in both men and women are asymptomatic.
- Up to 40% of untreated chlamydial cervicitis cases will ascend into the upper genital tract, where considerable tubal damage can occur with very few symptoms.
- All sexually active women under age 26 should be screened at least annually. Such screening has been demonstrated to reduce the incidence of upper tract infection.
- Mucopurulent cervicitis is treated with the same therapy as chlamydial cervicitis.

From: *Current Clinical Practice: Sexually Transmitted Diseases:*
A Practical Guide for Primary Care
Edited by: A. L. Nelson and J. A. Woodward © Humana Press, Totowa, NJ

PREVALENCE AND INCIDENCE

In 2000, the Centers for Disease Control and Prevention (CDC) required states to report all cases of chlamydia. Even with this requirement in place, it is believed that chlamydial infections are significantly underreported because of sporadic screening and the use of outdated (insensitive) tests. Local studies demonstrated that the prevalence of infected and untreated cases equals or exceeds the number of cases that were diagnosed and treated *(3)*. The CDC estimates that 2.8 million new cases occur in the United States each year *(4)*. Nearly 75% of cases occur in the 15- to 24-year-old age group *(5)*. The World Health Organization estimated that 92 million new infections with *C. trachomatis* occurred worldwide in 1999 *(6)*.

Women primarily are most likely to be diagnosed with infection and to suffer more severe, long-term consequences. Chlamydia infection rates were 3.3 times higher in women than men in 2004 in the United States. Of the 929,462 cases reported to the CDC in 2004, 78% were women *(4)*. Antibody testing demonstrates that nearly 50% of women have been exposed to *C. trachomatis* by age 30 *(7)*. The prevalence of active infection in sexually active, asymptomatic, non-pregnant women in the general population is between 3 and 5% *(8)*. The highest age-specific rates were reported in women age 15–26. Among men, the highest rate occurs in 20- to 24-year-olds *(1)*. The National Longitudinal Study of Adolescent Health tested the urine of more than 12,000 young adults ages 18–26 and found the overall prevalence of chlamydial infection was 4.19%, and ranged from 1.94 to 12.54%, depending on demographics *(9)*. Women in family planning clinics have a background rate of 2.8–9.4%, whereas patients in sexually transmitted disease (STD) clinics are found to have a 15–33% incidence *(8)*. About 9% of female military recruits *(10)*, 10.3% of Job Corps women *(11)*, 9.9–27% of teen women in juvenile detention centers *(11a,12)*, and 6% of women seeking elective abortions have acute chlamydial infections *(13)*.

In the general population, men have the same prevalence of chlamydial infections as women (3–5%). In STD clinics, the prevalence rates among men are 15–20%, which is slightly less than the rates among women *(8)*. Chlamydial infections are found in 13–15% of sexually active men in adolescent clinics. The prevalence of chlamydial infection in men who have sex with men (MSM) varies by anatomical site: rectal 7.9%, urethral 5.2%, and pharyngeal 1.4% *(14)*.

Chlamydia is often found as a co-infection with gonorrhea in both men and women. Between 30 and 50% of patients who have gonococcal infections also have infection with *C. trachomatis*. However, because the background incidence of gonorrhea is so much lower (< 0.5%), it is far less likely that a person infected with *C. trachomatis* will also have gonococcal infection. In the National Longitudinal Study, only 0.3% of young adults were co-infected *(9)*.

RISK FACTORS

Specific historical and behavioral factors place a patient at an increased risk for acquisition of *C. trachomatis*. The classic risk factors for chlamydial infection include age younger than 26, low socioeconomic status, minority group member, multiple sexual partners, and new partners. Age is an important risk factor because *C. trachomatis* typically infects the columnar cells of the cervix; in younger women, columnar cells are more likely to be on the ectocervix (ectopy), where they can be exposed to semen carrying the organism. As women age, the columnar cells are located higher in the cervical canal. Combination hormonal contraceptive use apparently increases cervical ectopy and has been a proposed risk factor chlamydial infection *(15)*. African-American women are disproportionately impacted by chlamydia. In 2004, the rate of chlamydia infection among black women was 7.5 times higher than in white women *(1)*.

INFECTIVITY AND TRANSMISSION

C. trachomatis is a relatively infectious agent. More than two-thirds of female partners of men with culture-positive chlamydial urethritis have chlamydial infection themselves *(8)*. The single exposure male-to-female transmission rate has been estimated to be 40%, and the female-to-male transmission rate has been estimated to be 32% *(8)*. Other investigators have found that transmission rates between sexes are equivalent *(16)*. Vertical transmission of *C. trachomatis* is more efficient than horizontal transmission. More than 60% of newborns who deliver through a chlamydia-infected cervix will acquire the infection *(8)*.

ETIOLOGY

C. trachomatis is one of four species of the genus *Chlamydia*. It is responsible for a wide range of infections, including trachoma (a chronic conjunctivitis, which is the leading preventable cause of blindness worldwide), newborn conjunctivitis, and genital infections in women and men. *C. trachomatis* is an obligate intracellular organism, dependent on the host cell's adenosine triphosphate (ATP) production. *C. trachomatis* has a unique life cycle, which differentiates it from all other microorganisms (*see* Fig. 1). Infection begins when elemental bodies (EBs) attach to specific receptors found on nonciliated columnar or cuboidal epithelium of the host. This type of epithelium is located in the endocervix, endometrium, fallopian tube, and urethra, making those sites vulnerable to infection.

The host cell ingests the organism by a chlamydia-specific phagocytic process. After phagocytosis, the EB exists within a cytoplasmic vacuole or phagosome, where it is protected from host defense systems. Within the phagosome, the EB transforms into a reticulate body (RB) in order to multiply. It multiplies

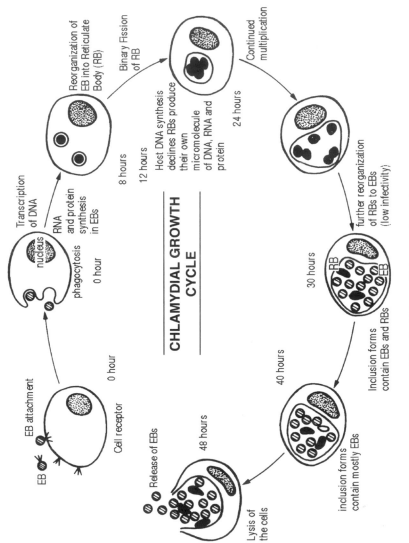

Fig. 1. Chlamydial growth cycle.

130

by binary fusion after duplicating its own DNA, RNA, and proteins by using host ATP. The RBs then reorganize back into EBs, the infectious form of the organism. Ultimately, the host cell undergoes either lysis or exocytosis with release of the EBs, which infect adjacent cells and restart the cycle. This process takes 2–3 days.

C. trachomatis has features of both bacteria and virus. *C. trachomatis* has a cell wall like Gram-negative bacteria but it cannot synthesize its own ATP or grow on artificial media, hence its similarity with a virus. Because of its unique developmental cycle, it is taxonomically classified in a separate order. The chemical composition of the cell wall of the EB is quite similar to that of Gram-negative bacteria. The cell wall of the RB contains less phospholipid than the EB; thus, RBs are highly labile and do not survive outside of the host cell. However, the EB is relatively stable in extracellular environments because its envelope is strengthened owing to cysteine proteins that are cross-linked by disulfide bonds, providing the EB structural integrity and resistance.

C. trachomatis is currently classified into 15 serotypes (serovars): A, B, Ba (AP-2), C, D, E, F, G, H, I, J, K, L1, L2, and L3. Classification is based on the major outer membrane protein using polyclonal and monoclonal antibodies. Typically, different serovars are associated with specific clinical diseases. The ocular disease trachoma is associated with serovars A, B, Ba, and C. Genital disease (exclusive of lymphogranuloma venereum), neonatal conjunctivitis, and pneumonia are associated with serovars of D through K. Serovars L1, L2, and L3 are associated with lymphogranuloma venereum. The different serovars of *C. trachomatis* within groups have not been shown to have different clinical courses *(17)*.

CLINICAL MANIFESTATIONS

The range of infections with *C. trachomatis* is impressive (*see* Table 1). The predominant infections are urethritis, cervicitis, and proctitis, but chlamydial infection can spread locally to the Bartholin glands, endosalpinges, or epididymis. In pregnancy, chlamydial infection is a risk factor for low-birth weight infants and preterm delivery. Postpartum, an infected woman is at increased risk for developing endometritis. Her newborn can develop conjunctivitis and pneumonia. Men who have chlamydial urethritis are at risk for developing Reiter's syndrome. Each of these clinical infections has a wide spectrum of initial presenting symptoms, ranging from no symptoms to noticeable discomfort and pain.

Infections in Women

CERVICITIS

The cervix is the most common site of infection for women. Women with chlamydial cervicitis generally are asymptomatic or report only nonspecific symptoms, such as vaginal discharge or postcoital spotting or bleeding. Two-

Table 1
Clinical Manifestations of *C. Trachomatis* Infection

Demonstrated		*Suggested*
Women		
• Cervicitis	• Perihepatitis	• Preterm labor
• Urethritis	• Conjunctivitis	• Preterm delivery
• Acute urethral	• Ectopic pregnancy	• Premature rupture
syndrome	• Infertility	of membranes
• Proctitis	• Chronic pelvic pain	• Postpartum
• Endometritis	• Reiter's syndrome	• endometritis
• Salpingitis		
Men		
• Urethritis	• Proctitis	
• Ependymitis	• Infertility	
• Prostatitis	• Conjunctivitis	
• Reiter's syndrome		
Newborns		
• Conjunctivitis	• Pneumonia	
• Otitis media		

thirds of infected women have no signs or symptoms. Furthermore, because the incubation period for *C. trachomatis* is 6–14 days, women may not relate their subtle symptoms to a distant exposure. Secondary or related infections (trichomoniasis or gonorrhea) are generally the etiology for complaints in women with symptoms.

On speculum exam, the chlamydia-infected cervix may appear entirely normal or may have a mucopurulent discharge and eroded friable appearance. *C. trachomatis* infects only columnar cells in the cervical squamocolumnar region or in the endocervix. In women with cervical ectopy and mucopurulent cervical discharge, *C. trachomatis* should be considered. The presence of leukocytes in endocervical samples studied under magnification is a better predictor of chlamydial infection, when other causes have been ruled out. Testing with sensitive laboratory-based tests (*see* the section on "Testing Techniques") is needed to confirm the diagnosis and distinguish it from mucopurulent cervicitis.

Bimanual exam should always be performed after appropriate specimens have been collected. Gentle exam for cervical motion tenderness should be performed to assess possible upper tract involvement (*see* the section on "Salpingitis"). Once chlamydial infection is suspected, concrete questions should be asked about sexual practices to identify other sites that might be involved.

URETHRITIS/URETHRAL SYNDROME

Women with chlamydial urethritis are generally asymptomatic. Those who have acute infections may complain of dysuria, slight discharge in urine, or urinary frequency. A woman with chlamydial urethritis/urethral syndrome will note that her symptoms are focused in the suprapubic area and start after she has finished voiding, which may help distinguish that infection from bacterial cystitis. Conventional urinalysis and culture testing will reveal sterile pyuria. Because only selective antibiotics will treat chlamydial infections, the symptoms will not resolve with typical antibiotic therapies for bacterial cystitis. The differential diagnosis includes infection with mycoplasma or ureaplasma, as well as urethral trauma and atrophic urethritis. Direct testing for *C. trachomatis* can be done on specimens obtained by urethral swabs or on urine from the first part of the stream. It is rare for chlamydial urethritis to exist independent of a cervical infection in a woman.

BARTHOLINITIS

The Bartholin's gland and ducts are lined with columnar epithelium and are susceptible to infection with *C. trachomatis*. It has been estimated that 30% of Bartholin infections are abscesses initiated by chlamydial infection, although the absolute contribution is not known *(18,19)*. Women with Bartholin's abscesses complain of acute onset of vulvar pain and swelling, which becomes quite intense as the abscess expands. The symptoms, rapid course of infection, and recommended treatments for chlamydial Bartholin's abscesses are similar to that with gonococcal abscesses (*see* Chapter 8).

SALPINGITIS

Ascending infection from the lower genital tract occurs in approximately 10% of patients with cervicitis. Sperm has been implicated in the transport of *C. trachomatis* into the upper genital tract in women. Symptoms may appear at any time during a woman's menstrual cycle, in contrast to gonococcal pelvic inflammatory disease (PID), which classically develops at the end of a woman's menses. The clinical presentation of chlamydial salpingitis is much more subtle than gonococcal salpingitis, because the fallopian tubes may not be distended with chlamydial infection even though the endosalpinges may suffer profound architectural damage because of chlamydial heat-shock proteins. Women with significant upper tract infection may be asymptomatic or have only mild flu-like discomforts that they attribute to other causes. Because of this very unremarkable clinical symptomatology and the relative paucity of clinical findings on examination and laboratory testing, the CDC revised its requirements for the criteria of pelvic inflammatory disease to lower the threshold for diagnosis. *See* Chapter 8 for more information about diagnosis and treatment.

Infections in Men

CHLAMYDIAL URETHRITIS

Nongonococcal urethritis is most commonly caused by *C. trachomatis*. The typical incubation period from exposure to infection is 1–2 weeks. Symptomatic men generally present with complaints of dysuria, urinary frequency, and urethral discharge. The discharge is greatest in the morning when it can be milked from the urethra. A diagnosis of nongonococcal urethritis is made when (1) a Gram-stain of the discharge demonstrates five or more white blood cells per field on high power (×1000) and there are no diplococci or (2) first voided urine has positive leukocyte esterase and microscopic examination reveals 10 or more white blood cells per high power field *(20,21)*. Urethritis is often asymptomatic; therefore, infected men are a major reservoir for infection of their sexual partners *(16)*.

PROSTATITIS

The symptoms associated with prostatitis are perineal pain, back pain, and pain with urination or ejaculation. Acute prostatitis in young men can occur with *C. trachomatis*. The role of *C. trachomatis* in chronic prostatitis is not as clear. More than one-fourth of men with nonbacterial chronic prostatitis were found to have chlamydial antigens and 80% showed cures after treatment with doxycycline *(22)*. More than one in five men with chronic prostatitis with inflammation seen on prostatic secretions had evidence of chlamydial infection *(23)*. These results suggest that *C. trachomatis* may be one of the causative agents of chronic prostatitis *(23)*.

EPIDIDYMITIS

Tenderness with swelling in the testicle is a sign of epididymitis. Acute epididymitis more commonly occurs in younger men. Other infectious etiologies for epididymitis include *Neisseria gonorrhea* and *Escherichia coli*. Chlamydial epididymitis has a milder course than other etiologies. Chronic epididymitis is defined as testicular pain persisting for at least 3 months. Because of the indolent nature of chlamydial infections, a patient with chronic epididymitis can also have a scrotal mass. Male infertility may be associated with chlamydial infections because the inflammatory process may damage the epididymis and the tubules. Men with fertility problems have been found by serology to have more likely had a previous infection of Chlamydia, but definitive proof is not yet been established *(24)*.

Infections in Men or Women

PROCTITIS

Chlamydial proctitis can occur in women and MSM who practice receptive anal intercourse. *C. trachomatis* was found in specimens from 5% of rectums and 13% of cervixes of 115 consecutive women presenting for examination. Rectal bleeding and microscopic evidence of proctitis without diarrhea was commonly found *(25)*. MSM are likely get infected from unprotected anal intercourse. Chlamydial proctitis has been found in 15% of asymptomatic MSM *(26)*. With symptomatic men and women, sigmoidoscopy and appropriate testing for infections organisms is required. Human immunodeficiency virus (HIV) antibody status should be established. If the patient is HIV-infected, uncommon pathogens need to be considered. With negative HIV tests, treatment for both gonorrhea and chlamydial infections is appropriate.

REACTIVE ARTHRITIS/REITER'S SYNDROME

Reactive arthritis is an inflammatory synovitis in which no viable organisms can be isolated from the joint and is precipitated by an immunological response to an infectious agent. Reiter's syndrome is composed of a triad of conjunctivitis, urethritis, and arthritis. Often individuals will not manifest all elements of the triad. Men are approximately nine times more likely to develop Reiter's syndrome than women are. Multiple joint involvement is common, usually affecting the knees or feet. Joint symptoms develop 2–4 weeks after urogenital infection, but 10% of affected individuals have no history of urethritis. Conjunctivitis and associated iritis and uveitis usually develop after the arthritis. A scaly skin rash (keratoderma blenorrhagica) on the palms or soles is also seen.

Many organisms have been implicated in reactive arthritis and Reiter's syndrome, including *C. trachomatis*. In genetically susceptible individuals, the immune system reacts to the infectious agent leading to the inflammatory response in the synovial surface *(27)*. Evidence of urogenital *C. trachomatis* was found in 36 to 61% of cases of Reiter's syndrome and chlamydial inclusions may be found in the fibroblast-like synovial cells *(28)*.

Chlamydial Infection in the Newborn

Neonatal chlamydial infection usually develops from vertical transmission. In one study, 6 out of 10 infants who delivered vaginally to mothers with infections had serological evidence of infection. The clinical manifestations varied; 18% of exposed infants developed neonatal conjunctivitis and 16% had pneumonia. Subclinical rectal and vaginal infections also occurred in the newborn *(29)*. Although the most common method of transmission is thought to be direct contact as the fetus delivers through an infected cervix, there have been reported instances where neonatal infection occurred with cesarean section delivery, with and without ruptured membranes *(30)*.

Chlamydial neonatal conjunctivitis has an incubation period of 10–14 days. The orbit of the eye swells and exudates are seen. *C. trachomatis* will be found in a high proportion of specimens. Because *C. trachomatis* can also be found in the nasopharynx, systemic treatment is required rather than a local ophthalmic solution. Twenty percent of untreated neonates will develop neonatal pneumonia without conjunctivitis *(31)*. Pneumonia occurs between the 4th and 12th week of life, with the majority of newborns becoming symptomatic by the 8th week. They may present with failure to thrive, decreased appetite, and some lethargy. More severely infected infants will present with tachypnea and a staccato-like cough. Upper respiratory symptoms include congestion and nasal passage obstruction without significant nasal discharge. Serious acute complications may require prolonged hospitalization and intubation with ventilator support. Diagnosis can be made by assessing *C. trachomatis* immunoglobulin (Ig)M antibody titers. Long-term complications of pneumonia can include abnormal pulmonary function tests and asthma *(32)*.

TESTING TECHNIQUES

Many tests are available today to detect *C. trachomatis* infection in a wide variety of specimens. Urogenital infections in women can be diagnosed by testing urine or swab specimens from the cervix or vagina. In men, urine tests or swabs of the urethra can be used. Rectal infection can be diagnosed by using rectal swabs. However, there are considerable differences in their respective abilities to detect infection. Selection of the appropriate test, and the need for possible confirmatory tests, depend in large part on the prevalence of the infection in local populations. Therefore, familiarity with the different tests and their properties is needed to enhance detection of infected individuals and to reduce false-positive results. *See* Table 2 for a summary of the different tests and testing sites by indication.

The most common tests used today are nonculture tests, although tissue culture tests are still required for some applications. Nonculture tests use a variety of techniques that bind tags to specific chlamydia proteins. The most sensitive and accurate of the nonculture tests are the nucleic acid amplification tests (NAATs). NAATs test for a unique nucleic acid (DNA or RNA) of the chlamydial organism or use a probe that is attached to the target nucleic acid. NAATs are very sensitive; they can detect a single gene copy. NAATs are also very specific.

There are several types of NAATs. The two most commonly used tests are the polymerase chain reaction (PCR) and ligase chain reaction (LCR) tests. PCR amplifies the nucleic acids found on the *C. trachomatis* elemental body (EB). PCR has a sensitivity of 90% and a specificity of 99–100%. PCR tests are approved for cervical, male urethral swabs, and male urine specimens. LCR has an overall sensitivity of 94% and a specificity of 99–100%. LCR can be used to test urethral and cervical swabs, as well as first-voided urine. More recently, LCR has been refined for use with liquid cytology specimens to test for *C. trachomatis* and *N. gonorrhoea*. Because NAATs detect DNA and RNA targets, they do not require viable organisms to detect infection. Therefore, if test of cure is needed, it should be delayed until all the chlamydial DNA/RNA has cleared, which usually takes more than 3 weeks.

Table 2
Recommendations for Test Selection for Common Chlamydial Infections

Endocervical swabs/urethral swabs

Indication for testing	*Test selection*

• Screening
   ◆ Females: when pelvic examination is indicated
   ◆ Males: urine might be more acceptable to asymptomatic males
• Endocervicitis
• Urethritis (males)
• Diseases at other anatomic locations possibly caused by sexually acquired *C. trachomatis* infection
   ◆ Pelvic inflammatory disease
   ◆ Urethral syndrome
   ◆ Bartholinitis
   ◆ Epididymitis
   ◆ Perihepatitis (Fitz-Hugh-Curtis syndrome) (females)
   ◆ Proctitis
   ◆ Reactive arthritis/Reiter's syndrome
   ◆ Conjunctivitis
   ◆ Not recommended for prepubertal children
	• Nucleic acid amplification tests (NAATs)
	   ◆ Preferred because of high sensitivity relative to other tests
	• Nonculture/non-NAAT
	   ◆ Recommended when a NAAT is not available or not economical
	• Culture
	   ◆ Preferred when an isolate is needed (e.g., sexual abuse or treatment failure)
	• Point-of-care tests
	   ◆ Recommended only when the patient is likely to be lost to follow-up and when the test will be performed while the patient waits for results and possible treatment
	• Additional testing is recommended after an initial positive screening test if a low positive predictive value can be expected or if a false-positive result would have serious psychosocial or legal consequences

Urethral swabs from women

Indication for testing	*Test selection*
• Used with endocervical swab to increase sensitivity of culture for screening • Urethral syndrome	• Culture • Nonculture tests are not recommended

(Continued on next page)

137

Table 2 (Continued)
Recommendations for Test Selection for Common Chlamydial Infections

Urine

Indication for testing	Test selection

• Females: screening or testing
• Males: screening
	• NAAT
	  ◆ Recommended on the basis of increased sensitivity and ease of use
	  ◆ For males, sensitivity with urine has been lower than with urethral swab in the majority of studies, but not all
	  ◆ Other tests are not recommended because of low sensitivity and, in the case of enzyme immunoassay (EIA) and lipopoly-saccharide (LPS)-specific direct fluorescent antibody (DFA) tests, lower specificity
	  ◆ Additional testing is recommended after an initial positive screening test if a low positive predictive value can be expected or if a false-positive result would have serious psychosocial or legal consequences

Rectal swabs

Indication for testing	Test selection

• Patients with history of receptive anal intercourse
• Proctitis
• Possible sexual abuse, children
	• Culture
	  ◆ Preferred when an isolate is needed (e.g., sexual abuse)
	  ◆ Sensitivity not well-defined; high specificity, especially if *C. trachomatis*-specific stain is used
	  ◆ Not readily available in most labs
	• DFA
	  ◆ FDA-cleared for use with rectal specimens
	  ◆ Limited evaluation in published studies
	  ◆ Sensitivity not well-defined; potentially high specificity if *C. trachomatis*-specific stain is used
	• Other tests are not recommended
	  ◆ NAAT
	    ■ Although crossreactivity with other rectal bacteria has not been reported for NAATs, they have received only limited evaluation in published studies
	    ■ Some non-commercial labs have initiated NAAT tests that meet CLIA standards

Pharyngeal swabs

Indication for testing	Test selection

• Patients concerned regarding exposure during fellatio or cunnilingus
• Newborns or infants (nasopharyngeal specimens)
  ◆ Neonatal conjunctivitis
  ◆ Pneumonia consistent with *C. trachomatis* etiology
• Possible sexual abuse, children
	• Culture
	  ◆ Preferred method
	  ◆ Necessary when an isolate is needed (e.g., sexual abuse)
	  ◆ Sensitivity not well-defined; high specificity, including if *C. trachomatis*-specific stain is used
	• DFA
	  ◆ FDA-cleared for use with pharyngeal specimens
	  ◆ Limited evaluation in published studies
	  ◆ Sensitivity not well-defined; potentially high specificity if *C. trachomatis*-specific stain is used
	• Other tests are not recommended
	  ◆ NAAT
	    ■ Although crossreactivity with other pharyngeal bacteria has not been reported for NAATs, they have received only limited evaluation in published studies

Conjunctivae swabs

Indication for testing	Test selection

• Conjunctivitis among adults
• Newborns or infants
  ◆ Neonatal conjunctivitis
  ◆ Pneumonia consistent with *C. trachomatis* etiology
	• Culture
	  ◆ Preferred, when available, because of high sensitivity and specificity
	• EIA, nucleic acid probe, and DFA tests
	  ◆ EIA, nucleic acid probe, and DFA tests that are FDA-cleared for use with conjunctival specimens have had uniformly high sensitivities with conjunctival specimens from newborns; evaluation studies are more limited for conjunctival specimens from adults with conjunctivitis
	  ◆ Specificities of tests on conjunctival specimens have also been high, although the potential for crossreaction with other bacteria exists for EIA and for culture and DFA if used with stains that are not specific for *C. trachomatis*
	• Other tests are not recommended

Source: From ref. 33.

The most common commercial test for *C. trachomatis* is the DNA probe, which uses nucleic acid hybridization to detect chlamydial DNA from urogenital swabs. The DNA probe detects an infection with specimens that have as few as 1000 EBs. It has a sensitivity of 85–90% and a specificity of 98–99% compared to culture, and has a sensitivity of 77–93% compared with NAATs *(8)*. Because the false-positive rates with DNA probes are high, the CDC recommends that positive DNA probe test results in low-prevalence populations be confirmed by a second test *(33)*. One very attractive feature of the DNA probe is that the swab that is used to collect the specimen from the urogenital tract to test for *C. trachomatis* can also be used to test for *N. gonorrhoea.*

Older nonculture diagnostic tests include direct fluorescent antibody (DFA) test and enzyme-linked immunoassay (EIA). DFA detects the outer membrane protein of EB and directly visualizes it with immunofluorescence. The sensitivity of DFA is only about 75%, but it has a specificity of 98%. At least 10 EBs are necessary to detect infection. Clinical skills are required to obtain specimens. The sensitivity of DFA is often reduced by blood on the sample. Today, DFA is used most frequently in the laboratory to confirm positive results of other nonculture tests.

One of the earliest nonculture tests developed was EIA. EIA detects a chlamydia lipoprotein antigen by attaching specific antibodies coupled with an enzyme to the antibody. A color change occurs when the enzyme, which remains after binding with the antibody, acts on a substrate. It takes approximately 10,000 EBs to cause an EIA to turn positive. The EIA has a sensitivity that varies from 62 to 75% and has a specificity of 97%. A major drawback of the older EIAs was that they bound to other Gram-negative organisms as well as *C. trachomatis*, which led to false-positive test results. This problem has been overcome in newer versions by the addition of blocking reagents or by using DFA tests to confirm EIA results. When either of these additional methods is used, specificity is increased to 99%. The antigen detection techniques are generally less expensive and easier to perform than NAATs. However, the antigen detection techniques have a lower sensitivity than NAATs, and they have lower positive predictive values. Therefore, if a antigen detection tests are used to screen a population with a 2–3% prevalence of infection, about half of the results will return falsely positive (an incorrect result). For this reason, routine confirmation is generally recommended for positive cases.

Chlamydial infections can also be diagnosed by culture. The specimen must be cultured in tissue culture because *C. trachomatis* is an obligate intracellular organism and, therefore, is unable to grow on artificial media. Culture allows for antibiotic sensitivity testing as well as genotyping, which may be important for public health reasons. In the past, the sensitivity of culture techniques was thought to be close to 100%. As a result, for many years, the culture was considered the gold standard. Today, however, it is recognized that at least 10–100 organisms are needed to result in a positive culture, but far fewer organisms can be detected by NAATs. Overall, it has been estimated that culture techniques have 65–85% sensitivity compared with NAATs. Tissue cultures cost more than NAATs, are technically difficult and labor-intensive, and take longer for results. However, in many courts, only the result of tissue culture may be introduced as evidence.

Regardless of the exact technology used to test for *C. trachomatis*, good specimen collection techniques are essential. In order to best detect the presence of *C. trachomatis*, infected cells should be collected. The scrapings from the endocervical area or the urethra are more apt to lead to detection of an infection than testing discharge. Using a cytobrush to collect cervical specimens improves the sensitivity of the culture and antigen-detection tests. The cytobrush can safely be used in pregnant women to collect specimens. When urine specimens are to be tested, sensitivity is acceptable only if the first drops of urine are collected, without significant dilution from additional urine. The patient should not have urinated for at least 1 hour before providing the specimen.

Cytology was used to detect chlamydial infections before more sensitive tests were developed. To make the diagnosis, specimens obtained from the genital tract were studied for the presence of inclusion bodies. The sensitivity of cytology testing is very low with only 20% cases being detected. However, NAATs can be used on cervical specimens collected by liquid cytology to detect low levels of chlamydial infection.

Antibodies for *C. trachomatis* can be assayed in serum. Serology for chlamydial antibodies is not useful in detection of acute infection because of poor specificity and reproducibility. In addition, serology and direct evidence of infection are not well correlated *(34)*. Therefore, serology cannot distinguish between active vs resolved infection. Serology may be helpful in assessing if possible tubal factors are a cause of a woman's infertility and help determine who might benefit from hysterosalpingography *(35)*.

SCREENING RECOMMENDATIONS

Targeted screening protocols are needed to control chlamydial infections for several reasons: the prevalence of *C. trachomatis* is relatively high, only a minority of women with chlamydial infections develop symptoms, and the sequelae of infection are potentially serious.

Routine screening of all sexually active women age 26 or younger is recommended whether or not the woman is pregnant. The frequency of subsequent testing of women under age 26 who are in stable mutually monogamous relationships after an initial negative test has not been determined. Screening of older women should be done only if these women are at increased risk (new or multiple sex partners, a prior history of a sexually transmitted infection [STI] and inconsistent use of condoms in high-risk relationships).

Routine screening of heterosexual men is not recommended, but testing is recommended for symptomatic men and those who are in settings with high prevalence of chlamydia (e.g., adolescent clinics, correctional facilities, and STD clinics). For sexually active MSM, the CDC recommends annual urethral/urine screening for chlamydia and rectal chlamydial cultures for MSM who have had receptive anal sex. The CDC recommends screening every 3–6 months for MSM at highest risk (those with multiple sexual partners, or those who use illicit drugs) *(21)*. Men who are sex partners of infected women or men do not require testing for chlamydia infection before initiation of therapy but might benefit from testing for public health reasons.

It is important to note that screening in low prevalence populations produces high false-positive test results. The positive predictive value using a DNA probe test, performed in a setting with a prevalence of 2%, is under 50%. Because over half of the positive test results are not true positives (the patient is not infected with *C. trachomatis*), a confirmatory test is required. This can be done either by retesting the original specimen automatically in the laboratory using a different testing technology or by performing a second test from the same or a different site in the patient.

DIAGNOSIS

Clinical syndromes, such as nongonococcal urethritis or mucopurulent cervicitis may be diagnosed based on clinical signs and symptoms if supported by microscopic findings of leukocytosis. However, chlamydial infections are often asymptomatic, so diagnosis generally requires chlamydia-specific laboratory test identification/confirmation. Care must be taken, particularly in low-risk patients and patients in low-prevalence populations, to confirm positive test results to reduce the risk of false-positivity.

In the face of laboratory-confirmed diagnosis of chlamydial cervicitis or urethritis, the patient should be evaluated for associated STIs. About 30% of women with chlamydial cervicitis have concomitant trichomonal vaginitis. Gonorrhea accompanies chlamydial infections, but because of relatively low population prevalence, treatment for gonorrhea should await laboratory confirmation in most geographic areas. Other STIs, such as HIV, hepatitis B virus, and syphilis, should be evaluated on the basis of local prevalence rates.

TREATMENT

Because of the unique intracellular characteristics of *C. trachomatis*, only certain antibiotics are effective in treatment. The CDC treatment guidelines for chlamydial infections are summarized in Table 3 *(21)*. Tetracycline and doxy-

Table 3
Chlamydial Infection—CDC STD Treatment Guidelines 2006

Recommended regimens

Adolescents and adults
Select one of the following:

Azithromycin [a]	1 g orally once
Doxycycline [c]	100 mg orally twice a day for 7 days

Pregnant women
Select one of the following:

Azithromycin	1 g orally in a single dose
Erythromycin base	500 mg orally four times a day for 7 days

Alternative regimens

Adolescents and adults
Select one of the following:

Erythromycin base [b]	500 mg orally four times a day for 7 days
Erythromycin ethylsuccinate [b]	800 mg orally four times a day for 7 days
Ofloxacin [d]	300 mg orally twice a day for 7 days
Levofloxacin [d]	500 mg orally daily for 7 days

Pregnant women
Select one of the following:

Erythromycin base [b]	500 mg orally four times a day for 7 days
Erythromycin base [b]	250 mg orally four times a day for 14 days
Erythromycin ethylsuccinate [b]	800 mg orally four times a day for 7 days
Erythromycin ethylsuccinate [b]	400 mg orally four times a day for 14 days

[a] Safety and efficacy among pregnant and lactating women has not been established (pregnancy category B).
[b] Erythromycin is less efficacious than either azithromycin or doxycycline, and gastrointestinal side effects frequently discourage patients from complying with this regimen. Test of cure should be done 3 weeks after completion of treatment with erythromycin.
[c] Contraindicated for pregnant and lactating women and for children younger than 8 years old.

Continued on next page

Table 3 (*Continued*)
Chlamydial Infection—CDC STD Treatment Guidelines 2006

Ophthalmia neonatorum caused by C. trachomatis

Erythromycin [b,e] base or ethylsuccinate   50 mg/kg/day orally divided into four doses daily for 14 days

Chlamydial infections among children who weigh ≤45 kg

Erythromycin [b] base or ethylsuccinate   50 mg/kg/day orally divided into four doses daily for 14 days

Chlamydial infections among children who weigh ≥45 kg but who are aged ≤8 years

Azithromycin [a]   1 g orally once

Chlamydial infections among children aged ≥8 years. Select on of the following:

Azithromycin [a]   1 g orally once

Doxycycline [c]   100 mg orally twice a day for 7 days

[a] Safety and efficacy among pregnant and lactating women has not been established (pregnancy category B).

[b] Erythromycin is less efficacious than either azithromycin or doxycycline, and gastrointestinal side effects frequently discourage patients from complying with this regimen. Test of cure should be done 3 weeks after completion of treatment with erythromycin.

[c] Contraindicated for pregnant and lactating women and for children younger than 8 years old.

[d] Contraindicated for pregnant and lactating women.

[e] An association between oral erythromycin and infantile hypertrophic pyloric stenosis (IHPS) has been reported in infants younger than 6 weeks who were treated with this drug. Infants treated with erythromycin should be followed for signs and symptoms of IHPS.

144

cycline inhibit bacterial protein synthesis by blocking the attachment of the transfer RNA-amino acid to the ribosome. Common alternatives to doxycycline are the macrolide antibiotics, erythromycin or azithromycin. Macrolide antibiotics inhibit protein synthesis by binding to the p site on 50S RNA molecule of the bacterial ribosome, blocking the exit of the growing peptide chain. Azithromycin has high tissue penetration levels and a very long half-life, allowing a single dosing regimen. Single-dose therapy enhances compliance and treatment success rates. Clinical cure rates for doxycycline and azithromycin are 96–99% and 97%, respectively *(36,37)*. Resistance to tetracycline and macrolide antibiotics has been reported *(38)*. Single-dose therapy with azithromycin is generally preferred when there is concern that multiple dose therapies will not be completed. In one study of patients prescribed 7-day therapies with doxycycline, only 25% of patients followed instructions completely, 24% took no drug, and the remaining 51% used some intermediate amount of the drug *(39)*.

Quinolone antibiotics act by targeting two enzymes, DNA gyrase and topoisomerase IV, which are necessary for DNA replication. Within this group of antibiotics, ofloxacin and levofloxacin are most effective. *C. trachomatis* has the potential to mutate leading to quinolone resistance when exposed to subinhibitory concentrations of antibiotics *(40)*. Patients should be encouraged to complete all medications for their full course of therapy.

Amoxicillin is no longer recommended for treatment. Other penicillin and all cephalosporin antibiotics have no role in the management of chlamydial infections *(41)*.

Patients should be instructed to abstain from all sexual contact until all of their sex partners have been treated. Treatment is considered complete 7 days after finishing medication. The need for this counseling was hightlighted by a study of 597 college women randomized to azithromycin vs doxycycline in which two pregnancies occurred during the 2-week study period *(37)*. Patients should also be counseled on future consistent use of condoms and other safer sex practices.

FOLLOW-UP

It is not necessary to perform a routine test of cure after therapy, except in women treated with erythromycin. It is recognized that erythromycin causes many side effects and that compliance is therefore often poor. Routine repeat testing of all non-pregnant women with chlamydial infection should be considered 3–4 months after treatment. This is particularly important for adolescent women who often return to the same high-risk environment from which they acquired their first infections. Routine repeat testing is also encouraged at every other examination done 3–12 months after treatment regardless of whether the patient believes that her sex partner(s) was treated.

COMPLICATIONS OF INFECTION

Infertility, ectopic pregnancy and pelvic pain are sequelae of both symptomatic and asymptomatic PID. In women with confirmed PID, infertility was seen in 16 vs 2.7% of controls. Ectopic pregnancy was 9.1 vs 1.4% and tubal factor infertility was 10.8 vs 0% (42). The risk of infertility increases with number of episodes and severity of the inflammation. In women who had had PID, hospital readmissions for abdominal and pelvic pain was significantly more likely and the risk for hysterectomy was six times greater than controls (43). Chronic pelvic pain after PID is associated with reduced physical and mental health (44).

PARTNER NOTIFICATION AND REPORTING REQUIREMENTS

Chlamydia is a reportable disease in all 50 states. All sexual contacts for the 60 days prior to onset of symptoms (or diagnosis of asymptomatic infections) should be evaluated, tested, and treated. It is important to note that it is *not* necessary to await positive test results for chlamydial infection to initiate partner therapy; therapy for chlamydial infection should be given to partners on an epidemiological basis. Treatment for other possible STIs not detected in the index case should await laboratory confirmation.

If there is a concern that a heterosexual sex partner will not seek care, the CDC suggests that the patient can provide the partner the treatment. In California, state law allows clinicians to treat sex partners of patients found to have laboratory-confirmed genital chlamydial infections without co-infection with gonorrhea or other complications. Under this law, treatment for chlamydia can be given without any contact or evaluation, even if the partner is not a patient of the clinician. This provision (patient-delivered partner therapy) is generally reserved for partners who are not expected not to seek care for the problem. The recommended treatment is azithromycin. Specialized instructions that explain the reason for the treatment and screen for macrolide allergy (e.g., erythromycin) accompany the medications. Also included in the packet is encouragement to seek professional care to be evaluated for other (as yet undiagnosed) STIs. Recently, research has demonstrated again that expedited treatment with patient-delivered partner therapy reduced the rates of persistent or recurrent gonorrhea and chlamydial infection, but gonorrhea reduction was more significant than chlamydia reduction (45). Patient-delivered partner therapy is not recommended for MSM because of the high risk of coexisting infections in that partner, especially HIV.

PREGNANCY-RELATED ISSUES

The association between chlamydial cervicitis and preterm rupture of membranes, preterm labor, and preterm delivery has been strongly suggested by two clinical trials, which served as a basis for CDC recommendation for screening in pregnancy *(46,47)*. However, no prospective placebo-controlled studies have verified this association. Given the strength of the association found in these earlier studies, however, it may not be ethical to conduct placebo-controlled trials. The role *C. trachomatis* plays in the etiology of postpartum endometritis is controversial, but the diagnosis should be considered when women present 2–3 weeks postpartum with fever, chills, purulent lochia, and a tender, boggy, enlarged uterus. Women infected with *C. trachomatis* at delivery were more likely to experience febrile complications after postpartum tubal ligation *(48)*. The association of chlamydial cervicitis and postabortal infection is clear. Estimates are that 10–35% of women who undergo elective abortion with chlamydial cervicitis will develop postabortal endometritis/PID. This observation has lead to the practice of routine antibiotic prophylaxis at the time of surgical abortion.

In pregnancy, the optimal testing scheduled has not been established but the CDC recommends testing prenatal patients under 25 and other high-risk women depending on local prevalence rates. Early testing could reduce pregnancy risks associated with infection, such as low birth weight and premature delivery. Testing late in pregnancy can decrease transmission to the infant and diminish the risk of postpartum maternal infections. Combined testing has not been evaluated.

Doxycycline should not be used in pregnancy. In pregnant women, test of cure is routinely recommended by the CDC, although some experts do not deem it necessary if the patient was treated with azithromycin. It is important to wait 3 weeks from the completion of therapy to do test of cure, because some tests may detect *C. trachomatis* remnants even after the organisms have been eradicated. Infected women should be retested in the third trimester.

PREVENTION

A National Institutes of Health panel performed a comprehensive review of the literature in 2000 and concluded that there was not sufficient evidence to allow an accurate assessment of the degree of protection against chlamydia offered by correct and consistent condom use (*see* Chapter 15) *(49)*. The CDC now recommends condom use to reduce the spread of chlamydia *(50)*. A recent study with a case-crossover design suggested that correct and consistent condom use was associated with a 50% reduction in chlamydial infection. The investigators were also able to indentify a dose–response relationship.

In 2004, a review of studies published after the NIH conference found that the literature in that time period supported the conclusion that condom use was associated with a statistically significant protection for men and women from chlamydia infections *(51)*. An analysis of 45 studies published between 1966–2004 concluded that most studies found that condom use was associated with a reduced risk of chlamydia in both men and women *(52)*.

CASE STUDY

Robert calls your office because a short-term female partner notified him that he has been exposed to chlamydia. He says that she gave him four antibiotic tablets to take, but he did not use this medication yet because he has no symptoms. He takes tetracycline 250 mg daily for acne treatment. He wants to know if it is safe to take these tablets.

Questions

1. What pills did his partner give him?
2. Should he be treated without any other evaluation?
3. Should he be treated without a test showing that he is infected?
4. Will his daily tetracycline be adequate therapy?
5. What if he says that he used condoms when he had sex with her?

Answers and Teaching Points

1. California allows providers to give patients who have chlamydial cervicitis azithromycin to treat their partners, especially if the woman doubts her partner will seek professional care. This is called patient-delivered partner therapy.
2. Robert should be advised that he needs to be seen immediately and tested for related STIs. All anatomical sites where he had sexual contact with her should be tested. All of his subsequent sexual contacts need testing and treatment.
3. Robert should take the azithromycin therapy based only on his partner's infection.
4. His tetracycline dose is too low to provide treatment for his chlamydial infection.
5. If he used condoms before any genital contact with the infected woman, his treatment may be held awaiting the test results unless he had other sexual contact with her not protected by condoms.

REFERENCES

1. Centers for Disease Control and Prevention. Trends in reportable sexually transmitted diseases in the United States, 2004: national surveillance data for chlamydia, gonorrhea and syphilis. Atlanta, GA: Centers for Disease Control and Prevention, 2005. Available from: http://www.cdc.gov/std/stats/. Accessed Nov. 24, 2006.
2. Washington AE, Johnson RE, Sanders LL Jr. *Chlamydia trachomatis* infections in the United States. What are they costing us? JAMA 1987; 257:2070–2072.
3. Turner CF, Rogers SM, Miller HG, et al. Untreated gonococcal and chlamydial infection in a probability sample of adults. JAMA 2002; 287:726–733.
4. Centers for Disease Control and Prevention. Sexually transmitted disease surveillance, 2004. Atlanta, GA: US Department of Health and Human Services, 2005. Available from: http://www.cdc.gov/std/stats/. Accessed Nov. 24, 2006.
5. Groseclose SL, Zaidi AA, DeLisle SJ, Levine WC, St Louis ME. Estimated incidence and prevalence of genital *Chlamydia trachomatis* infections in the United States, 1996. Sex Transm Dis 1999; 26:339–344.

 6. World Health Organization. Global prevalence and incidence of selected curable sexually transmitted infections: overview and estimates. Geneva: World Health Organization, 2001.
 7. Stamm WE. *Chlamydia trachomatis* infections of the adult. In: Holmes KK, Mårdh PA, Sparlin PF, et al., eds., *Sexually Transmitted Diseases*, 3rd Ed. New York, NY: Mc-Graw Hill, 1999, pp. 407–422.
 8. Sweet RL., Gibbs RS. Chlamydial infections. In: Sweet RL, Gibbs RS, eds., *Infectious Diseases of the Female Genital Tract*, 4th Ed. Philadelphia, PA: Lippincott Williams & Wilkins, 2002, pp. 57–100.
 9. Miller WC, Ford CA, Morris M, et al. Prevalence of chlamydial and gonococcal infections among young adults in the United States. JAMA 2004; 291:2229–2236.
10. Howell MR, Gaydos JC, McKee KT Jr, Quinn TC, Gaydos CA. Control of *Chlamydia trachomatis* infections in female army recruits: cost-effective screening and treatment in training cohorts to prevent pelvic inflammatory disease. Sex Transm Dis 1999; 26:519–526.
11. Joesoef MR, Mosure DJ. Prevalence trends in chlamydial infections among young women entering the national job training program, 1998–2004. Sex Transm Dis 2006; 33:571–575.
11a. Bernstein KT, Chow JM, Ruiz J, et al. *Chlamydia trachomatis* and *Neisseria gonorrhea* infections among men and women entering California prisons. Am J Public Health 2006; 96:1826–1866.
12. Centers for Disease Control and Prevention. High prevalence of chlamydial and gonococcal infection in women entering jails and juvenile detention centers—Chicago, Birmingham, and San Francisco, 1998. MMWR Morb Mortal Wkly Rep 1999; 48:793–796.
13. Cameron ST, Stewart S, Sutherland S. Can a busy abortion service cope with a screen-and-treat policy for *Chlamydia trachomatis* infection? Int J STD AIDS 2003; 14:50–54.
14. Kent CK, Chaw JK, Wong W, et al. Prevalence of rectal, urethral, and pharyngeal chlamydia and gonorrhea detected in 2 clinical settings among men who have sex with men: San Francisco, California, 2003. Clin Infect Dis 2005; 41:67–74.
15. Jacobson DL, Peralta L, Graham NM, Zenilman J. Histologic development of cervical ectopy: relationship to reproductive hormones. Sex Transm Dis 2000; 27:252–258.
16. Quinn TC, Gaydos C, Shepherd M, et al. Epidemiologic and microbiologic correlates of *Chlamydia trachomatis* infection in sexual partnerships. JAMA 1996; 276:1737–1742.
17. Morre SA, Rozendaal L, van Valkengoed IG, et al. Urogenital *Chlamydia trachomatis* serovars in men and women with a symptomatic or asymptomatic infection: an association with clinical manifestations? J Clin Microbiol 2000; 38:2292–2296.
18. Davies JA, Rees E, Hobson D, Karayiannis P. Isolation of *Chlamydia trachomatis* from Bartholin's ducts. Br J Vener Dis 1978; 54:409–413.
19. Saul HM, Grossman MB. The role of *Chlamydia trachomatis* in Bartholin's gland abscess. Am J Obstet Gynecol 1988; 158:76–77.
20. Batteiger BE, Jones RB. Chlamydial infections. Infect Dis Clin North Am 1987; 1:55–81.
21. Centers for Disease Control and Prevention. Sexually transmitted diseases treatment guidelines, 2006. MMWR Recomm Rep 2006; 55(RR-11):38–42. Available from: http://www.cdc.gov/std/treatment/. Accessed Nov. 24, 2006.
22. Mutlu N, Mutlu B, Culha M, Hamsioglu Z, Demirtas M, Gokalp A. The role of *Chlamydia trachomatis* in patients with non-bacterial prostatitis. Int J Clin Pract 1998; 52:540–541.
23. Ostaszewska I, Zdrodowska-Stefanow B, Badyda J, Pucilo K, Trybula J, Bulhak V. *Chlamydia trachomatis*: probable cause of prostatitis. Int J STD AIDS 1998; 9:350–353.
24. Ness RB, Markovic N, Carlson CL, Coughlin MT. Do men become infertile after having sexually transmitted urethritis? An epidemiologic examination. Fertil Steril 1997; 68:205–213.
25. Thompson CI, MacAulay AJ, Smith IW. *Chlamydia trachomatis* infections in the female rectums. Genitourin Med 1989; 65:269–273.

26. Wexner SD. Sexually transmitted diseases of the colon, rectum, and anus. The challenge of the nineties. Dis Colon Rectum 1990; 33:1048–1062.

27. Silveira LH, Gutierrez F, Scopelitis E, Cuellar ML, Citera G, Espinoza LR. Chlamydia-induced reactive arthritis. Rheum Dis Clin North Am 1993; 19:351–362.

28. Hanada H, Ikeda-Dantsuji Y, Naito M, Nagayama A. Infection of human fibroblast-like synovial cells with Chlamydia trachomatis results in persistent infection and interleukin-6 production. Microb Pathog 2003; 34:57–63.

29. Schachter J, Grossman M, Sweet RL, Holt J, Jordan C, Bishop E. Prospective study of perinatal transmission of Chlamydia trachomatis. JAMA 1986; 255:3374–3377.

30. Bell TA, Stamm WE, Kuo CC, Wang SP, Holmes KK, Grayston JT. Risk of perinatal transmission of Chlamydia trachomatis by mode of delivery. J Infect 1994; 29:165–169.

31. Jain S. Perinatally acquired Chlamydia trachomatis associated morbidity in young infants. J Matern Fetal Med 1999; 8:130–133.

32. Weiss SG, Newcomb RW, Beem MO. Pulmonary assessment of children after chlamydial pneumonia of infancy. J Pediatr 1986; 108:659–664.

33. Johnson RE, Newhall WJ, Papp JR, et al. Screening tests to detect Chlamydia trachomatis and Neisseria gonorrhoeae infections—2002. MMWR Recomm Rep 2002; 51:1–38.

34. Rabenau HF, Kohler E, Peters M, Doerr HW, Weber B. Low correlation of serology with detection of Chlamydia trachomatis by ligase chain reaction and antigen EIA. Infection 2000; 28:97–102.

35. Akande VA, Hunt LP, Cahill DJ, Caul EO, Ford WC, Jenkins JM. Tubal damage in infertile women: prediction using chlamydia serology. Hum Reprod 2003; 18:1841–1847.

36. Martin DH, Mroczkowski TF, Dalu ZA, et al. A controlled trial of a single dose of azithromycin for the treatment of chlamydial urethritis and cervicitis. The Azithromycin for Chlamydial Infections Study Group. N Engl J Med 1992; 327:921–925.

37. Thorpe EM Jr, Stamm WE, Hook EW III, et al. Chlamydial cervicitis and urethritis: single dose treatment compared with doxycycline for seven days in community based practises. Genitourin Med 1996; 72:93–97.

38. Somani J, Bhullar VB, Workowski KA, Farshy CE, Black CM. Multiple drug-resistant Chlamydia trachomatis associated with clinical treatment failure. J Infect Dis 2000; 181: 1421–1427.

39. Augenbraun M, Bachmann L, Wallace T, Dubouchet L, McCormack W, Hook EW III. Compliance with doxycycline therapy in sexually transmitted diseases clinics. Sex Transm Dis 1998; 25:1–4.

40. Dessus-Babus S, Bebear CM, Charron A, Bebear C, de Barbeyrac B. Sequencing of gyrase and topoisomerase IV quinolone-resistance-determining regions of Chlamydia trachomatis and characterization of quinolone-resistant mutants obtained In vitro. Antimicrob Agents Chemother 1998; 42:2474–2481.

41. Ridgway GL. Treatment of chlamydial genital infection. J Antimicrob Chemother 1997; 40: 311–314.

42. Westrom L, Joesoef R, Reynolds G, Hagdu A, Thompson SE. Pelvic inflammatory disease and fertility. A cohort study of 1,844 women with laparoscopically verified disease and 657 control women with normal laparoscopic results. Sex Transm Dis 1992; 19:185–192.

43. Buchan H, Vessey M, Goldacre M, Fairweather J. Morbidity following pelvic inflammatory disease. Br J Obstet Gynaecol 1993; 100:558–562.

44. Haggerty CL, Schulz R, Ness RB; PID Evaluation and Clinical Health Study Investigators. Lower quality of life among women with chronic pelvic pain after pelvic inflammatory disease. Obstet Gynecol 2003; 102:934–939.

45. Golden MR, Whittington WL, Handsfield HH, et al. Effect of expedited treatment of sex partners on recurrent or persistent gonorrhea or chlamydial infection. N Engl J Med 2005; 352:676–685.

46. Ryan GM Jr, Abdella TN, McNeeley SG, Baselski VS, Drummond DE. *Chlamydia trachomatis* infection in pregnancy and effect of treatment on outcome. Am J Obstet Gynecol 1990; 162:34–39.

47. Cohen I, Veille JC, Calkins BM. Improved pregnancy outcome following successful treatment of chlamydial infection. JAMA 1990; 263:3160–3163.

48. Todd CS, Jones RB, Golichowski A, Arno JN. *Chlamydia trachomatis* and febrile complications of postpartum tubal ligation. Am J Obstet Gynecol 1997; 176:100–102.

49. National Institute of Allergy and Infectious Diseases. Workshop Summary. Scientific evidence on condom effectiveness for sexually transmitted disease (STD) prevention. National Institutes of Health, Department of Health and Human Services, 2001. Available from: http://www.niaid.nih.gov/dmid/stds/condomreport.pdf. Accessed Nov. 24, 2006.

50. Centers for Disease Control and Prevention. Fact sheet for public health personnel: male latex condoms and sexually transmitted diseases. Centers for Disease Control and Prevention, National Center for HIV, STD and TB Prevention, 2004. Available from: http://www.cdc.gov/nchstp/od/latex.htm. Accessed Nov. 24, 2006.

51. Holmes KK, Levine R, Weaver M. Effectiveness of condoms in preventing sexually transmitted infections. Bull World Health Organ 2004; 82:454–461.

52. Warner L, Stone KM, Macaluso M, Buehler JW, Austin HD. Condom use and risk of gonorrhea and Chlamydia: a systematic review of design and measurement factors assessed in epidemiologic studies. Sex Transm Dis 2006; 33:36–51.

7

Gonorrheal Infections

Anita L. Nelson

INTRODUCTION

Gonorrhca was one of the most recognized medical conditions in ancient times. It was described in Chinese writings dating 2500 years ago, in the Papyrus of Ebers, and by Hippocrates. It was named by Galen in 130 AD, who confused the purulent discharge seen with its urethritis for semen and named it "gonorrhea" for "flow of seed." Its more common name, "clap," derives from the Middle French word "clapoir" for "bubo." Understanding of its unique etiology and its impact on women occurred only in the recent times. Historically, *Neisseria gonorrhoeae* was the second bacterial pathogen ever identified.

FAST FACTS

1. Gonorrhea is the second most commonly reported bacterial STD in the United States.
2. Gonorrheal infections among women now exceed the rates seen in men.
3. Infections in women are most often asymptomatic.
4. Sensitive nucleic acid amplification tests (NAATs) tests are now available to reduce testing costs and improve accuracy.
5. Gonococcal resistance to fluoroquinolones (QRNG) changed treatment recommendations for infections in MSM or in those with a history of recent foreign travel or partner's travel, infections acquired in Hawaii or California, or infections acquired in the other areas of QRNG.

PREVALENCE/INCIDENCE

Gonorrhea remains a significant public health problem in the United States. In 2004, there were 330,132 cases reported (*1*). However, because of the high rate of under-reporting, the Centers for Disease Control and Prevention (CDC) estimates that the actual number of cases was at least double the number of reported

From: *Current Clinical Practice: Sexually Transmitted Diseases:*
A Practical Guide for Primary Care
Edited by: A. L. Nelson and J. A. Woodward © Humana Press, Totowa, NJ

cases. In the past few years, infection rates increased from historical lows with relaxation of safer sex practices, especially among men who have sex with men (MSM). US rates are much higher than the rates in Canada and Western Europe.

The prevalence of gonorrhea infections peaked in 1975 when there were nearly 1 million infections. Since 1975, the numbers of infections have declined but the *patterns* of infections have changed *(2)*. In the mid-1960s, gonorrhea was predominantly a man's infection; the male to female ratio was 3:1. Now, gonorrheal infection is more gender-neutral; by 1996, the incidence of new infections in women equaled those in men. In 2004, the reported rate among women (116.5 per 100,000) was higher than in men (110 per 100,000). The clinical setting in which infection is being diagnosed has also changed. Gonorrhea has become more mainstream; today, only about 30% of all cases are diagnosed in sexually transmitted disease (STD) clinics *(2a)*. Prevalence among young adults is 0.43% *(3)*.

There are significant differences in infection rates by geography, age, and ethnic groups. The highest incidence of gonorrheal infection in the United States is in the southern states. Nearly 80% of new cases occur in men and women 15–29 years of age. For men, the incidence peaks in the 20–24 age group, whereas women have the highest infection rates between ages 15 and 19. Infection rates are highest in African-Americans, but they are also high among Hispanic and Native American groups.

However, among the general population, the incidence of gonorrhea is less than 1%, so routine screening of low-risk people, even in pregnancy, is not recommended. Screening is reserved for high-risk groups. Among MSM, it has been estimated that 64% of gonococcal infections would be missed without routine rectal and pharyngeal screening.

RISK FACTORS

The CDC has identified several classic risk factors for infection, including multiple or new sex partners, inconsistent condom use, living in urban areas with high prevalence, being an adolescent woman, low socioeconomic status, using drugs (including alcohol), and exchanging sex for drugs or money. Blacks have rates of gonorrhea infections 18-fold higher than whites. The CDC attributes the recent increases in gonorrhea to less adherence of safer sex practices, use of some illegal drugs such as "crystal meth" before sex, and the practice of finding sex partners through the Internet *(4)*. Antibiotic therapies are available to cure infections, but the cost to society is impressive.

INFECTIVITY AND TRANSMISSION

Gonorrhea is a highly infectious bacterial infection. Transmission in adults is almost exclusively by sexual activity, with exposure to infectious cervical/vaginal secretions or ejaculate during oral, vaginal, or anal sex. One ejaculate from an infected man contains approximately 6 million live bacteria *(5)*. Incubation time is usually 3–5 days, but it may be as short as 24 hours or longer than 30 days *(6)*. Infectivity varies by gender and different sexual practices. With single exposure by genital-to-genital intercourse, an uninfected woman has a 60–80% chance of acquiring the infection from an infected man. Men are at less risk, facing a 20% chance of acquiring an infection with a single act of coitus, but they have a cumulative risk of 60–80% with four or more exposures *(7)*. Precise estimates of transmission rates for rectal infections are not available, but the organism is known to be quite infectious in that setting too. Pharyngeal gonococcal infection is readily acquired by fellatio, but is less likely by cunnilingus *(8)*. *N. gonorrhoeae* has been detected and demonstrated to survive in both fresh and frozen semen. A vaginally delivered neonate has 30–35% chance of developing conjunctivitis or positive of gastric aspirate if the mother has a cervical infection. One case has demonstrated transmission by formite—in this case an inflatable doll used by sailors.

Infection with *N. gonorrhoeae* increases a woman's susceptibility to human immunodeficiency virus (HIV) infection. Infection in the man may increase HIV transmission because it may increase viral shedding.

ETIOLOGY

N. gonorrhoeae is an oxidase-positive, Gram-negative, spherical or ovoid, encapsulated, generally nonmotile diplococcus measuring 0.6–2.0 µm. *N. gonorrhoeae* is a fastidious organism with very specific media and environmental requirements, which determine the conditions in which it must be cultured. *N. gonorrhoeae* can be distinguished from other similarly shaped *Neisseria* by its ability to grow on selective media, reduce nitrites, and utilize glucose in culture but not maltose, sucrose, or lactose *(9)*.

Humans are the only natural host for *N. gonorrhoeae*. The organism preferentially infects columnar or pseudo-stratified (transitional) epithelia, such as those found in mucous membranes. This explains why the urogenital tract is the most common site of infection, although mucous membranes at other sites are also susceptible.

The physical composition of the organism allows it to attach to the surface of a target cell to enable it to adapt to the host and evade its immune response. There are many colony types. Those with pili to facilitate attachment to epithelial cells (P$^+$ colonies) are able to produce infections, whereas those shown lacking pili (P$^-$ colonies) are not infectious. Pili also interfere with phagocytosis by host neutrophils. *N. gonorrhoeae* has a cell envelope with three layers, including an inner cytoplasmic membrane, a middle peptidoglycan cell wall, and an outer membrane with lipooligosaccharide (LOS) phospholipids and several types of proteins *(9)*. The organism is able to vary its surface antigens (proteins) to avoid both detection and attack by the host immune system. The opacity-associated (Opa) proteins promote cell adhesion to other *N. gonorrhoeae* and to a variety of host cells. The porins (Por) proteins are cofactors that enable the organism to penetrate into the host cell by facilitating endocytosis of *N. gonorrhoeae* by host mucosal cells. Reduction modifiable protein is needed for transmission to sexual partners because it can stimulate blocking antibodies that reduce host serum bactericidal activity against *N. gonorrhoeae*. Immunoglobulin A protease destroys host immunoglobulin A in the cervical mucus. The LOSs in the outer cell layer have endotoxin activity and can kill adjacent uninfected cells.

Given all these factors, the *N. gonorrhoeae* adheres to mucosal cells lining the genitourinary tract using both the pili and surface proteins. Attachment releases endotoxins from gonococcal LOS, which damage vulnerable cells such as those lining the fallopian tube. Pinocytosis, which is a process utilized by host cells to destroy invading organisms, actually allows the *N. gonorrhoeae* to enter into the target cell and move into submucosal layers.

CLINICAL MANIFESTATIONS

The range of infection varies by gender but, in general, can vary from isolated self-limited infections to serious, even life-threatening systemic infections. In men, gonococcal infections may cause urethritis, proctitis, epididymitis, pharyngeal and tonsillar infection, conjunctivitis, and disseminated gonococcal infections (DGI). DGI is characterized by bacteremia, arthritis, meningitis, and endocarditis. Women have virtually the same nongenital infections but usually have cervicitis as their preliminary infection. The cervical infection can ascend into the upper genital tract and cause a very characteristic pelvic inflammatory disease (PID). Infected pregnant women are at risk for premature rupture of membranes, chorioamnionitis, and postpartum endometritis; their fetuses/newborns are at risk for amniotic infection syndrome, prematurity, intrauterine growth retardation, neonatal sepsis, and conjunctivitis. Prepubertal girls are more likely to manifest vulvar and vaginal infections. Young boys are more likely to have pharyngeal or rectal infections.

In women, the primary site of infection is the endocervical canal and the transformation zone on the ectocervix. Colonization of the female urethra is common (40–90%). It is also possible for infection to occur in the periurethral (Skene's) glands, in the Bartholin's glands, and in the anorectal area. About 35–50% of women with endocervical infections have rectal infections, but only 5% of cases have the rectum as the sole site of infection. Anorectal infection occurs by perineal contamination even in women who do not practice rectal sexual intercourse. The most obvious risk factor for pharyngeal infections is oral–genital sex. Estimates are that 10–20% of women and MSM with gonorrheal infections have pharyngeal involvement, whereas 3–7% of heterosexual men with gonococcal infections have such pharyngeal involvement. Only 5% of men and women have a solo infection of the pharynx, but that number may increase as sexual practices change.

Genital Infections in Women

Gonorrheal infections in women are quite likely (40–60%) to be asymptomatic. Another 20–40% of infected women have symptoms that are initially so slight that they are ignored by the woman *(6)*. When a woman has symptoms, those symptoms generally develop within 10 days of exposure. The most common symptoms of genital infection in women include vaginal discharge, dysuria, lower abdominal pain, dyspareunia, and abnormal uterine bleeding (such as intermenstrual bleeding, postcoital bleeding, or menorrhagia). Women with rectal infections have a wide spectrum of complaints from mild pruritus with a mucous discharge to severe proctitis. Most pharyngeal infections cause no symptoms, but if present, symptoms vary from a mild sore throat to purulent pharyngitis with lymphadenopathy and ulcerations in the pharynx, tonsils, and oral cavity.

Signs of infection are also quite variable. In women, nonspecific inguinal adenopathy may be noted. The woman's urethra and Skene's glands may be involved in the infection. She may have only a slight painless edema but at the other extreme, she may have a grossly enlarged, tender urethral meatus with erythema and spontaneous mucopurulent discharge. On bimanual exam, the urethra should be palpated ("milked") to determine if there is any tenderness or expressible purulent material. The bladder should be compressed to establish the baseline tenderness and to see if cystitis may also be on the differential diagnosis. At her introitus, there may be copious vaginal discharge. Her Bartholin's glands may also be acutely infected (*see* the section on "Abscesses of Female External Genitalia"). On rectal exam, a mucopurulent discharge may be found inside and around the external anal sphincter. In more complicated cases, anal fissures may be apparent. On speculum exam, the vaginal vault may be filled with purulent discharge or may demonstrate only a slight collection of fluid. Classically, the cervix will appear edematous, erythematous, and friable, and possibly have areas of erosion and mucopurulent exudate. On isolated compression of the cervix, tenderness may be noted. However, this presentation is not diagnostic; virtually every type of cervical infection has similar findings.

Women with cervical infection need to be gently but thoroughly examined to rule out upper tract involvement. The classic test to perform on bimanual examination is a test for cervical motion tenderness (CMT). With the vaginal examining fingers grasping the cervix between them, the cervix is gently pivoted to the patient's right and left sides with care *not* to cause any contact with peritoneal surfaces. This means that during the exam for CMT, the examiner should apply no pressure against the abdomen and there should only be slow lateral movement of the cervix; no anterior–posterior motion of the cervix or uterus should be allowed. The principle behind this maneuver is that, because each fallopian tube is a hollow viscous, distention of the tube will cause the patient pain (much a gas distention causes extreme discomfort in people with postoperative ileus). When the woman's cervix is pivoted to her right, the fundus of her uterus is rotated to her left side, which stretches her right fallopian tube. When the tube is stretched, its internal diameter is reduced. Anything inside the tube exerting outward pressure will exert even more pressure when the internal diameter is reduced. This will cause the patient to experience pain. This is why a woman with an ectopic pregnancy in her right fallopian tube will complain of pain when her cervix is moved to her right side, but may not have discomfort when it is moved to her left side. In a woman with gonococcal PID, the infection invariably involves both fallopian tubes, so she should have CMT bilaterally. She may have notable uterine tenderness when that organ is compressed between the examining fingers of the abdominal and vaginal hands. Careful adnexal examination during the digital examination is needed to rule out pelvic abscesses. In a woman who is too tender to permit a thorough pelvic examination, a rectal examination may reveal a large, indurated mass filling the cul-de-sac. A transvaginal ultrasound exam can be helpful to determine the presence of such pelvic abscesses, often called tubo-ovarian abscesses. For more details about PID, *see* Chapter 8.

With pharyngeal infections, the pharynges will appear injected with some purulent material around the tonsils. Cervical lymphadenopathy may be impressive.

Genital Infections in Men

Gonococcal urethritis is almost always a symptomatic condition; the infection is noted by 90–99% of infected men. However, asymptomatic cases (1–10%) constitute an important reservoir in the population for spreading the infection. Symptoms progress rapidly. Dysuria may become quite severe and may cause urinary retention. Infected men usually have a urethral discharge that contains *N. gonorrhoeae*. That discharge varies from a scanty, mucoid secretion to a copious and grossly purulent discharge, which can also be blood-stained. Edema of the meatus is common. Edema of the distal penile shaft and prepuce may be complicated by thrombosis of the penile dorsal veins and lymphangitis. Painful lymph gland enlargement is reported in 15% of cases. Folliculitis or cellulitis on the thigh or abdomen rarely develop. If the urethritis is not treated, the infection will spontaneously resolve after several weeks. Postgonococcal strictures of the urethra occur in only 1 out of 200 cases (0.5%). Other rare complications of initial gonococcal urethritis include penile edema, penile lymphangitis, gangrenous balanitis, and periurethral abscess.

Acute proctitis is most commonly acquired by anal intercourse. Anoreceptive MSM can develop acute proctitis with or without urethritis or pharyngitis. The rectum is the sole infection in 40% of such cases. Most cases are asymptomatic. If noted, symptoms are often mild; patients may complain of anal irritation, pruritus, painful defecation, constipation, and scant rectal spotting. Stool may be coated with a white, yellow, or blood-stained discharge. More severe infections induce tenesmus. On exam, anal dampness, with perianal mucoid or purulent discharge, may be noted. On anoscopy, the mucosa may appear normal or it may have localized infection. In severe cases, blood-stained purulent discharge may be found on the mucosal folds. Longer-term complications of anorectal infection include fistulas. The most common complication is unilateral or bilateral epididymitis, but even this complication is uncommon in developed countries. Testicular pain and swelling and epididymal tenderness associated with epididymitis often develop after the signs and symptoms of urethritis have resolved.

Other Gonococcal-Related Syndromes

Gonococcal infections can spread by direct, contiguous spread or hematological pathways and result in a number of disparate syndromes.

ABSCESSES OF FEMALE EXTERNAL GENITALIA

Skene's gland infection is common with gonococcal cervicitis. The Skene's glands are located around the urethral meatus. Abscesses may form when the duct is obstructed. This type of abscess is quite painful and often causes severe dysuria.

Bartholin's abscess is one of the most frequent manifestations of gonococcal infection in women; however, not all Bartholin's abscesses are due to a sexually transmitted infection (STI). The Bartholin glands are two rounded, nonpalpable glands located deep in the perineum about 2 cm above the hymenal ring at 5 and 7 o'clock. The Bartholin ducts are lined with transitional epithelium and run from the gland to the duct opening just above the hymenal ring in the posterior lateral walls of the vagina. The duct is easily obstructed at its distal orifice. Because the gland continues to secrete fluid, ductal obstruction leads to cystic dilation of the duct. When that cyst becomes infected, an abscess develops very rapidly. Symptoms include extreme vulvar pain, pain with movement and, if coitus is attempted, dyspareunia.

On exam, the infected labium is erythematous, exquisitely tender, and fluctuant. A mass extending into distal portion of the vagina can be seen and palpated. There may be cellulitis in the surrounding tissue, which is particularly concerning in women with immunocompromising conditions, such as diabetes. Most abscesses rupture in 3–4 days. However, earlier diagnosis and treatment can permit not only more rapid recovery, but can also reduce the risk of re-occurrence. Even if the initial infection was caused by gonorrhea, the abscess generally contains a mixture of predominantly anaerobic organisms with some aerobic and facultative aerobic organisms. If the abscess fluid is cultured, it may return sterile, reflecting the fact that most organisms are dead. However, culture of a sample of the abscess wall will yield more information about the organisms responsible for the infection.

All abscesses require drainage. Bartholin's abscesses also respond to incision and drainage. However, there are two special features of Bartholin's abscesses that require different techniques and follow-up procedures than are usually implemented in the management of other types of abscesses. First, the incision is *not* placed where the abscess may be pointing, but is made just inside the hymen at the site of normal duct opening. This is important because the goal of therapy is not only to cure the acute abscess, but also to permit resumption of gland function after the infection resolves. The incision should be modest in size: just large enough to permit introduction of small forceps to break up all loculations within the cavity. After the abscess is completely drained, the patient should be comfortable enough to tolerate careful palpation of the affected area to insure there are no undrained areas within the abscess. Then a Word catheter is placed inside the cavity and the balloon at its tip is inflated with sterile water to keep the abscess cavity from collapsing and reforming recurrent cysts or abscesses. The distal end of the catheter is tucked inside her vagina.

The patient is often too tender at this moment to tolerate a speculum exam, so urine tests for gonorrhea and chlamydia should be sent. As mentioned, do not rely on culture of the abscess fluid to determine if the patient has an STI. If her history of sexual activity suggests this abscess may be the result of an STI, empiric antibiotic therapy may be prudent. This is particularly relevant if the patient's ability to follow up for routine visits in the near future is at all questionable. In general, other antibiotic therapy is not needed in treatment of isolated Bartholin's abscesses in healthy women. However, women who have diabetes, pregnant women, and those who are immunocompromised may require antibiotic therapy. If the patient has significant cellulitis surrounding the abscess, antibiotics targeting STIs, staphylococcal and streptococcus organisms, and anaerobes should be given. Close follow-up is mandatory. Immunocompromised women with such cellulitis and women with signs of sepsis must be hospitalized for intravenous antibiotic therapy and close observation. Subcutaneous infections and even necrotizing fascitis are possible, especially in women with diabetes.

Patients treated on an outpatient basis must be re-examined within 48 hours of initial incision and drainage. Generally, the erythema and edema will have resolved. The Word catheter balloon may be decompressed somewhat at this time; only enough fluid is retained in the balloon to keep the catheter inside the cavity. The patient can be more thoroughly examined to rule out other vaginal infections and cervical infections. She should be reminded to avoid all sexual activity until the duct has re-epithelized around the catheter in 4–6 weeks and the Word catheter is removed.

After removal of the Word catheter, some women can experience recurrent abscess (generally because of re-infection) or formation of a Bartholin's cyst (because of non-infectious scarring of the duct). Women with recurrent Bartholin's abscesses and cysts generally are treated with marsupialization of the abscess or the cyst to develop a more permanent fistulous tract from the duct to the introitus. In this case, a larger incision is made at the level of the old duct opening. The cyst/abscess is drained and the edges of the duct or abscess are everted over themselves and sutured to the surrounding skin. This creates an epithelialized drainage pouch. Recurrence occurs after marsupialization in only 5–10% of cases (10). Excision of the gland is indicated only for persistent deep infections in younger women or in women over age 40 to determine if they have adenocarcinoma of the Bartholin's gland.

CONJUNCTIVITIS

Gonococcal conjunctivitis in adults can result from direct sexual contact, but usually results from auto-inoculation. In the newborn, the infection, which is called *ophthalmia neonatorum*, can be more devastating. It can result from amniotic fluid infection or contaminated fingers, but generally results from exposure to an infected cervix during delivery. About one-third of exposed newborns acquire gonorrhea during vaginal delivery. Before the introduction of routine silver nitrate prophylaxis, ophthalmia neonatorum from all causes was seen in almost 10% of US infants (11) and was the most common cause of blindness (9). Half of these cases were owing to *N. gonorrhoeae*. Clinical manifestations usually develop 2–5 days after birth, however, the incubation time may be up to 21 days. There is an acute onset of purulent conjunctivitis with copious purulent secretion and extensive inflammation involving one or both eyes. The newborn becomes photophobic and its eyelids become swollen. If untreated, the infection can progress to involve the cornea and cause either ulceration with permanent scarring or perforation with formulation of synechiae. At the extreme, the eye may be lost.

DISSEMINATED GONOCOCCAL INFECTION

DGI is a relatively rare complication, which develops in less than 1% of gonococcal mucosal infections. However, women are more likely to develop systemic infections; the female to male ratio is 4:1. There may be predisposing conditions that render some individuals more vulnerable. People who are deficient in late complement factor may not be able to clear *N. gonorrhoeae* because they cannot kill or lyse the organisms (9). Similarly, certain strains of *N. gonorrhoeae* are resistant to bacteriocidal activity of human serum and are, therefore, able to disseminate more readily.

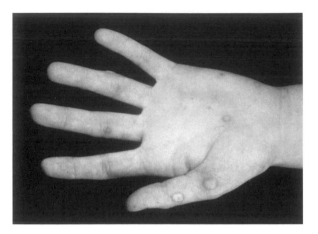

Skin lesions resulting from gonococcal emboli.

There are two clinical stages of DGI. The early stage is associated with initial bacteremia and is characterized by chills, fevers (38–39°C), typical skin lesions, malaise, asymmetric joint involvement, and tenosynovitis. During this stage, about half of blood cultures will be positive for *N. gonorrhoeae*. The skin lesions, which are the most common manifestation, result from gonococcal emboli. They may start as small vesicles that develop into pustules, but lesions with characteristic hemorrhagic bases with central necrosis rapidly follow. The lesions may be found on any part of the body, but the volar aspects of the arms, hands, and legs, especially near the small joints of the hands and feet, are most often involved. These skin lesions are transitory; they heal spontaneously without scarring after a few days. Asymmetric joint involvement occurs in 30–40% of cases and presents as septic arthritis and migratory polyarthralgia. The knees are the most common joint infection, but elbow, ankle, and metacarpophalangeal and interphalangeal joints are other frequent sites. The arthritis is often migrating and typically involves two or more joints. The majority of septic arthritis in US adults is caused by the *N. gonorrhoeae*.

In the late stage of DGI, the arthritis progresses and many other systems are compromised. Such arthritis in the knees, ankles, and wrist joints generally results in permanent joint damage. Endocarditis is reported to complicate 1–3% of cases of DGI. It more commonly occurs in men. There is progressive valvular damage, most commonly in the aortic valve. The victim experiences weeks of febrile illness with weakness, weight loss, and fatigue. Regurgitant murmurs usually develop, reflecting valvular insufficiency. Other serious manifestations of systemic gonococcal infections include meningitis, pericarditis, osteomyelitis, severe sepsis accompanied by Waterhouse-Friderichsen syndrome, and adult respiratory distress syndrome.

Infections in Children

Young sexually abused children demonstrate less classic infections. Prepubescent girls are more likely to have vulvovaginitis (rather than cervical infection), vaginal discharge (purulent or crusted), dysuria, odor, irritation, and vulvar pruritus. However, the risk of ascent into the upper reproductive tract is higher for prepubescent girls than those in the reproductive age group *(12)*. Young boys most frequently have anorectal or pharyngeal infection; urethritis is rare.

TESTING AND DIAGNOSIS

In order to diagnose any infection confidently, it is necessary to identify the organism at the site of infection. There are numerous testing modalities for gonococcal infections including Gram stain, culture, immunochemical, and molecular detection. Each has its strengths, drawbacks, and appropriate applications (*see* Table 1). It is also important to establish who should be tested and when.

The classic test for gonococcal infections has been Gram stain of the urethral material obtained from men who present with urethral discharge and dysuria. If Gram-negative diplococci are seen within or closely associated with polymorphonuclear leukocytes, the diagnosis is relatively secure. Gram stain in this situation is estimated to be 90–95% sensitive and 95–100% specific *(13)*. However, the test is not 100% sensitive, so it is generally recommended that symptomatic men be cultured even if the Gram stain is negative. There are serovars of *Neisseria* (1B02, 1A05, 1A21, B08) that are mostly undetected with microscopy, making them more likely to spread within the community *(14)*. It should be noted that the Gram stain is not an appropriate test for the cervix of a woman or for the pharynx or rectum of either women or men. In women with gonococcal cervicitis, Gram stain has only 60% sensitivity. Blind anorectal swabs detect only 40–60% of infections.

Culture in selective media has several advantages. It is low cost, suitable for a variety of infection sites, and may be the only evidence accepted in some legal jurisdictions. Culture also permits testing for antibiotic susceptibility. The two most commonly used media are Thayer-Martin and Martin-Lewis media, which contain vancomycin or ristocetin, colistin or polymyxin B, and nystatin or amphotericin B with or without trimethoprim (to control Proteus). Proper handling of the culture medium and the specimen is imperative during collection, transport, and in the lab. The organisms do not tolerate drying; they are temperature-sensitive (only growing between 35 and 37°C) and require an enriched CO_2 environment (3–10% CO_2). To collect the specimen, a sterile cotton-tipped swab should be introduced into the cervix, urethra, or tonsillar area and pharynx behind the uvula.

(The section "Testing and Diagnosis" will continue on page 169 after Table 1 concludes.)

Table 1

CDC—Indications for *Neisseria gonorrhoeae* Testing and Test Selection by Specimen Type

Readers are cautioned to refer to the manufacturers' test kit inserts for specific details. Information in this table represents general conditions for comparative purposes.

Endocervical swabs/urethral swabs from males

Indication for testing	Test selection
• Screening	• Gram-stained smear as a point-of-care test for males with urethral discharge
◆ Females: when pelvic examination is indicated	◆ For males with urethral discharge, the sensitivity and specificity are similar to culture with oxidase testing and Gram-staining of any colonies with *N. gonorrhoeae* morphology
◆ Males: urine might be more acceptable to asymptomatic males	◆ Culture after a positive Gram-stained smear might be useful for quality assurance, but additional testing is not usually otherwise indicated
• Endocervicitis	• Culture
• Urethritis (males)	◆ Preferred if ambient conditions during holding and transport of inoculated media are adequate to maintain the viability of organisms; sensitivity and specificity of culture with additional testing approaches or surpasses that of other tests
• Diseases at other anatomic locations possibly caused by sexually acquired *N. gonorrhoeae* infection	
◆ Pelvic inflammatory disease	◆ A culture isolate should be tested for antimicrobial resistance if a patient fails therapy
◆ Urethral syndrome	◆ Culture allows monitoring for antimicrobial resistance
◆ Bartholinitis	• Nucleic acid amplification tests (NAATs) or nucleic acid hybridization tests
◆ Epididymitis	
◆ Perihepatitis (Fitz-Hugh-Curtis syndrome) (females)	◆ Recommended when conditions during holding and transport of inoculated culture media are not adequate to maintain the viability of organisms
◆ Proctitis	
◆ Disseminated gonococcal infections	◆ Commercial polymerase chain reaction (PCR) and strand displacement assays have cross-reacted with nongonococcal *Neisseria*; such cross-reactivity has not been reported for commercial ligase chain reaction (LCR) and unamplified probe assays
◆ Conjunctivitis	
• Not recommended for prepubertal children	

Urine

Indication for testing

- Females: screening when pelvic examination is not indicated
- Males: screening

Test selection

- NAATs
  - ◆ Sensitivity with urine might be lower than with urethral (males) or endocervical swabs
  - ◆ Other tests are not recommended because of low sensitivity
  - ◆ Additional testing is recommended after an initial positive screening test if a low positive predictive value can be expected because of a low prevalence or if a false-positive result would have serious psychosocial or legal consequences for a person

(continued from previous) Additional testing is recommended after an initial positive screening test if a low positive predictive value can be expected or if a false-positive result would have serious psychosocial or legal consequences

Vaginal swabs, postmenarcheal adolescents and adults

Indication for testing

- Screening/testing of women when pelvic examination is not otherwise indicated

Test selection

- No test is recommended for use with vaginal swab specimens
  - ◆ The Food and Drug Administration (FDA) has not cleared any nonculture test for use with vaginal specimens
  - ◆ NAAT
    - ▪ Additional review is needed before a recommendation can be made; however, in one study, sensitivity and specificity with a provider or client collected vaginal swab was similar to screening with endocervical or urine specimens
    - ▪ Additional testing is recommended after an initial positive screening test if a low positive predictive value can be expected or if a false-positive result would have serious psychosocial or legal consequences
  - ◆ Culture
    - ▪ Not recommended for adults because of suboptimal sensitivity
  - ◆ Other tests are not recommended because of low sensitivity

Continued on next page

165

Table 1 (*Continued*)

CDC—Indications for *Neisseria gonorrhoeae* Testing and Test Selection by Specimen Type

Readers are cautioned to refer to the manufacturers' test kit inserts for specific details. Information in this table represents general conditions for comparative purposes.

Vaginal swabs, prepubescent children

Indication for testing	Test selection

• Possible sexual abuse, children	• Culture
	   ◆ Preferred for possibly sexually abused children because of presence of vaginal epithelium that is susceptible to *N. gonorrhoeae* infection, high specificity, and ability to retain isolate for additional testing
	   ◆ The FDA has not cleared any nonculture test for use with vaginal specimens
	• NAATs
	   ◆ When culture is not available, certain specialists support use of a NAAT if a positive result can be verified by another NAAT
	• Other tests are not recommended because of low sensitivity and specificity

Rectal Swabs

Indication for testing	Test selection

• Patients with history of receptive anal intercourse
• Proctitis
• Possible sexual abuse, children
	• Culture
	   ◆ The sensitivity of culture is not well-defined; isolates that are oxidase-positive and Gram-negative diplococci should receive additional testing to verify an initial presumptive *N. gonorrhoeae* diagnosis, if a false-positive result would have serious medical, psychosocial, or legal consequences
	   ◆ A culture isolate should be tested for antimicrobial resistance if a patient fails therapy
	• Other tests are not recommended

Pharyngeal swabs

Indication for testing	Test selection

• Patients concerned regarding exposure during fellatio or cumilingus
• Newborns or infants (nasopharyngeal specimens)
  ◆ Neonatal conjunctivitis
• Possible sexual abuse, children
	• Culture
	  ◆ Sensitivity of culture for pharyngeal specimens is not well-defined
	  ◆ Isolates that are oxidase-positive and contain Gram-negative diplococci should receive additional testing to verify an initial presumptive *N. gonorrhoeae* diagnosis because of the common occurrence of nongonococcal *Neisseria* in the pharynx
	  ◆ A culture isolate should be tested for antimicrobial resistance if a patient fails therapy
	• Other tests are not recommended

Conjunctival swabs

Indication for testing	Test selection

• Conjunctivitis among adults
• Newborns or infants
  ◆ Neonatal conjunctivitis
	• Gram stain as point-of-care test
	  ◆ Recommended to establish a presumptive diagnosis of *N. gonorrhoeae* during a patient's visit for conjunctivitis
	  ◆ Adequate sensitivity because of high concentration of organisms
	  ◆ Gram stain should be followed by laboratory-based testing because Gram-negative diplococci other than *N. gonorrhoeae* are occasionally isolated from conjunctiva
	• Culture
	  ◆ Preferred
	    ▪ High sensitivity because of high concentration of organisms
	    ▪ Oxidase-positive and Gram-stain-positive bacteria other than *N. gonorrhoeae* occasionally isolated from conjunctiva
	    ▪ Inoculation onto nonselective media might increase sensitivity
	• Only a limited number, if any, nonculture tests are FDA-cleared for conjunctival specimens

Continued on next page

Table 1 (*Continued*)

CDC—Indications for *Neisseria gonorrhoeae* Testing and Test Selection by Specimen Type

Readers are cautioned to refer to the manufacturers' test kit inserts for specific details. Information in this table represents general conditions for comparative purposes.

	Test selection

Diagnosing disseminated gonococcal infection, adults or neonates	• Gram stain as point-of-care test
	   ♦ Recommended on any synovial fluid and cerebrospinal fluid collected for other tests and on endocervical and urethral swab specimens
	   ♦ Gram stain should be followed by laboratory-based testing that is more sensitive and specific
	• Culture
	   ♦ Blood, synovial fluid from affected joints, and, if indicated, cerebrospinal fluid specimens should be inoculated onto nonselective as well as selective media
	   ♦ Swab specimens from the endocervix (adult female), vagina (neonate), urethra (adult male), rectum, and pharynx should be inoculated onto selective media
	   ♦ Additional testing recommended after an initial positive test to verify diagnosis
	• No other tests are recommended

The swab should be kept in place for 15–30 seconds to permit organisms to be absorbed by capillary action. A single swab in those areas has 80–90% sensitivity. Adding a second swab increases sensitivity by 7–10%. A second rectal swab achieves 93% sensitivity. In a woman without a cervix, a swab of her urethra has the highest yield. One investigator recently reported that KY jelly may have inhibitory impact on the growth of *N. gonorrhoeae (15)*. The specimen must be immediately placed onto the medium, which must not be cold. The plate must be placed in a CO_2 incubator or candle jar or CO_2-generating tablets may be placed inside the collection plate to create an adequate concentration of CO_2.

The specimen must be processed in the lab within 24 hours. Many of the popular transport media lose 10–79% of isolates after 24 hours and even the use of an environmental chamber has been associated with 7–22% loss of colonies after 1 day *(2)*. This presents challenges for many practice sites, especially on weekends and holidays.

Within the lab, there are several tests used. *N. gonorrhoeae* demonstrates typical growth on selective media when incubated at 35–36.5° in an atmosphere supplemented with 5% CO_2 *(16)*. A presumptive diagnosis can be made from specimens grown in colonies on the basis of a Gram-stain morphology (Gram-negative diplococcus), a positive oxidase reaction, and selective fermentation reactions (the organism ferments glucose but not sucrose, maltose, or lactose). Testing of isolates with direct fluorescent antibody tests or DNA probes (AccuProbe, PACE 2) enables rapid laboratory identification of presumptive isolates. It is required that antibiotic sensitivity be performed on all isolates.

To screen larger, generally asymptomatic populations for infection of gonorrhea and/or *Chlamydia trachomatis* (CT), nonculture assays have been developed. Older technologies used for screening of syphilis and other STIs do not work for gonococcal testing. These include serological tests (not available for gonorrhea), direct fluorescent antibody tests (not available outside the lab), and enzyme immunoassay (not cost-competitive with culture for *N. gonorrhoeae*). In general, the tests that are used can be classified as being non-NAATs or NAATs.

The non-amplified DNA probe tests use single-stranded DNA probes, which hybridize to the ribosomal RNA of *N. gonorrhoeae* or to *C. trachomatis*. Compared with culture tests, these tests are less affected by transport conditions and may provide more timely results. Overall, the sensitivity of available tests is reported to be 89–97% with a specificity of 99%. A 98.4% concordance with cultures has been reported *(17)*. The Food and Drug Administration (FDA) has approved tests (such as PACE 2 System [GenProbe] and Digene Hybrid Captive or Capture II assay) for testing the endocervix of women and the urethra of men. However, these tests are not FDA-approved for pharyngeal, rectal, or urine testing. A negative test result rules out gonococcal and chlamydia infection. However, a positive test does not distinguish between the two organisms.

Additional follow-up tests need to be performed to provide organism-specific results.

The second category of tests used to test for gonococcal and chlamydial infections is NAATs. All NAATs have proven to be superior to *N. gonorrhoeae* culture *(18)*. There are many different versions of NAATs but they share the ability to produce a positive test result from as little as a single copy of target DNA or RNA. Most amplified tests are approved for endocervical and male urethral specimens. Most are effective in detecting both gonorrheal and chlamydial infections using either male or female urine specimens. However, none are approved for rectal or oropharyngeal infection testing. One common NAAT used today is the ligase chain reaction (LCR) test (such as Abbott LCx), which detects a 48 base-pair sequence in the *Opa* gene. LCR's sensitivity is 95–98%. When used on a first-voided urine specimen, the LCR is as sensitive in detecting infection as culture of the endocervix. Another newer application for LCR is to use it to test liquid cytology specimens for cervical infection. In comparative trials, sensitivity of this test was 86% vs endocervical culture and 89% of that of polymerase chain reaction (PCR) of cervical swabs. A distinct advantage of this application is the stability of the specimen. Liquid cytology uses methanol-based fixatives, which preserve the organism and its DNA for up to 7 days at room temperature *(19)*. Of course, there should never be an intentional delay in diagnosis of any STI, but this stability is important in many practice settings.

Other NAATs use other markers of infection. PCR tests (such as Amplicor® CT/NG Test, Roche Molecular Diagnostics, Pleasanton, CA) target a 201 base-pair sequence within the cytosine methyltransferase gene *M:NgoPll*. Transcription-mediated amplification tests (such as APTIMA Combo 2® Assay, Gen-Probe Incorporated, San Diego, CA) identify a 16S ribosome RNA of *N. gonorrhoeae*. Strand displacement amplification (SDA) tests (such as BD ProbeTec™ ET system, Becton-Dickinson Diagnostic Systems, Sparks, MD) search for a DNA sequence found in the "pilin" gene-inverting protein homolog of *N. gonorrhoeae*.

As specific as these NAATs are, they do have limitations. One problem is that some test specimens may contain host amplification inhibitors, which causes false-negative results. NAATs are also subject to higher false-positive rates than non-NAAT tests because of cross-contamination. These false-positive results are particularly problematic in low-prevalence populations *(20)*. It has been suggested that repeat testing of specimens, preferably with a different sensitive assay be performed to reduce the possibility of false-positive results *(21)*. The CDC recommends that additional confirmatory testing may be needed in low-prevalence populations or when other factors reduce the positive predictive value to below 90% *(16)*. Another approach is to use nucleic acid genetic transformation tests, such as Gonostat (Sierra Diagnostics, Sonora, CA). This test uses a mutant of gonorrhea that grows only when transformed by DNA extracted from a swab specimen containing gonorrhea. Unfortunately, Neisseria meningitis can cause a false-positive result. There has been some evidence that some of these tests (such as SDA, LCR, and PCR) may be able to detect gonococcal infection based on a vaginal swab, which might permit self-collected specimens in the future *(22–24)*.

In general, the choice of test to be used should be individualized and is determined by local factors (such as transport challenges) and specimen availability. For women, the CDC recommends that culture-based tests in the endocervix be performed unless there are transport problems, to monitor for development of antibiotic resistance *(16)*. NAAT or nucleic acid hybridization from endocervical specimens are the choices in that situation. The second choice will be urine NAATs because they are less sensitive. In men, the first choice is either culture of intra-urethral swabs (to obtain information about antibiotic sensitivity), NAATs, or nucleic acid hybridization of intra-urethral specimen. A second choice would be a urinary NAAT. Throat and rectal infections are best tested by culture *(16)*. In children (especially young girls), it has been recommended that sequential testing is the most sensitive. The sequence of tests is important. The first test should be the most sensitive (nonculture method) followed by culture tests. This reduces the false-positive rate to 0% and the false-negative rate is 0.8% *(25)*.

Knowing who to test and when and where to perform it is as important as knowing which technology to use. Recently, it has been demonstrated in US jails that the presumptive treatment of symptomatic female infection without testing may be the most prudent approach, because gonococcal testing is not cost-effective for women unless there is a high prevalence of the infection in the population *(26)*. For sexually active MSM, the CDC treatment guidelines recommend annual urethral/urine screening for *N. gonorrhoeae*, pharyngeal cultures for MSM with oral–genital exposure, and rectal cultures for MSM who have had receptive anal sex. Screening should be done every 3–6 months for MSM at highest risk (e.g., those with multiple sexual partners or illicit drug users) *(16)*.

When obtaining a sexual history to assess the need to test for STIs, it is important to define terms clearly to patients and ask very concrete questions about their sexual practices (*see* Chapter 13). Terms such as "sexually active" are different for STI purposes than for pregnancy prevention. The wide range of vulnerable activities is not generally appreciated. In a recent survey of college students, "abstinence" was defined by the students to permit penile–anal intercourse (19%) and oral–genital contact (59%) *(27)*. All of these people would have denied having any sexual activity if asked only that question. In a related study of high school virgins, it was found that 9% of them admitted to engaging in heterosexual fellatio sex with ejaculation, 10% engaged in heterosexual cunnilingus, and 1% engaged in heterosexual anal intercourse *(28)*.

All states have statutes allowing minors to receive services related to STI testing and treatment without parental consent or involvement, however, those laws may specify the age at which minors can begin to consent for such care *(29)*. Because the peak years for gonococcal infection in women is 15–24 years of age, at an age when a young woman's sexual activity may not be known to her parents, confidentiality issues can present significant barriers to teens in accessing diagnosis. In a recent survey, 92% of sexually active teens said they would be tested for STIs if they could be reassured that their parents would not find out; that rate plummeted to 38% if there was *any* chance that their parents might find out *(30)*.

People who are found to have gonococcal infections should be tested for other common STIs including chlamydia, HIV, trichomoniasis, and in endemic areas, syphilis. They should also be tested for hepatitis B infection and receive vaccination unless they have proof of prior vaccination.

TREATMENT

The 2006 CDC treatment guidelines for gonococcal infections are displayed in Table 2. Treatments for gonorrhea require constant updating because of the development of antibiotic resistance. For many years after the discovery of penicillin, most experts believed that the scourge of gonorrhea (and syphilis) was coming to an end. All cases were easily treated with the wonder drug. Then, in the 1960s, penicillinase-producing *N. gonorrhoeae* were reported almost simultaneously in the United States, western Europe, Philippines, and western Africa. Both chromosomal and plasma-mediated types of gonococcal resistance occur *(9)*. Plasmids of different types produce β lactamase. In some areas of Africa and Asia, more than one-half of infections are now penicillinase-producing *N. gonorrhoeae*. In urban areas in the United States, 15–20% of strains are so affected.

N. gonorrhoeae has also developed resistance to other antibiotics. It has been estimated that, worldwide, at least 20–30% of gonococcal infections are resistant to some antibiotic and 18% are resistant to penicillin, tetracycline, or both. More recently, gonococcal infections in certain areas have demonstrated decreased sensitivity to fluoroquinolones, which are included in the CDC recommended treatments (ciprofloxacin, ofloxacin, and levofloxacin) as well as those in the alternate regimen lists (gatifloxacin, norfloxacin, and lomefloxacin). Because of this documented resistance, the CDC revised its treatment guidelines and recommended that the fluoroquinolones should no longer be used as first-line treatment of infections in MSM or in those with a history of recent foreign travel or partner's travel, infections acquired in California or Hawaii, or infections acquired in other areas of QRNG prevalence *(31)*. MSM have been identified as a high-risk group because resistance in this group is 12 times the heterosexual rate and now exceeds the 5% threshold level. Inner cities of other states may have pockets of high incidence of resistance *(32)*.

(The section "Treatment" will continue on page 176 after Table 2 concludes.)

Table 2
Gonococcal Infection—CDC STD Treatment Guidelines 2006

Uncomplicated infections of the cervix, urethra, or rectum in non-pregnant women

Recommended regimens—*select one of the following:*

Ceftriaxone [b,c,h]	125 mg IM in a single dose
Cefixime [h]	400 mg orally in a single dose
Ciprofloxacin [d,e]	500 mg orally in a single dose
Ofloxacin [d,e,f]	400 mg orally in a single dose
Levofloxacin [d,e,f]	250 mg orally in a single dose

Plus, *if chlamydial infection is not ruled out—*
select one of the following:

Azithromycin [c]	1 g orally in a single dose
Doxycycline [g]	100 mg orally twice a day

Alternative regimens—*select one of the following:*

Spectinomycin [a]	2 g IM in a single dose
Ceftizoxime	500 mg IM in a single dose
Cefoxitin with Probenecid	2 gram IM in a single dose 1 g orally in a single dose
Cefotaxime	500 mg IM in a single dose
Gatifloxacin [d,e]	400 mg orally in a single dose
Norfloxacin [d,e]	800 mg orally in a single dose
Lomefloxacin [d,e]	400 mg orally in a single dose for 7 days

Plus, *if chlamydial infection is not ruled out—*
select one of the following:

Azithromycin [c]	1 g orally in a single dose
Doxycycline [g]	100 mg orally twice a day

Uncomplicated infections of the pharynx

Recommended regimens—*select one of the following:*

Ceftriaxone [b,c]	125 mg IM in a single dose
Ciprofloxacin [d,e]	500 mg orally in a single dose

Plus, *if chlamydial infection is not ruled out—*
select one of the following:

Azithromycin [c]	1 g orally in a single dose
Doxycycline [g]	100 mg orally twice a day for 7 days

Alternative regimen

Spectinomycin [a]	2 g IM in a single dose (for allergy, intolerance, or adverse reactions; only 52% effective— needs test of cure)

Plus, *if chlamydial infection is not ruled out—*
select one of the following:

Azithromycin [c]	1 g orally in a single dose
Doxycycline [g]	100 mg orally twice a day for 7 days

(Continued on next page)

Table 2 (*Continued*)
Gonococcal Infection—CDC STD Treatment Guidelines 2006

Uncomplicated infections in pregnant women

Recommended regimens—select one of the following:

		Alternative regimen—select one of the following:
Cefixime	400 mg orally in a single dose	Spectinomycin[a] 2 g IM in a single dose
Ceftriaxone [b,c]	125 mg IM in a single dose	
Ceftizoxime or cefotaxime	500 mg IM in a single dose	
Cefoxitin with probenecid	2 g IM in a single dose 1 g orally in a single dose	

Plus, if chlamydial infection is not ruled out—
select one of the following:

Chlamydia treatment for pregnant women

Gonococcal conjunctivitis in adults

Recommended regimens

Ceftriaxone [b,c]	1 g IM in a single dose. Consider lavage of the infected eye with saline solution once.

Ophthalmia neonatorum prophylaxis

Recommended regimens—select one of the following:

Erythromycin	(0.5%) ophthalmic ointment
Tetracycline	(1%) ophthalmic ointment

Instill in a single applicator into both eyes as soon as possible after delivery

Source: ref. *16*.

a Spectinomycin is expensive, inactive against *T. pallidum*, and relatively ineffective against gonococcal pharyngeal infection. Useful to treat patients who cannot tolerate cephalosporins and quinolones.

b Ceftriaxone may treat incubating syphilis.

c Safety and efficacy among pregnant and lactating women have not been established (pregnancy category B).

d Contraindicated for pregnant and lactating women.

e Quinolones should not be used for infections. In MSM or in those with a history of recent foreign travel or partner's travel, infections acquired in California or Hawaii, or infections acquired in other areas of QRNG resistance.

f Ofloxacin and levofloxacin provide coverage for both *N. gonorrhoeae* and *C. trachomatis*, except as noted in Note *e*.

g Contraindicated for pregnant and lactating women and for children under 8 years old.

h Recommended for treatment of infections in MSM or heterosexual with a history of recent foreign travel or partner's travel, infections acquired in California or Hawaii, or infections acquired in other areas of QRNG resistance.

For uncomplicated gonococcal infections in the cervix, urethra, and rectum in adults, ceftriaxone is the cornerstone of therapy, curing 98.9% of infections. Cefixime 400 mg is another recommended option, but it is available only in liquid form in the United States. This agent does not provide as high or as sustained bactericidal levels as ceftriaxone. Several cephalosporins listed in the alternative regimens are reasonably effective, although none of the cephalosporins offers any advantage over ceftriaxone. These agents can all be relied on to achieve more than 97% cure rate. Patients who are allergic to or intolerant of cephalosporins or quinolones should be treated with spectinomycin. Pregnant women with uncomplicated cervical or urethral infections should not be treated with quinolones or tetracyclines, but should be given cephalosporin. Women who cannot tolerate cephalosporins may be treated with spectinomycin 2 g intramuscularly in a single dose.

Gonococcal pharyngitis is more difficult to treat. Few antibiotic therapies can reliably cure more than 90% of those infections (16). Spectinomycin only clears pharyngitis in 52% of cases. If spectinomycin is used to treat pharyngeal infection, a repeat culture should be performed 3–5 days after treatment to document a cure. It should be noted that proctitis in women may also be resistant to treatment and may cause re-infection of the urethra and cervix.

Gonococcal conjunctivitis in adults should be treated with ceftriaxone 1 g intramuscularly in a single dose. Newborns with ophthalmic neonatorum are best treated with ceftriaxone 25–50 mg/kg intravenously or intramuscularly in a single dose not to exceed 125 mg. Treatment of other infant gonococcal-related infections requires hospitalization for parenteral therapy, as well as epidemiology treatment of the mother and her sexual contacts. When gonococcal infection is found in children, sexual abuse must be ruled out.

Because of high co-infection rates with chlamydia, all treatment guidelines for gonorrhea also include antibiotic therapy for chlamydia unless there is laboratory evidence that the patient does *not* have chlamydia. Women are nearly four times more likely to have chlamydia when they are diagnosed with gonococcal infection than men. In two recent analysis of subjects being treated for *N. gonorrhoeae* infections, 38–42% of the women and 20–24% of the men were co-infected with chlamydia (33,34). The CDC recommends treatment with azithromycin or doxycycline in adults and adolescents.

Patients and their partners should abstain from intercourse (and all other sexual contacts) until treatment is completed and until they and all their partners no longer have symptoms. Each should be encouraged to practice safer sex practices. This is often challenging. A recent survey of primary care physicians in the United States revealed that 70% believe that their counseling of patients about STIs was ineffective. Nearly half reported that their medical school STI training was inadequate or that they felt that they were not responsible for STI preventive services. They also complained that their contracts limited their ability to provide these services *(35)*. There may be some basis for their pessimism. In a 1991 national survey of men with a history of STIs, 25% reported they had sex while infected and 29% did not modify behavior subsequent to their diagnosis. Of those who did make changes, 10% adopted abstinence and 33% stopped having sex with a partner they did not know well, whereas only one in five changed his practice of multiple sex partners or initiated condom use *(36)*.

No formal test of cure is needed for initial treatment of *N. gonorrhoeae* (except as noted for treatment for pharyngeal infection). Patients who have symptoms that persist after treatment should be tested by culture for *N. gonorrhoeae* and tested for antibiotic susceptibility. Many studies have demonstrated high re-infection rates. In one study of more than 200 sexually active teens who were followed for 1–2 years, the rates of initial gonococcal infection (11.6%) were lower than for chlamydia (23.2%), but initial infection with *N. gonorrhoeae* was found to be a risk factor for subsequent infection with chlamydia and gonorrhea. Less than 10% of the population (with recurrent cervicitis) accounted for one-third of all episodes of cervicitis identified during the study *(37)*. As a result, the CDC advises clinicians to recommended that all patients with gonorrhea to be retested 3 months after treatment.

PARTNER NOTIFICATION
AND REPORTING REQUIREMENTS

All others with whom the infected person has had sexual contact in the 60 days before the onset of symptoms or diagnosis of *N. gonorrhoeae* must be treated for gonococcal and chlamydial infections and tested for other related STIs. If the infected person denies any sexual contact within that 60-day time frame, the last person with whom the patient had sexual contact must be treated epidemiologically and evaluated for other STIs. Research has found that patient-delivered partner therapy to sex partners who themselves are unlikely to seek care can be a safe and effective way to reach those patients *(37a)*. However, patient education materials must always accompany such prescriptions. Clinicians should consult state laws to verify that such practices are legal in their areas.

All states require that persons with gonococcal infections be reported to public health authorities by the clinician, laboratory, or both.

PREGNANCY-RELATED ISSUES

Gonococcal infection during pregnancy can result in postabortal/postpartum gonococcal endometritis and salpingitis. In the early part of the first trimester of pregnancy, the fallopian tubes are still patent and susceptible to ascending infection with *N. gonorrhoeae*. It is unclear if gonococcal infection is directly responsible for many of the adverse outcomes seen in infected pregnancies or if the infection is a marker for other risk factors. However, infected women can experience premature rupture of membranes with subsequent amniotic infection syndrome (placental, fetal membrane, and umbilical cord inflammation), premature delivery, intrauterine growth retardation, higher rates of infant morbidity and mortality, chorioamnionitis, and neonatal infections, such as conjunctival, pharyngeal, respiratory, and anal infections.

Pregnant women do not need routine screening for gonococcal infection, but at-risk women should be tested at the first prenatal visit. At-risk women include adolescents; women in high-prevalence areas; women who are partners of men with gonococcal urethritis; women who have other STDs, multiple sex partners, or other high-risk sex practices; intravenous drug users; and women who have PID by clinical presentation. Other risk factors include admission to jail or other detention facilities, military recruits, and Job Corp volunteers. Testing for gonococcal infection should be repeated in the third trimester in these women. Pregnant women should not be treated with quinolones or tetracyclines. Cephalosporins are the drug of choice for treating pregnant women with gonococcal infections. Women with an inability to tolerate a cephalosporin should be administered a single 2 g intramuscular dose of spectinomycin to treat cervical infections. Appropriate therapy should be given for presumptive or diagnosed chlamydial infection.

PREVENTION

Correct and consistent use of condoms has been shown to reduce the risk of gonorrheal infection in men, but the available evidence at the time of the NIH conference did not allow for an accurate assessment of the degree of protection in women (38). Subsequently newer studies and meta-analyses have shown that use of male condoms is associated with a significate reduction in the risk of gonorrhea for both men and women (38a).

CASE STUDY

Joe, age 16, complains of 4 days of penile discharge and burning since returning from a trip to San Francisco. He requests confidentiality regarding the reason for his visit. He tried two antibiotic pills that he found in his mother's medicine cabinet without relief; he can't remember the name of these pills. He denies involuntary sexual activity.

Questions

1. What additional history would you like?
2. What tests are needed?
3. What treatments should be started?
4. What follow-up is needed?

5. What about his partner(s)?
6. What kind of confidentiality can you offer?

Answers and Teaching Points

1. Is he having any other symptoms, such as painful defecation or sore throat? Does he have testicular pain or difficulty starting a stream of urine? Has he noticed any rashes on his penis or other areas that were exposed? In addition to obtaining more information about his specific sex practices, it would be important to learn how many sex contacts he has had in the last 60 days or at least since the time that he contracted the infection. Has he been vaccinated against hepatitis B?

2. The tests that are needed depend on the sexual activities in which he engaged. Were they same sex or heterosexual? Which anatomical sites were exposed to infection? At a minimum, a Gram stain of his urethral discharge obtained by a urethral swab should be performed to provide rapid results. If it reveals Gram-positive diplococci intracellularly, treatments should be started for both *N. gonorrhoeae* and *C. trachomatis*. Confirming NAATs can be performed on the first drops of urine that are collected more than 60 minutes after last urination. If other areas were contacted, culture of these areas may be needed, especially pharyngeal tests. He should also be tested now for HIV.

3. If he is found to have gonococcal urethritis, he should be treated with ceftriaxone. The quinolones are not appropriate because he contracted the infection in California. He should also be treated presumptively for chlamydia. Other treatments should await test results. If he had been exposed to syphilis, ceftriaxone will cure that infection.

4. He needs to be retested in 3 months for HIV if the initial test was nonreactive.

5. All sexual contacts since the trip to San Francisco should be contacted and urged to seek medical evaluation and presumptive treatment for gonorrhea and chlamydia.

6. Confidentiality is important to him because he does not want his parents to know what he did in San Francisco. If these tests cannot be offered confidentially in your office, refer him to a site (e.g., Planned Parenthood, health department) where confidentiality can be provided if state laws permit. Work out a system to contact him with the results confidentially. Either use a name that will trigger him to call the office or obtain a cell phone number to which he has exclusive access.

REFERENCES

1. Centers for Disease Control and Prevention. Summary of notifiable diseases—United States, 2003. MMWR Recomm Rep 2003; 52:7.
2. Sweet RL, Gibbs RS. Sexually transmitted diseases. In: *Infectious Diseases of the Female Genital Tract*. Philadelphia, PA: Lippincott Williams & Wilkins, 2002, pp. 122–131.

2a. Centers for Disease Control and Prevention. Sexually Transmitted Disease Surveillance, 2004. Atlanta, GA: US Department of Health and Human Services. Available from: http://www.cdc.gov/STD/stats/. Accessed Nov. 24, 2006.

 3. Miller WC, Ford CA, Morris M, et al. Prevalence of chlamydial and gonococcal infections among young adults in the United States. JAMA 2004; 291:2229–2236.

3a. Kent CK, Chaw JK, Wong W, et al. Prevalence of rectal, urethral, and pharyngeal chlamydia and gonorrhea detected in 2 clinical settings among men who have sex with men: San Francisco, California, 2003. Clin Infect Dis. 2005; 41(1):67–74.

 4. Stephenson J. Rise in drug-resistant gonorrhea cases: spurs new treatment advice for gay, bisexual men. JAMA 2004; 291:2420.

 5. Isbey SF, Alcorn TM, Davis RH, Haizlip J, Leone PA, Cohen MS. Characterisation of *Neisseria gonorrhoeae* in semen during urethral infection in men. Genitourin Med 1997; 73: 378–382.

 6. Wisdom A, Hawkins DA. In: *Diagnosis in Color: Sexually Transmitted Diseases*, 2nd Ed. St. Louis, MO: Mosby, 1997, pp. 124–129.

 7. Hooper RR, Reynolds GH, Jones OG, et al. Cohort study of venereal disease. I: the risk of gonorrhea transmission from infected women to men. Am J Epidemiol 1978; 108:136–144.

 8. Centers for Disease Control and Prevention (CDC). Self-Study STD Module—Gonorrhea, 2003. Available from: http://www2a.cdc.gov/stdtraining/self-study/default.asp. Accessed Nov. 24, 2006.

 9. Schwartz DA, Lack EE. Neisserial Infections: Gonorrhea. In: Connor DH, Chandler FW, Schwartz DA, Mantz HJ, Lack EE, eds., *Pathology of Infectious Diseases*. Stamford, CT: Appleton & Lange, 1997, 1: pp. 681–690.

10. Stenchever MA, Droegemueller W, Herbst AL, Mishell DR. *Comprehensive Gynecology*, 4th Ed. St. Louis, MO: Mosby, 2001, pp. 645.

11. Rothenberg R. Ophthalmia neonatorum due to *Neisseria gonorrhoeae*: prevention and treatment. Sex Transm Dis 1979; 6:187–191.

12. World Health Organization (WHO). Guidelines for management of sexually transmitted diseases. Geneva: WHO, 2003. Available from http://www.who.int/reproductive-health/publications/rhr_01_10mngt_stis/index.html. Accessed Nov. 24, 2006.

13. Hook EW, Hansfield HH. Gonococcal infections in adults. In: Holmes KK, Sparling PF, Mardh PA, Wiesner PJ, eds., *Sexually Transmitted Diseases*, 3rd Ed. New York, NY: McGraw-Hill, 1999, pp. 451–466.

14. Manavi K, Young H, Clutterbuck D. Sensitivity of microscopy for the rapid diagnosis of gonorrhoea in men and women and the role of *Gonorrhoea serovars*. Int J STD AIDS 2003; 14:390–394.

15. Holliman RE, Johnson JD, Davidson F. Inhibition of *Neisseria gonorrhoeae* by vaginal lubricants. Sex Transm Infect 2002; 78:468.

16. Centers for Disease Control and Prevention. Sexually transmitted diseases treatment guidelines, 2006. MMWR Recomm Rep 2006; 55(RR-11):38–42. Available from: http://www.cdc.gov/std/treatment/. Accessed Nov. 24, 2006.

17. Stary A, Kopp W, Zahel B, Nerad S, Teodorowicz L, Horting-Muller I. Comparison of DNA-probe test and culture for the detection of *Neisseria gonorrhoeae* in genital samples. Sex Transm Dis 1993; 20:243–247.

18. Van Dyck E, Ieven M, Pattyn S, Van Damme L, Laga M. Detection of *Chlamydia trachomatis* and *Neisseria gonorrhoeae* by enzyme immunoassay, culture, and three nucleic acid amplification tests. J Clin Microbiol 2001; 39:1751–1756.

19. Koumans EH, Black CM, Markowitz LE, et al. Comparison of methods for detection of *Chlamydia trachomatis* and *Neisseria gonorrhoeae* using commercially available nucleic acid amplification tests and a liquid pap smear medium. J Clin Microbiol 2003; 41:1507–1511.

20. Culler EE, Caliendo AM, Nolte FS. Reproducibility of positive test results in the BDProbeTec ET system for detection of *Chlamydia trachomatis* and *Neisseria gonorrhoeae*. J Clin Microbiol 2003; 41:3911–3914.

21. Zenilman JM, Miller WC, Gaydos C, Rogers SM, Turner CF. LCR testing for gonorrhoea and chlamydia in population surveys and other screenings of low prevalence populations: coping with decreased positive predictive value. Sex Transm Infect 2003; 79:94–97.

22. Cosentino LA, Landers DV, Hillier SL. Detection of *Chlamydia trachomatis* and *Neisseria gonorrhoeae* by strand displacement amplification and relevance of the amplification control for use with vaginal swab specimens. J Clin Microbiol 2003; 41:3592–3596.

23. Garrow SC, Smith DW, Harnett GB. The diagnosis of chlamydia, gonorrhoea, and trichomonas infections by self obtained low vaginal swabs, in remote northern Australian clinical practice. Sex Transm Infect 2002; 78:278–281.

24. Wiesenfeld HC, Lowry DL, Heine RP, et al. Self-collection of vaginal swabs for the detection of *Chlamydia*, gonorrhea, and trichomoniasis: opportunity to encourage sexually transmitted disease testing among adolescents. Sex Transm Dis 2001; 28:321–325.

25. Palusci VJ, Reeves MJ. Testing for genital gonorrhea infections in prepubertal girls with suspected sexual abuse. Pediatr Infect Dis J 2003; 22:618–623.

26. Kraut-Becher JR, Gift TL, Haddix AC, Irwin KL, Greifinger RB. Cost-effectiveness of universal screening for chlamydia and gonorrhea in US jails. J Urban Health 2004; 81:453–471.

27. Sanders SA, Reinisch JM. Would you say you "had sex" if...? JAMA 1999; 281:275–277.

28. Schuster MA, Bell RM, Kanouse DE. The sexual practices of adolescent virgins: genital sexual activities of high school students who have never had vaginal intercourse. Am J Public Health 1996; 86:1570–1576.

29. American College of Obstetricians and Gynecologists (ACOG) Committee on Adolescent Health Care. ACOG committee opinion #301: sexually transmitted diseases in adolescents. Obstet Gynecol 2004; 104:891–898.

30. Ford CA, Best D, Miller WC. Arch Pediatr Adolesc Med 2001; 155:1072–1073.

31. Centers for Disease Control and Prevention (CDC). Increases in fluoroquinolone-resistant *Neisseria gonorrhoeae* among men who have sex with men—United States, 2003, and revised recommendations for gonorrhea treatment, 2004. MMWR Morb Mortal Wkly Rep 2004; 53:335–338.

32. Kilmarx PH, Knapp JS, Xia M, et al. Intercity spread of gonococci with decreased susceptibility to fluoroquinolones: a unique focus in the United States. J Infect Dis 1998; 177:677–682.

33. Creighton S, Tenant-Flowers M, Taylor CB, Miller R, Low N. Co-infection with gonorrhoea and chlamydia: how much is there and what does it mean? Int J STD AIDS 2003; 14:109–113.

34. Lyss SB, Kamb ML, Peterman TA, et al. *Chlamydia trachomatis* among patients infected with and treated for *Neisseria gonorrhoeae* in sexually transmitted disease clinics in the United States. Ann Intern Med 2003; 139:178–185.

35. Ashton MR, Cook RL, Wiesenfeld HC, et al. Primary care physician attitudes regarding sexually transmitted diseases. Sex Transm Dis 2002; 29:246–251.

36. Payn B, Tanfer K, Billy JO, Grady WR. Men's behavior change following infection with a sexually transmitted disease. Fam Plann Perspect 1997; 29:152–157.

37. Oh MK, Cloud GA, Fleenor M, Sturdevant MS, Nesmith JD, Feinstein RA. Risk for gonococcal and chlamydial cervicitis in adolescent females: incidence and recurrence in a prospective cohort study. J Adolesc Health 1996; 18:270–275.

37a. Golden MR, Whittington WL, Handsfield HH, et al. Effect of expedited treatment of sex partners on recurrent or persistent gonorrhea or chlamydial infection. N Engl J Med. 2005; 352(7):676–685.

38. National Institute of Allergy and Infectious Diseases. Workshop summary: scientific evidence on condom effectiveness for sexually transmitted disease (STD) prevention. Washington, DC: National Institutes of Health, Department of Health Services, July 20, 2001. Available from: http://www.niaid.nih.gov/dmid/stds/condomreport.pdf. Accessed Nov. 24, 2006.

38a. Holmes KK, Levine R, Weaver M. Effectiveness of condoms in preventing sexually transmitted infections. Bull World Health Organ 2004; 82:454–461.

8

Upper Genital Tract Infections in Women

Frances E. Likis

INTRODUCTION

Female upper genital tract infections can occur in the endometrium (endometritis), uterine wall (myometritis), the uterine serosa and broad ligaments (parametritis), the fallopian tubes (salpingitis), the ovary (oophoritis), and the pelvic peritoneum (peritonitis). Because it may not be possible to identify the site of infection precisely, the term *pelvic inflammatory disease* (PID) is often used when one or more of these organs are involved. The terms *upper genital tract infections* and *PID* are used interchangeably in this chapter. Salpingitis is the most common form of PID. These infections can result from ascent of cervical sexually transmitted infections (STIs) or other pathogens or from complications of surgery. Direct medical costs of upper genital tract infections and their sequelae are estimated to be nearly $2 billion annually in the United States *(1)*.

FAST FACTS

- More than 1 million cases of upper genital tract infections occur in women each year.
- The classic clinical presentation with high fevers, extreme pain, and tenderness with obvious laboratory abnormalities is more commonly associated with gonococcal (GC) PID.
- The more prevalent form of PID is more subtle. All that is needed to diagnose PID is either cervical motion tenderness or uterine tenderness or adnexal tenderness with no other ethology.
- If a woman does not have mucopurulent cervicitis and excessive white blood cells (WBCs) on microscopic examination of vaginal secretions, the likelihood of PID is low.

From: *Current Clinical Practice: Sexually Transmitted Diseases:*
A Practical Guide for Primary Care
Edited by: A. L. Nelson and J. A. Woodward © Humana Press, Totowa, NJ

- Most cases of upper genital tract infection in women can be managed on an outpatient basis, but compliance is often suboptimal.
- The rates of PID can be reduced by screening high-risk populations for cervical infection.

PREVALENCE AND INCIDENCE

The exact incidence and prevalence of upper genital tract infections are unknown because these conditions are not reportable in every health jurisdiction. It is estimated that there are more than 1 million cases of PID in the United States per year, but this is likely an underestimate because of the number of unrecognized cases *(1)*. It has been estimated that about 150,000 surgical procedures are performed annually for complications of PID *(2)*. PID is the most common cause of gynecological hospitalizations and emergency room visits among women of reproductive age *(3,4)*.

RISK FACTORS

STI-related PID is almost exclusively seen in sexually active, reproductive-aged women and is rare in women who are not menstruating *(5)*. Younger women are at particular risk, as noted above. Other risk factors include a previous history of PID, multiple sexual partners, not using contraception (particularly not using barrier methods), living in an area with a high prevalence of STIs, bacterial vaginosis, recent onset of menses, sexual intercourse during menstruation, douching, lower socioeconomic status (SES), substance abuse, and cigarette smoking *(5–7)*. The association between douching and PID has been called into question. Currently available IUDs increase the risk of upper genital tract infections only slightly (1:1000), and only in the first few weeks of use. Prolonged IUD use (more than 5 years) has been associated with a slightly increased risk of actinomycotic PID. Risks factors vary with different gynecological surgeries, but include lower SES, obesity, immunocompromise, long duration of the procedure, shaving skin, indwelling catheter, and prolonged pre-operative hospitalization. In obstetrical cases, additional risk factors include prolonged labor, prolonged or premature rupture of membranes, and multiple vaginal exams. Surgically related infection rates may also be increased in the face of cervical infection or bacterial vaginosis.

Because teens are at highest risk for acquiring STIs involved in PID, adolescents have the highest age-specific rates of upper genital tract infections. Approximately one in eight sexually adolescent females will develop PID *(8,9)*. This high rate of PID has been attributed to behavioral and biological factors. Adolescents often have higher risk sexual practices, such as multiple or new sex partners and lack of contraceptive use, and biological factors, such as larger areas of cervical ectopy that may predispose them to some STIs. Other adolescent risk factors for

PID include having an older partner, earlier age at first sex, use of alcohol, previous suicide attempt, and a history of involvement with a child protection agency *(10)*.

ETIOLOGY

Slightly more than half of the upper genital tract infections result from STIs of the cervix that ascend to the upper tract. A portion of such infections result from surgical procedures or manipulations, such as hysterectomy, Cesarean section, dilation and curettage, and vaginal delivery. Some of these latter cases of PID may result from iatrogenic spread of STI-related cervical infections or may result from seeding of vaginal flora into the upper tract.

MICROBIOLOGY

PID is a polymicrobial infection that involves many different organisms including sexually transmitted organisms, such as *Nesseria gonorrhoeae* and *Chlamydia trachomatis*, as well as mycoplasma. In addition, aerobic and anaerobic bacteria from the vagina, such as *Bacteroides* (*Prevotella*), *Peptostreptococcus, Escherichia coli, Haemophilus influenza*, and aerobic streptococci are found in PID infections. Anaerobes and aerobes were associated with two out of three of cases of acute PID *(11)*. Other pathogens have been associated with acute salpingitis (such as cytomegalovirus and herpes simplex virus) but causation has not been verified. Although there are great similarities in the impacts of PID caused by different pathogens, different microbiological causes have different pathological processes and different clinical presentations (Fig. 1).

In order to ascend through the cervix into the endometrium, the organisms must be able to overcome the host defenses in the endocervical canal and mucous plug. Once in the endometrium, the pathogens need to survive the normal clearance mechanisms of the ciliated cells in the endometrium and fallopian tubes.

Infection of the cervix with *C. trachomatis* or *N. gonorrhoeae* or other organisms could cause breakdown of the mucous plug or cause damage to the cells in the endocervical canal, which would permit entry of vaginal and cervical pathogens into the endometrial cavity. Hormonal changes associated with the menstrual cycle have profound effects on the mucous plug. At menses, the plug is lost and microorganisms can easily gain access to upper genital tract. Retrograde flow of menses may explain the spread of pathogens from the endometrium into the fallopian tubes. At the time of ovulation, the estrogen-primed mucus may actively facilitate ascension of microbes alone or those carried by sperm. Instrumentation and/or manipulation of the cervix can cause iatrogenic spread of the pathogens into the upper genital tract.

N. gonorrhoeae generally ascends directly from the cervix into the endometrium and out into the salpinges during menses, when many important

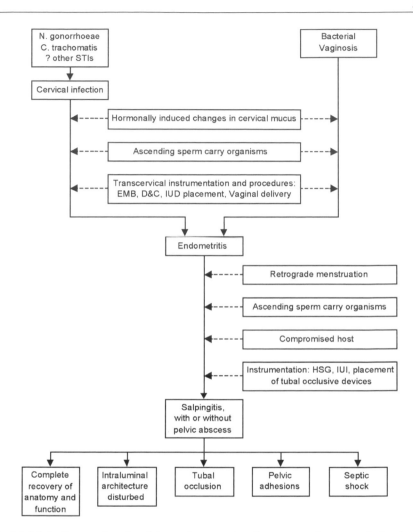

Fig. 1. Multiple factors involved in pathogenesis of upper genital tract infection and associated outcomes. (Modified from ref. *16*).

changes may facilitate such infection. The bacteriostatic features of the cervical mucus are lowest at the beginning of the menstrual cycle, and the elements in the endometrium that can protect against bacteria slough during menses. The menstrual blood flow itself is an excellent culture medium. Gonococci attach to the mucosal cells lining the endosalpinges, penetrate those cells, and cause their destruction. In fallopian tube cultures exposed to *N. gonorrhoeae*, ciliary motility is lost in 2–7 days. The fimbria of the fallopian tubes close off, causing tubal distention and architectural distortion.

C. trachomatis is also a cause of PID. After the organism ascends into the salpinges, it attaches to the tubal epithelium and is taken up into those cells by endocytosis. This permits the organism to replicate within the cells, generally protected from host defenses. In contrast to *N. gonorrhoeae*, which causes direct cellular damage, the damage caused by *C. trachomatis* is caused by the host response to the infection. Primary chlamydial infection is associated with a mild-to-moderate inflammation, which causes a cell-mediated immune response directed against the chlamydial heat shock protein 60. This causes a delayed hypersensitivity reaction, which in turn leads to destruction of the mucosal cells lining the tube—rendering the tube denuded, functionless, and possibly obstructed.

Sweet et al. have found that in one-third of women who were hospitalized for acute salpingitis, only anaerobes and aerobes could be isolated from specimens obtained by laparoscopy *(12)*. Several investigators have noted the similarity between the organisms in PID and the organisms found in bacterial vaginosis (BV). They have postulated that BV may either predispose or directly cause PID. In particular, one study of 84 patients with laparoscopically confirmed PID, 100% of the anaerobes isolated from the upper genital tract were microorganisms of BV *(13)*. Interestingly, human immunodeficiency virus (HIV)-infected women have an even higher association between PID and BV than do immunocompetent women *(14,15)*.

Actinomyces is a slowly duplicating enteric organism, which often colonizes the vagina, especially with prolonged IUD use.

Surgically related upper genital tract infection can result from iatrogenic transport of cervical infections into the endometrium, fallopian tubes, and peritoneal cavity (e.g., dilation and curettage) or from infection caused by contamination of the surgical field during laparoscopy. Interestingly, the organisms involved in these infections include the same enteric and anaerobic organism involved in STI-related PID.

INFECTIVITY AND TRANSMISSION

Upper genital tract infections that result from an infection of the cervix are primarily sexually transmitted. Of women with cervical infection with *N. gonorrhoeae*, 10–17% will develop upper genital tract infection *(16)*. With chlamydial cervicitis, the risk of PID is about 10%. Procedures, such as IUD insertion, abortion, endometrial sampling, endocervical curettage, vaginal hysterectomy, and even vaginal birth carry higher risk for infection if performed through an infected cervix.

Although PID can occur early in pregnancy, PID cannot be transmitted between a mother and her fetus or infant, but the most common causative organisms, *C. trachomatis* and *N. gonorrhoeae*, can be vertically transmitted with potentially serious sequelae. (*See* Chapters 6 and 7 for information about fetal and neonatal complications.)

CLINICAL MANIFESTATIONS

Initial symptoms and the clinical presentation of PID vary greatly by etiology. Much of what we have learned about the signs and symptoms of PID derive from GC-induced PID. In GC-induced PID, the tubal fimbriae are clubbed (closed) early in the clinical course. The lumen of the fallopian tubes fill with purulent material and become distended. The distention and inflammation cause significant pain. Symptoms usually start at the end of menses. These symptoms can include fever, chills, abdominal pain, dysuria, vaginal discharge, dyspareunia, postcoital bleeding, nausea, and vomiting. The classic picture is a woman bent forward slightly, clutching her lower abdomen, and sliding—rather than lifting—her feet to decrease the pain that walking can cause. This motion is known as the "PID shuffle." The abdominal finding of rebound tenderness mimics an acute abdomen caused by appendicitis, except it is bilateral. Pelvic exam can help make the diagnosis when the patient has bilateral cervical motion tenderness, as well as uterine and adnexal tenderness. She may have pelvic masses consistent with tubo-ovarian abscesses (TOAs). She usually has sheets of WBCs and clue cells on microscopic evaluation of her vaginal smear. Elevated WBC count and sedimentation rates are also the rule.

On the other hand, the symptoms of chlamydial PID are more insidious and subtle. They are often mild and nonspecific and can be similar to those seen numerous other gynecological, gastrointestinal, and urinary conditions. The terms "unrecognized," "subclinical," and "silent" PID are also used to refer to asymptomatic infections. These upper genital tract infections can be extremely difficult to diagnose.

When a woman is suspected to have PID, ask about recent history, previous history of sexually transmitted diseases (STDs) and PID, sexual history, and contraceptive use. Vital signs should be taken and any fever noted. Observe the woman for visible evidence of pain, such as the change in gait described previously. Complete abdominal and pelvic exams should be performed with particular attention to areas of palpable tenderness. On bimanual exam, assess for cervical motion tenderness (CMT) by grasping the cervix between your fingers and moving it from side to side. A classic finding on exam with gonorrheal PID is known as the "chandelier" sign. This is severe CMT that causes the woman to leap from the table toward the ceiling; although it is highly unlikely one would find a chandelier in a modern exam room. CMT with chlamydial PID is less impressive. Be certain to examine the upper right quadrant of the abdomen and to carefully palpate the adnexae for masses in order to assess for Fitz-Hugh-Curtis syndrome and tubo-ovarian absess respectively (these conditions are discussed in the section "Complications").

TESTING TECHNIQUES

There is no single laboratory test that can be used to detect upper genital tract infections. Testing for cervical chlamydia and gonorrhea should be performed (*see* Chapters 6 and 7 for testing techniques), but negative results do not rule out their presence in the upper genital tract. Other laboratory tests that are commonly performed include the wet mount, erythrocyte sedimentation rate (ESR), C-reactive protein(CRP), and WBC count. The examination of vaginal secretions for WBCs using a saline wet mount has demonstrated high sensitivity (78–90.9%) and negative predictive value (94.5%), but low specificity (26.3%) and low positive predictive value (17.1%) *(17,18)*. An elevated ESR has 75–81% sensitivity and 25–57% specificity, whereas an elevated CRP has 74–92% sensitivity and 50–90% specificity *(19)*. Less than 50% of women with PID have an elevated WBC count; this test may support the diagnosis but is not a necessary for diagnosing PID *(5,20)*.

Procedures that can be used in the evaluation of upper genital tract infections are ultrasound, magnetic resonance imaging (MRI), endometrial biopsy, and laparoscopy. Transvaginal ultrasound is specific (67–97%) but not sensitive (30–32%) for the diagnosis of PID *(21,22)*. It is helpful in visualizing abscesses and ruling out other pelvic pathology. One study demonstrated superior sensitivity (95%) and specificity (89%) of MRI in a comparison with ultrasound *(23)*. Endometrial biopsy has sensitivity as high as 92% and specificity as high as 87% *(24)*, but the time required to obtain the results makes this test impractical on a routine basis. Laparoscopy is considered the gold standard for the diagnosis of upper genital tract infections, but its use is limited by the cost and invasive nature of the procedure.

DIAGNOSIS

The differential diagnosis for severe, symptomatic PID includes acute surgical emergencies, such as appendicitis, torsion, or ruptured endometrioma, and serious bowel and genitourinary problems such as diverticulitis, renal calculi, cystitis, or severe constipation. Other gynecological pathology, such as ectopic pregnancy, septic abortion, ruptured hemorrhagic corpus luteum cyst, endometriosis, or necrosing leiomyoma must be considered. In older women, consideration must be given to superinfection of an underlying neoplasm, especially carcinoma. For this reason, the first step in diagnosing PID is to rule out these other conditions by history and physical findings. Basic laboratory tests, such as a urinalysis or urine pregnancy test are quite useful. Occasionally, imaging studies may be needed. Ultrasound is particularly helpful in ruling out adnexal torsion, ovarian masses, and appendicitis.

Often, however, PID presents with subtle symptoms. Upper genital tract infections are usually diagnosed clinically using the criteria found in Table 1.

Table 1
Criteria for Diagnosis of PID (CDC, 2006)

Minimum criteria (at least one of the following):

- Cervical motion tenderness.
- Uterine tenderness.
- Adnexal tenderness.

Additional criteria:

- Oral temperature over 101°F (38.3°C).
- Abnormal cervical or vaginal mucopurulent discharge.
- Presence of abundant numbers of white blood cells (WBCs) on saline microscopy of vaginal secretions.
- Elevated erythrocyte sedimentation rate.
- Elevated C-reactive protein.
- Laboratory documentation of cervical infection with *N. gonorrhoeae* or *C. trachomatis.*

Other:

Most women with PID have either mucopurulent cervical discharge or evidence of WBCs on a microscopic evaluation of a saline preparation of vaginal fluid. If the cervical discharge appears normal and no WBCs are found on the wet prep, the diagnosis of PID is unlikely, and alternative causes of pain should be investigated.

The most specific criteria for diagnosing PID include the following:

- Endometrial biopsy with histopathological evidence of endometritis.
- Transvaginal sonography or magnetic resonance imaging techniques showing thickened, fluid-filled tubes with or without free pelvic fluid or tubo-ovarian complex.
- Laparoscopic abnormalities consistent with PID.

A diagnostic evaluation that includes some of these more extensive studies may be warranted in certain cases.

PID, pelvic inflammatory disease; CDC, Centers for Disease Control and Prevention. Source: From ref. *20.*

The physical findings needed to diagnose PID are minimal. All that is needed to make the diagnosis is either CMT or adnexal tenderness or uterine tenderness without other etiology. The reason that the threshold for diagnosis is set so low is that the symptoms of tubal infection can be subtle, however, the damage done by untreated infection can be extensive. The Centers for Disease Control and Prevention (CDC) cautions that if the patient's cervix appears normal and abundant numbers of WBCs are not found in microscopic evaluation of a vaginal specimen, the diagnosis of PID is unlikely and alternate causes of pain should be assessed. Most of the diagnostic effort is spent in ruling out other etiologies, especially in lower risk women. The diagnosis of PID can be made more securely if additional criteria are met, including fever, elevated sedimentation rate, or laboratory documentation of cervical infection *N. gonorrhoeae* or *C. trachomatis*. Requiring multiple findings to make the diagnosis may improve the positive predictive value of the diagnosis (by excluding those who do not have PID), but it will reduce the overall sensitivity of diagnosis (by reducing the numbers of women who have PID being diagnosed with that condition).

The most specific criteria for the diagnosis of PID are endometrial biopsy with histopathological evidence of endometritis; transvaginal sonography or MRI techniques showing thickened, fluid-filled tubes with or without free pelvic fluid or tubo-ovarian complex; and laparoscopic abnormalities consistent with PID *(20)*. These methods of diagnosis are not used routinely but may be warranted in certain circumstances, such as treatment failure.

Providers are now urged to have a low threshold for diagnosis *(20)*. A recent prospective cohort study of incarcerated adolescents at high risk for STDs found that using the diagnostic criteria listed in Table 1 doubled the prevalence and more than tripled the incidence of PID, as compared with diagnosis with the old criteria *(25)*. This must be balanced, however, with the recognition that many of these cases may be overdiagnosed. The CDC notes that the positive predictive value of clinical diagnosis of PID depends on the population and practice setting and ranges from 65 to 90% compared with laparoscopy *(20)*. In some instances, the accuracy of clinical diagnosis is even lower. In one study of women diagnosed clinically as having recurrent PID, only 30% of the cases were found to have PID at the time of laparoscopy. The most common finding was a normal pelvis *(26)*.

TREATMENT

Treatment for upper genital tract infections must be effective against the broad spectrum of microbiological etiologies. Most importantly, both enteric organisms (e.g., *E. coli*) and anaerobic pathogens must be covered. Early studies with animal models showed that in untreated cases septic shock was a common manifestation; survivors were noted to have pelvic abscesses. Treatment directed against the enteric organisms alone prevented septic shock, but not the abscess formation. Treatment against anaerobic organism did not prevent sepsis but reduced abscesses. Thus, a two-pronged approach is necessary.

Most cases of PID are now treated on an outpatient basis with close follow-up. A randomized controlled trial of 831 women with mild to moderate PID found no difference in short-term improvement and long-term reproductive outcomes (e.g., pregnancy rates, PID recurrence, chronic pelvic pain, and ectopic pregnancy) between those treated in inpatient and outpatient settings *(27)*.

Table 2
Oral Outpatient Treatments for Pelvic Inflammatory
Disease [a] CDC STD Treatment Guidelines 2006

Oral regimen A	
Levofloxacin [c,d,e]	500 mg orally once daily for 14 days
Or	
Ofloxacin [c,d,e]	400 mg orally twice a day for 14 days
With or without	
Metronidazole [f]	500 mg orally twice a day for 14 days

Oral regimen B	
Ceftriaxone [b,c]	250 mg IM in a single dose
Or	
Ccfoxitin	1 g orally administered concurrently in a single dose
And	
Probenecid	1 g orally administered
Or	
Other parenteral third-generation cephalosporin (e.g., ceftizoxime or cefotaxime)	
Plus Doxycycline [b]	100 mg orally twice a day for 14 days
With or without	
Metronidazole [f]	500 mg orally twice a day for 14 days

Oral regimen follow-up	
A follow-up examination should be performed within 72 hours. If the patient has not improved, hospitalization for parenteral therapy and further evaluation are recommended.	

CDC, Centers for Disease Control and Prevention; STD, sexually transmitted disease. Source: From ref. *20*.

[a] Because of the high risk for maternal morbidity, fetal loss and abortion, and preterm delivery, pregnant women who have suspected PID should be hospitalized and treated with parenteral antibiotics.

[b] Ceftriaxone may treat incubating syphilis.

[c] Safety and efficacy among pregnant and lactating women have not been established (pregnancy category B).

[d] Quinolones should not be used for infections. Quinolones should not be used in MSM or persons with a history of recent foreign travel or partner's travel, infections acquired in California or Hawaii, or infections acquired in other areas with increased QRNG prevalence.

[e] Ofloxacin and levofloxacin provide coverage for both *N. gonorrhoeae* and *C. trachomatis*, except as noted above.

[f] Patients should be advised to avoid consuming alcohol during treatment with metronidazole and for 24 hours thereafter.

Outpatient treatment recommendations with oral therapies for PID can be found in Table 2. Some clinical conditions require hospitalization (*see* Table 3) and parenteral therapy (*see* Table 4). Parenteral therapy can be discontinued 24 hours after a patient improves clinically. The patient should then be given oral antibiotics to complete a 14-day treatment. Treatment recommendations are subject to change as new evidence becomes available. The most current edition

Table 3
Criteria for Hospitalization of Women With PID (CDC, 2006)

- Surgical emergencies (e.g., appendicitis) cannot be excluded.
- The patient is pregnant.
- The patient does not respond clinically to oral antimicrobial therapy.
- The patient is unable to follow or tolerate an outpatient oral regimen.
- The patient has severe illness, nausea and vomiting, or high fever.
- The patient has a tubo-ovarian abscess.

CDC, Centers for Disease Control and Prevention; PID, pelvic inflammatory disease. Source: From ref. 20.

of the CDC STD treatment guidelines should be consulted when developing a management plan for PID. IUD users with PID may be treated with IUD in place.

It is important to encourage women to initiate and complete the entire course of antibiotic therapy. One study in a public hospital emergency room found that less than 72% of women filled their prescriptions within 48 hours and only 31% took all their antibiotics for the recommended treatment period (28). Surgical therapies are recommended only for those who do not respond to medical therapy (see Short-Term Complication section).

PREGNANCY-RELATED ISSUES

The cervical mucous plug that forms during pregnancy provides some protection from upper genital tract infections. When PID does occur during pregnancy, there is a high risk for maternal morbidity, spontaneous abortion, stillbirth, and preterm birth. Therefore, hospitalization and parenteral antibiotics are recommended (20). The parenteral regimens for treatment can be found in Table 4. As with any pharmacological treatment during pregnancy, medications with the least teratogenic potential should be selected.

PARTNER NOTIFICATION
AND REPORTING REQUIREMENTS

Male partners of women who have PID should be examined and treated presumptively on an epidemiological basis. Gonorrheal and chlamydial infections are common in these men, even though they are likely to be asymptomatic (29). It is recommended that all sex contacts in the previous 60 days be treated with regimens that are effective against both *N. gonorrhoeae* and *C. trachomatis*, regardless of the etiology of the woman's infection (20). The likelihood of asymptomatic infection necessitates careful explanation of why treatment is important because male partners may not feel it is necessary to take medication

Table 4
Parenteral Treatments for Pelvic Inflammatory Disease (PID)[a]
CDC STD Treatment Guidelines 2006

Parenteral regimen A

Cefotetan	2 g IV every 12 hours
Or	
Cefoxitin	2 g IV every 6 hours plus
Plus Doxycycline	100 mg orally or IV every 12 hours [b]

Note: Parenteral therapy may be discontinued 24 hours after a patient improves clinically, and oral therapy with doxycycline[b] (100 mg twice a day) should continue to complete 14 days of therapy. When tubo-ovarian abscess (TOA) is present, many health care providers use clindamycin or metronidazole with doxycycline for continued therapy rather than doxycycline alone to provide more effective anaerobic coverage.

Parenteral regimen B

Clindamycin	900 mg IV every 8 hours
Plus Gentamicin	Loading dose IV or IM (2 mg/kg of body weight) followed by a maintenance dose (1.5 mg/kg) every 8 hours. Single daily dosing may be substituted.

Note: Parenteral therapy can be discontinued 24 hours after a patient improves clinically and continuing oral therapy should consist of doxycycline [b] 100 mg orally twice a day or clindamycin 450 mg orally four times a day to complete a total of 14 days of therapy. When TOA is present, many health care providers use clindamycin for continued therapy rather than doxycycline to provide more effective anaerobic coverage.

Alternative parenteral regimens

Levofloxacin [c,d,e]	500 mg orally once daily for 14 days
Or	
Ofloxacin [c,d,e]	400 mg orally twice a day for 14 days
Or	
Ampicillin/sulbactam	3 g IV every 6 hours plus
Plus Doxycycline [b]	100 mg orally or IV every 12 hours
With or without	
Metronidazole[f]	500 mg orally twice a day for 14 days

Note: Parenteral therapy can be discontinued 24 hours after a patient improves clinically, and oral therapy should be given with the agents listed in either parenteral regimen A or B to complete 14 days of therapy.

CDC, Centers for Disease Control and Prevention; STD, sexually transmitted disease.

[a] Because of the high risk for maternal morbidity, fetal loss or abortion, and preterm delivery, pregnant women who have suspected PID should be hospitalized and treated with parenteral antibiotics.

[b] Contraindicated for pregnant and lactating women and for children under 8 years old.

[c] Contraindicated for pregnant and lactating women.

[d] Quinolones should not be used for infections. Quinolones should not be used in MSM or persons with a history of recent foreign travel or partner's travel, infections acquired in California or Hawaii, or infections acquired in other areas with increased QRNG prevalence.

[e] Ofloxacin and levofloxacin provide coverage for both *N. gonorrhoeae* and *C. trachomatis*, except as noted above.

[f] Patients should be advised to avoid consuming alcohol during treatment with metronidazole and for 24 hours thereafter.

if they are not experiencing symptoms themselves. General STI prevention education is also warranted. In some health districts, PID is a reportable disease.

FOLLOW-UP

Women should have clinical improvement, including defervescence, reduced abdominal tenderness, and reduced uterine, adnexal, and cervical motion tenderness, within 3 days of beginning treatment. Women receiving outpatient treatment should have a follow-up examination within 48–72 hours to verify that they have initiated antibiotic therapy and started to improve clinically. If there is no improvement, hospitalization is recommended for parenteral therapy and further evaluation. Women who have had *C. trachomatis* should be rescreened at 3–4 months, especially if they are adolescents.

RECURRENCE OF DISEASE

Approximately 25% of women experience recurrence of PID *(5)*. Recurrent infections increase the likelihood of long-term sequelae. For these reasons, it is crucial to educate women diagnosed with PID about STD prevention. Condom use after an episode of PID decreases the risk not only of recurrence, but also of subsequent pelvic pain and infertility *(30)*.

COMPLICATIONS

Upper genital tract infections are associated with numerous short- and long-term sequelae that can cause both morbidity and mortality. The potential short-term complications are TOAs and Fitz-Hugh-Curtis syndrome. One in four women with PID experiences long-term complications, which include infertility, ectopic pregnancy, and chronic pelvic pain. These long-term sequelae are associated with both physical and emotional distress and are the leading cause of non-HIV STD morbidity in the United States *(31)*. In addition, they are the source of significant health care costs *(1,31)*.

Short-Term Complications

Tubo-Ovarian Abscess

Pelvic TOA is an inflammatory mass of the fallopian tube and ovary that often involves adjacent structures, such as the bowel and pelvic peritoneum. These pelvic abscesses are usually bilateral. The exact incidence of pelvic abscess is unknown, but it has been reported in as many as one-third of women who were hospitalized with PID *(32)*. Higher rates of TOA have recently been reported in women with stage III and IV endometriosis *(33)*. Pelvic abscesses are usually polymicrobial and contain anaerobic organisms. It is rare to culture *N. gonorrhoeae* and *C. trachomatis* from the actual abscess. The clinical presentation of pelvic abscesses is similar to that of the other upper genital tract infections and does not necessarily cause more severe symptoms than uncomplicated PID. An adnexal mass may or may not be palpable on exam, but ultrasound can be helpful in making the diagnosis. Parenteral therapy is required for treatment of pelvic abscess; patients must be hospitalized for at least 24 hours after they respond clinically to therapy. After discharge from hospital, they require continued oral therapy for a total of 14 days of antibiotic therapy. Clindamycin is generally indicated in lieu of doxycycline to provide better coverage for anaerobic organisms with oral therapies (20).

For infections that are resistant to parenteral therapy, surgical procedures traditionally have been recommended. The surgeries have varied from surgical incision and drainage to salpingo-oophorectomy to complete "pelvic sweep" with removal of the uterus, fallopian tubes, and ovaries, the most frequently performed procedure (34). Rupture of an abscesses can provide temporary symptom relief, but is followed by acute onset of peritonitis and septic shock; it requires immediate surgical intervention. Each of these surgeries is much more complicated and associated with higher risk for surgical complication when it is performed while the pelvis is infected than when the surgical field is not acutely inflamed (34). Investigators have demonstrated the safety of aspirating the abscesses under radiographic guidance when medical therapy alone has failed (35,36). Real-time ultrasound-guided transvaginal and transrectal aspiration of the abscess and continued antibiotic therapy cured about 90% of these women and eliminated their need for immediate surgery (37,38). Others have demonstrated that computed tomography (CT)-guided procedures are also feasible although they are associated with greater discomfort and radiation exposure. Increasing age is associated with antibiotic therapy failure requiring surgical intervention (39).

A special case of pelvic abscess is the actinomycoses-related abscess. This is a relatively rare occurrence, but may present with unilateral TOA. Diagnosis may be suspected if IUD scrapings have sulfur granules on cytological exam. Abscesses may be unilateral. The infection can spread throughout the abdominal cavity and form multiple abscesses, which can cause life-threatening bowel obstruction. Medical therapy for this infection differs from other types of pelvic abscesses. The cornerstone of therapy is high-dose penicillin, which may need to be continued for 30 days, because Actinomyces is a slow-growing organism.

FITZ-HUGH-CURTIS SYNDROME

Fitz-Hugh-Curtis syndrome or perihepatitis occurs in 4–14% percent of adult women with upper genital tract infections and is associated with both *C. trachomatis* and *N. gonorrhoeae* (40). One study of adolescents with salpingitis found a higher rate (27%) rate of this condition than reported in studies of adults (41). The cause of the liver capsule inflammation of Fitz-Hugh-Curtis syndrome is not well understood, but the most likely theories are the spread of organisms via the peritoneum or an exaggerated immune response to *C. trachomatis*. The primary symptom of Fitz-Hugh-Curtis syndrome is right upper quadrant pain that may be referred to the right arm or shoulder. Symptoms of PID are usually present. Other associated symptoms include nausea, vomiting, fever, chills, night sweats, malaise, and headache. Physical examination reveals marked tenderness of the right upper quadrant that may be accompanied by guarding, splinting, and a friction rub along the anterior costal margin. In addition to history and physical examination, diagnostic imaging and laboratory tests may be helpful in establishing the diagnosis and ruling out other etiologies for the pain. Abnormalities on examination with both ultrasonography and CT have been reported with Fitz-Hugh-Curtis syndrome. The liver enzymes are typically normal or minimally elevated, and the ESR and WBC count may be normal or elevated *(42)*. Definitive diagnosis is made by laparoscopy, but surgery is not necessary unless treatment is ineffective. The treatment regimens for PID (*see* Tables 2 and 4) are also used for Fitz-Hugh-Curtis syndrome, and the same criteria should be used to determine the need for inpatient treatment (Table 3). Typically, Fitz-Hugh-Curtis syndrome resolves without sequelae, but it can result in perihepatic adhesions requiring lysis for pain relief.

Long-Term Complications

Infertility can result from tubal occlusion and tubal, ovarian, and perihepatic adhesions caused by upper genital tract infections. Westrom et al. *(43)* found that the risk of tubal factor infertility increased with subsequent episodes of PID and ranged from 8% after one episode to 40% after three episodes. A smaller study demonstrated a 40% rate of infertility after a single episode of PID *(44)*. In addition to the number of episodes, severity of disease also affects fertility. A prospective cohort study found that the cumulative proportion of women with a live birth 12 years after PID was 90% for women with mild disease, 82% for women with moderate disease, and 57% for women with severe disease *(45)*. Evidence of prior untreated upper genital tract infection—as demonstrated by laparoscopy, tissue culture, direct antigen detection, or serology—is found in many women who do not report a history of upper genital tract infections or symptoms *(11,46–50)*. Most women with PID consider future infertility to be a significant issue *(51)*.

Ectopic pregnancy after upper genital tract infections occurs because of tubal damage. The rate of ectopic pregnancy is increased 7- to 10-fold in women with a history of PID *(9,52)*. Westrom et al. *(43)* found ectopic pregnancy rates of 9.1% among women who had a history of salpingitis and 1.4% among controls. Reduction in the incidence of PID is strongly associated with a subsequent decrease in ectopic pregnancies *(53)*. Ectopic pregnancy can result in maternal mortality and is associated with future recurrences and infertility.

Chronic pelvic pain is usually defined as pain that has lasted 6 months or more. One-fifth to one-third of women with PID will experience chronic pelvic pain later in life *(30,54)*. The exact mechanisms that cause chronic pelvic pain after upper genital tract infections are unknown *(55)*. A follow-up study of women hospitalized with PID found that these women were much more likely to have subsequent hospitalizations for abdominal pain, gynecological pain, endometriosis, and hysterectomy than were women without a history of PID *(56)*. Women with chronic pelvic pain after PID report reductions in both their mental and physical health *(57)*.

More recently, the PID Evaluation and Clinical Health study found that with clinically suspected mild to moderate PID treated with standard antibiotics, upper genital tract infection was not associated with increases in chronic pelvic pain or recurrent PID *(58)*.

POTENTIAL FOR VACCINES AND OTHER PREVENTIVE AND/OR THERAPEUTIC MEASURES

Primary prevention of PID is achieved by the same strategies used for other STDs, such as the use of barrier contraceptives and limiting the number of sexual partners. The evidence regarding the ability of hormonal contraceptive methods to prevent upper genital tract infections is conflicting. Combined oral contraceptives (OCs) have shown a protective effect in some studies but not in others *(59)*. The consensus is that OCs reduce the risk of hospitalization with gonorrhea-related PID. Progestin-only contraceptives (i.e., pills, injections, implants, and the levonorgestrel IUD) thicken the cervical mucus and could theoretically decrease the risk of PID, but demonstration of this effect has not been consistent in clinical trials *(59–61)*.

Secondary prevention of upper genital tract infections involves attempts to prevent lower genital tract infections from ascending. Early detection and treatment of chlamydial and gonorrheal infections can reduce the risk of PID by more than 50% *(20,62)*. Appropriate screening for gonorrhea and chlamydia is imperative, and the importance of treatment and follow-up should be stressed to patients diagnosed with these infections. The association of bacterial vaginosis with PID makes it theoretically plausible that identification and treatment of this condition could prevent PID, however, there are no studies to date that support this proposition *(20)*.

Tertiary prevention calls for prompt diagnosis of STI and PID, effective therapy, and treatment of sex partners. Another important component is to achieve good patient compliance with therapy for cervicitis to prevent the development of PID *(63)*. Educating patients about PID is crucial as demonstrated by a study that found 33% of the participants were unaware of the condition and more than 75% could not identify the associated subsequent sequelae *(64)*.

CASE STUDY

Paula is a 17-year-old who is recalled to your office because routine screening revealed that she has chlamydial cervicitis. Her last menstrual period was about 32 days earlier. She reports she has noticed postcoital spotting since her Pap smear and has had some deep-thrust dyspareunia. She denies any fever, chills, or significant pelvic pain. On exam, she is noted to have some mild CMT and uterine tenderness but no pronounced adnexal tenderness or obvious masses. Her vaginal wet mount reveals numerous leukocytes and clue cells.

Questions

1. What is in your differential diagnosis?
2. Are there any other tests you want to order?
3. Should ultrasound imaging of her pelvis be performed?
4. What treatment do you want to prescribe?
5. What follow-up is needed and why?
6. Does her infection need to be reported to the local health department?
7. What about her former partner(s)?

Answers

1. Although upper tract infection is the most likely diagnosed, other etiologies of her symptoms must be ruled out. She may have an early pregnancy complicated by her chlamydial cervicitis or an ectopic pregnancy. Other causes such as a persistent corpus luteum cyst may have delayed her menses, but have been ruled out by the digital examination. A urinalysis may help to rule out cystitis as a cause of her deep-thrust dyspareunia.
2. The most important test needed is a sensitive urine pregnancy test. She has no gastrointestinal complaints or upper right quadrant pain, so liver function tests are not needed. A baseline complete blood count is not needed because a normal white blood count would not rule out PID. Similarly, ESR is not necessary and does not contribute to her diagnosis. Tests for other STIs are very important. She should be offered HIV testing (unless she had the test within the month), and hepatitis B virus (HBV) surface antigen test (unless she has previously been vaccinated). If she to lives in an area of high prevalence of syphilis, a reactive plasma reagin (RPR) should also be drawn.
3. There is no indication for an ultrasound study at the time. If she were pregnant, the location of the pregnancy cannot be determined this early. There was no suggestion of pelvic masses that need better characterization.
4. She should be offered outpatient management for her PID. She may also need HBV vaccination. She will need condoms and counseling about avoiding risky sex. She should be counseled about the long-term potential complications of her infection including infertility, ectopic pregnancy, and pain. She should avoid sexual contact unless she and her partners have completed therapy.

5. She should return in 48–73 hours to confirm she is taking and responding to her antibiotic therapy. She also needs to be retested for chlamydia in 3–4 months.
6. Many local health departments list PID as a separate disease.
7. Her sex contacts in the last 60 days need to be treated for chlamydia and tested for other STIs. The partners who are not HBV vaccinated should be offered immunization.

REFERENCES

1. Rein DB, Kassler WJ, Irwin KL, Rabiee L. Direct medical cost of pelvic inflammatory disease and its sequelae: decreasing, but still substantial. Obstet Gynecol 2000; 95:397–402.
2. Washington AE, Cates W Jr, Zaidi AA. Hospitalizations for pelvic inflammatory disease. Epidemiology and trends in the United States, 1975 to 1981. JAMA 1984; 251:2529–2533.
3. Velebil P, Wingo PA, Xia Z, Wilcox LS, Peterson HB. Rate of hospitalization for gynecologic disorders among reproductive-age women in the United States. Obstet Gynecol 1995; 86:764–769.
4. Curtis KM, Hillis SD, Kieke BA Jr, Brett KM, Marchbanks PA, Peterson HB. Visits to emergency departments for gynecologic disorders in the United States, 1992–1994. Obstet Gynecol 1998; 91:1007–1012.
5. Stenchever MA, Droegemueller W, Herbst AL, Mishell DR. Infections of the upper genital tract: endometritis, acute and chronic salpingitis. In: *Comprehensive Gynecology*, 4th Ed. St. Louis, MO: Mosby, 2001, pp.707–739.
6. Beigi RH, Wiesenfeld HC. Pelvic inflammatory disease: new diagnostic criteria and treatment. Obstet Gynecol Clin North Am 2003; 30:777–793.
7. Dallabetta G, Kamenga MC, Field ML. Infections of the female pelvis including septic abortion. In: Cohen J, Powderly WG, Berkley SF, et al., eds. *Infectious Diseases*, 2nd Ed. Edinburgh, Scotland: Mosby, 2004, pp. 693–700.
8. Bell TA, Holmes KK. Age-specific risks of syphilis, gonorrhea, and hospitalized pelvic inflammatory disease in sexually experienced U. S. women. Sex Transm Dis 1984; 11:291–295.
9. Westrom L. Incidence, prevalence, and trends of acute pelvic inflammatory disease and its consequences in industrialized countries. Am J Obstet Gynecol 1980; 138:880–892.
10. Suss AL, Homel P, Hammerschlag M, Bromberg K. Risk factors for pelvic inflammatory disease in inner-city adolescents. Sex Transm Dis 2000; 27:289–291.
11. Thejls H, Gnarpe J, Lundkvist O, Heimer G, Larsson G, Victor A. Diagnosis and prevalence of persistent chlamydia infection in infertile women: tissue culture, direct antigen detection, and serology. Fertil Steril 1991; 55:304–310.
12. Sweet RL, Gibbs RS. *Infectious Diseases of the Female Genital Tract*, 4th Ed. Philadelphia, PA: Lippincott Williams & Wilkins, 2002.
13. Soper DE, Brockwell NJ, Dalton HP, Johnson D. Observations concerning the microbial etiology of acute salpingitis. Am J Obstet Gynecol 1994; 170:1008–1017.
14. Bukusi EA, Cohen CR, Stevens CE, et al. Effects of human immunodeficiency virus 1 infection on microbial origins of pelvic inflammatory disease and on efficacy of ambulatory oral therapy. Am J Obstet Gynecol 1999; 181:1374–1381.
15. Hillier SL, Kiviat NB, Hawes SE, et al. Role of bacterial vaginosis-associated microorganisms in endometritis. Am J Obstet Gynecol 1996; 175:435–441.
16. Sweet RL, Gibbs RS. Pelvic Inflammatory disease. In: *Infectious Diseases of the Female Genital Tract*, 4th Ed. Philadelphia, PA: Lippincott Williams & Wilkins, 2002, pp. 368–412.
17. Peipert JF, Boardman L, Hogan JW, Sung J, Mayer KH. Laboratory evaluation of acute upper genital tract infection. Obstet Gynecol 1996; 87:730–736.

18. Yudin MH, Hillier SL, Wiesenfeld HC, Krohn MA, Amortegui AA, Sweet RL. Vaginal poly-morphonuclear leukocytes and bacterial vaginosis as markers for histologic endometritis among women without symptoms of pelvic inflammatory disease. Am J Obstet Gynecol 2003; 188: 318–323.

19. Kahn JG, Walker CK, Washington AE, Landers DV, Sweet RL. Diagnosing pelvic inflam-matory disease. A comprehensive analysis and considerations for developing a new model. JAMA 1991; 266:2594–2604.

20. Centers for Disease Control and Prevention. Sexually transmitted diseases treatment guide-lines, 2006. MMWR Recomm Rep 2006; 55(RR-11):56–61. Available from: http://www. cdc.gov/std/treatment/. Accesssed Nov. 24, 2006.

21. Boardman LA, Peipert JF, Brody JM, Cooper AS, Sung J. Endovaginal sonography for the diagnosis of upper genital tract infection. Obstet Gynecol 1997; 90:54–57.

22. Gaitan H, Angel E, Diaz R, Parada A, Sanchez L, Vargas C. Accuracy of five different diagnostic techniques in mild-to-moderate pelvic inflammatory disease. Infect Dis Obstet Gynecol 2002; 10:171–180.

23. Tukeva TA, Aronen HJ, Karjalainen PT, Molander P, Paavonen T, Paavonen J. MR imaging in pelvic inflammatory disease: comparison with laparoscopy and US. Radiology 1999; 210: 209–216.

24. Kiviat NB, Wolner-Hanssen P, Eschenbach DA, et al. Endometrial histopathology in patients with culture-proved upper genital tract infection and laparoscopically diagnosed acute salpin-gitis. Am J Surg Pathol 1990; 14:167–175.

25. Risser WL, Cromwell PF, Bortot AT, Risser JM. Impact of new diagnostic criteria on the prevalence and incidence of pelvic inflammatory disease. J Pediatr Adolesc Gynecol 2004; 17: 39–44.

26. Cibula D, Kuzel D, Fucikova Z, Svabik K, Zivny J. Acute exacerbation of recurrent pelvic inflammatory disease. Laparoscopic findings in 141 women with a clinical diagnosis. J Reprod Med 2001; 46:49–53.

27. Ness RB, Soper DE, Holley RL, et al. Effectiveness of inpatient and outpatient treatment strategies for women with pelvic inflammatory disease: results from the Pelvic Inflammatory Disease Evaluation and Clinical Health (PEACH) Randomized Trial. Am J Obstet Gynecol 2002; 186:929–937.

28. Brookoff D. Compliance with doxycycline therapy for outpatient treatment of pelvic inflam-matory disease. South Med J 1994; 87:1088–1091.

29. Kamwendo F, Johansson E, Moi H, Forslin L, Danielsson D. Gonorrhea, genital chlamydial infection, and nonspecific urethritis in male partners of women hospitalized and treated for acute pelvic inflammatory disease. Sex Transm Dis 1993; 20:143–146.

30. Ness RB, Randall H, Richter HE, et al. Condom use and the risk of recurrent pelvic inflam-matory disease, chronic pelvic pain, or infertility following an episode of pelvic inflamma-tory disease. Am J Public Health 2004; 94:1327–1329.

31. Yeh JM, Hook EW 3rd, Goldie SJ. A refined estimate of the average lifetime cost of pelvic inflammatory disease. Sex Transm Dis 2003; 30:369–378.

32. Landers DV, Sweet RL. Current trends in the diagnosis and treatment of tuboovarian abscess. Am J Obstet Gynecol 1985; 151:1098–1110.

33. Chen MJ, Yang JH, Yang YS, Ho HN. Increased occurrence of tubo-ovarian abscesses in women with stage III and IV endometriosis. Fertil Steril 2004; 82:498–499.

34. Hager WD. Follow-up of patients with tubo-ovarian abscess(es) in association with salpin-gitis. Obstet Gynecol 1983; 61:680–684.

35. Perez-Medina T, Huertas MA, Bajo JM. Early ultrasound-guided transvaginal drainage of tubo-ovarian abscesses: a randomized study. Ultrasound Obstet Gynecol 1996; 7:435–438.

36. Corsi PJ, Johnson SC, Gonik B, Hendrix SL, McNeeley SG Jr, Diamond MP. Transvaginal ultrasound-guided aspiration of pelvic abscesses. Infect Dis Obstet Gynecol 1999; 7:216–221.

37. Nelson AL, Sinow RM, Renslo R, Renslo J, Atamdede F. Related Articles, Endovaginal ultrasonographically guided transvaginal drainage for treatment of pelvic abscesses. Am J Obstet Gynecol 1995; 172:1926–1932.

38. Nelson AL, Sinow RM, Oliak D. Transrectal ultrasonographically guided drainage of gynecologic pelvic abscesses. Am J Obstet Gynecol 2000; 182:1382–1388.

39. Halperin R, Levinson O, Yaron M, Bukovsky I, Schneider D. Tubo-ovarian abscess in older women: is the woman's age a risk factor for failed response to conservative treatment? Gynecol Obstet Invest 2003; 55:211–215.

40. Wang SP, Eschenbach DA, Holmes KK, Wager G, Grayston JT. *Chlamydia trachomatis* infection in Fitz-Hugh-Curtis syndrome. Am J Obstet Gynecol 1980; 138:1034–1038.

41. Litt IF, Cohen MI. Perihepatitis associated with salpingitis in adolescents. JAMA 1978; 240:1253–1254.

42. Peter NG, Clark LR, Jaeger JR. Fitz-Hugh-Curtis syndrome: a diagnosis to consider in women with right upper quadrant pain. Cleve Clin J Med 2004; 71:233–239.

43. Westrom L, Joesoef R, Reynolds G, Hagdu A, Thompson SE. Pelvic inflammatory disease and fertility. A cohort study of 1,844 women with laparoscopically verified disease and 657 control women with normal laparoscopic results. Sex Transm Dis 1992; 19:185–192.

44. Pavletic AJ, Wolner-Hanssen P, Paavonen J, Hawes SE, Eschenbach DA. Infertility following pelvic inflammatory disease. Infect Dis Obstet Gynecol 1999; 7:145–152.

45 Lepine LA, Hillis SD, Marchbanks PA, Joesoef MR, Peterson HB, Westrom L. Severity of pelvic inflammatory disease as a predictor of the probability of live birth. Am J Obstet Gynecol 1998; 178:977–981.

46. Hubacher D, Grimes D, Lara-Ricalde R, de la Jara J, Garcia-Luna A. The limited clinical usefulness of taking a history in the evaluation of women with tubal factor infertility. Fertil Steril 2004; 81:6–10.

47. Miettinen A, Heinonen PK, Teisala K, Hakkarainen K, Punnonen R. Serologic evidence for the role of *Chlamydia trachomatis*, *Neisseria gonorrhoeae*, and *Mycoplasma hominis* in the etiology of tubal factor infertility and ectopic pregnancy. Sex Transm Dis 1990; 17:10–14.

48. Rosenfeld DL, Seidman SM, Bronson RA, Scholl GM. Unsuspected chronic pelvic inflammatory disease in the infertile female. Fertil Steril 1983; 39:44–48.

49. Sellors JW, Mahony JB, Chernesky MA, Rath DJ. Tubal factor infertility: an association with prior chlamydial infection and asymptomatic salpingitis. Fertil Steril 1988; 49:451–457.

50. Wolner-Hanssen P. Silent pelvic inflammatory disease: is it overstated? Obstet Gynecol 1995; 86:321–325.

51. Songer TJ, Lave JR, Kamlet MS, Frederick S, Ness RB; Pelvic Inflammatory Disease Evaluation and Clinical Health (PEACH) Study. Preferences for fertility in women with pelvic inflammatory disease. Fertil Steril 2004; 81:1344–1350.

52. Westrom L, Bengtsson LP, Mardh PA. Incidence, trends, and risks of ectopic pregnancy in a population of women. Br Med J (Clin Res Ed) 1981; 282:15–18.

53. Kamwendo F, Forslin L, Bodin L, Danielsson D. Epidemiology of ectopic pregnancy during a 28 year period and the role of pelvic inflammatory disease. Sex Transm Infect 2000; 76:28–32.

54. Westrom L. Effect of acute pelvic inflammatory disease on fertility. Am J Obstet Gynecol 1975; 121:707–713.

55. American College of Obstetricians and Gynecologists (ACOG). ACOG practice bulletin no. 51: chronic pelvic pain. Washington, DC: ACOG, 2004.

56. Buchan H, Vessey M, Goldacre M, Fairweather J. Morbidity following pelvic inflammatory disease. Br J Obstet Gynaecol 1993; 100:558–562.
57. Haggerty CL, Schulz R, Ness RB; PID Evaluation and Clinical Health Study Investigators. Lower quality of life among women with chronic pelvic pain after pelvic inflammatory disease. Obstet Gynecol 2003; 102:934–939.
58. Haggerty CL, Ness RB, Amortegui A, et al. Endometritis does not predict reproductive morbidity after pelvic inflammatory disease. Am J Obstet Gynecol 2003; 188:141–148.
59. Ness RB, Soper DE, Holley RL, et al. Hormonal and barrier contraception and risk of upper genital tract disease in the PID Evaluation and Clinical Health (PEACH) study. Am J Obstet Gynecol 2001; 185:121–127.
60. Hatcher RA, Zieman M, Cwiak C, Darney PD, Creinen MD, Stosur HR. *Managing Contraception: 2004–2005*. Tiger, GA: Bridging the Gap Foundation, 2004.
61. Hubacher D, Grimes DA. Noncontraceptive health benefits of intrauterine devices: a systematic review. Obstet Gynecol Surv 2002; 57:120–128.
62. Scholes D, Stergachis A, Heidrich FE, Andrilla H, Holmes KK, Stamm WE. Prevention of pelvic inflammatory disease by screening for cervical chlamydial infection. N Engl J Med 1996; 334:1362–1366.
63. Washington AE, Cates W Jr, Wasserheit JN. Preventing pelvic inflammatory disease. JAMA 1991; 266:2574–2580.
64. Whiteside JL, Katz T, Anthes T, Boardman L, Peipert JF. Risks and adverse outcomes of sexually transmitted diseases. Patients' attitudes and beliefs. J Reprod Med 2001; 46:34–38.

9

Syphilis

Carolyn Sutton

INTRODUCTION

Syphilis has been the defining sexually transmitted disease in the history of western Europe and the Americas since the late 1490s. Fear of syphilis motivated the development and use of male condoms more than fear of pregnancy. Syphilis was a particularly horrifying infection that periodically recurred in its victims with increasingly devastating manifestations over time. In the early 20th century, syphilis was still a major health problem. More than one in five patients in US mental institutions in the 1920s had tertiary syphilis (general paresis) *(1)*. In 1937, the US Surgeon General predicted that 10% of Americans would be infected with syphilis during their lives *(2)*.

Syphilis is a chronic systemic infection that is often categorized as a genital ulcerative disease. If left untreated, the infection progresses in stages, with varied and often subtle clinical manifestations, which can result in serious and potentially life-threatening cardiovascular and neurological disease (*see* Fig. 1). Syphilis causes fetal and perinatal death in 40% of affected pregnancies and major anomalies among newborn survivors *(3)*. Syphilis also doubles the risk of the transmission of human immunodeficiency virus (HIV) and is important in contributing to HIV transmission in those parts of the country where, and in those populations in which, rates of both infections are high *(3)*. Syphilis is preventable with safer sex practices and treatable with inexpensive antibiotics. Recently, the numbers of individuals with syphilis has increased, especially in the South, among men of have sex with men (MSM), and among those who use methamphetamines *(3)*.

After the introduction of antibiotics, the prevalence of this infection was low for so many decades that professional experience and training about its clinical manifestations diminished over time. In this chapter, because of the profound direct and indirect consequences of syphilis, detailed descriptions will be provided for each of its presentations in adults.

From: *Current Clinical Practice: Sexually Transmitted Diseases:*
A Practical Guide for Primary Care
Edited by: A. L. Nelson and J. A. Woodward © Humana Press, Totowa, NJ

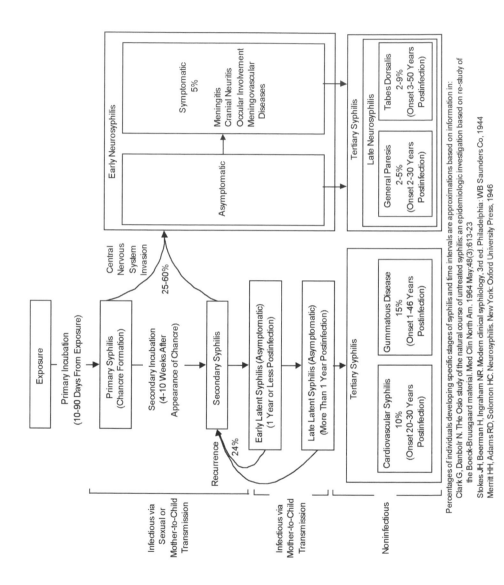

Percentages of individuals developing specific stages of syphilis and time intervals are approximations based on information in:

Clark G, Danbolr N. The Oslo study of the natural course of untreated syphilis: an epidemiologic investigation based on re-study of the Boeck-Bruusgaard material. Med Clin North Am. 1964 May;48(3):613-23

Stokes JH, Beerman H, Ingraham NR. Modern clinical syphilology, 3rd ed. Philadelphia: WB Saunders Co, 1944

Merritt HH, Adams RD, Solomon HC. Neurosyphilis. New York: Oxford University Press, 1946

FAST FACTS

- More than 50% of the new cases of syphilis occur in only 16 areas of the country.
- The number of cases of primary and secondary syphilis has been increasing.
- Syphilis is known as a great imitator, because its clinical presentations mimic so many other conditions.
- More than 80% of cases of congenital syphilis occurred in women who were not tested or treated.
- All prenatal women infected with syphilis should be treated with penicillin. Desensitization protocols should be used for those with penicillin allergy.

PREVALENCE AND INCIDENCE

Although the statistics for primary and secondary syphilis reported in the general population were very bleak in the early part of the 20th century, after the introduction of antibiotics and public health measures, the picture changed. The infection was almost entirely eliminated by 1957. Since then, there have been cyclic national epidemics every 7–10 years. The last peak occurred in 1990. Rates then steadily declined until 2000 when the rate was the lowest since reporting began in 1941 *(3)*. The prevalence of primary and secondary syphilis varies greatly by geographical area; in 2004, 79.3% of US counties reported no cases of syphilis. Rates are highest in the South, in large urban centers outside the South (especially in Baltimore, MD; Danville, VA; and St. Louis, MO), in heterosexual African-Americans, and in individuals in their early 20s–30s. In 1999, the CDC developed a national plan to eliminate syphilis because the cases were so geographically concentrated. In 2004, the CDC reported that the remaining numbers of primary and secondary syphilis increased 11.2% to 7980, but total cases decreased 2.6% to 33,401. Estimates are that 64% of all primary and secondary syphilis occurred in MSM; rates of infection in Afro-American men were 14.1/100,000, whereas in Hispanic men rates were 5.5/100,000 *(3)*.

Fortunately, the national trends in primary and secondary syphilis among reproductive age women has decreased, and so have the rates of pregnancy complications associated with syphilis. In 2003–2004, the rate of congenital syphilis was 8.8 cases per 100,000 live births *(3)*. In 2000, adolescent mothers who delivered at or less than 19 years of age had the highest rate of infants with congenital syphilis. Also, among the cases of congenital syphilis reported in 2002, 73.8% occurred because the mother had no documented treatment or had received inadequate treatment of syphilis before or during pregnancy *(4)*.

Fig. 1. *(opposite page)* Natural history of untreated syphilis in immunocompetent individuals. (From ref. *30.*)

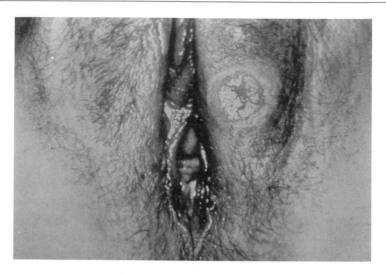

Vulvar syphilis chancre.

RISK FACTORS

Relatively small groups (4–15%) of high-risk individuals (core transmitters) can maintain syphilis in a larger community of low-to-moderate risky behaviors *(4a,4b)*. Populations at increased risk for contracting and transmitting syphilis in the US include those who engage in high-risk behaviors, those who are diagnosed with other sexually transmitted diseases (including HIV infection), MSM, commercial sex workers, those who exchange sex for drugs, incarcerated individuals, and those who are contacts of an individual with active syphilis *(3)*. The local incidence of syphilis in the community and the number of sex partners reported by an individual should also be considered in identifying persons at high risk of infection. Lack of prenatal care, late or limited prenatal care, and maternal use of illicit drugs, including crack cocaine and methamphetamines, are associated with congenital syphilis *(5)*. In a review of cases of early syphilis, jail screening identified the cases of women who were most likely to spread the disease, whereas testing in STD clinics identified women who were not likely to transmit the infection *(5a)*.

INFECTIVITY AND TRANSMISSION

Treponema pallidum is spread through contact with infected lesions or body fluids. The disease is most commonly transmitted through direct contact with moist mucosal or cutaneous lesions during anal, vaginal, or oral–genital sex. Kissing a person who has primary or secondary syphilitic lesions on the lips or in the oral cavity can transmit the infection—especially if the kiss is moist. Infection cannot be transmitted by inanimate objects (fomites).

It has been estimated that 3 to 10% of individuals acquire the infection from a single sexual encounter with an infected partner. Patients are most infectious during the first year of infection, when the rate of transmission is 90% *(6)*. Transmission by intimate sexual contact drops dramatically after that; by the second year, transmission is 5%, and by the end of the fourth year, syphilis can no longer be contracted by sexual contact. In untreated populations, 50–75% of sex partners of people diagnosed with primary or secondary syphilis are infected. In addition, of the remaining contacts (those without initial clinical or serological evidence of infection), 30% developed syphilis if not treated *(7)*. Since the introduction of antibiotic therapy, the prevalence of syphilis among sex partners of index cases has varied between 10 and 60%, with an average of about 33% in early syphilis *(1)*. *T. pallidum* can penetrate intact mucous membranes or enter through epithelial defects.

Vertical transmission (maternal–fetal) can occur either through transplacental spread or at the time of delivery from direct contact with the syphilitic lesions of the mother. Transplacental infection generally occurs after 18 weeks of gestation because of the relative immunocompetence before that gestational age *(8)*. It can occur at any time in the course of infection, even during latent period. However, fetal infection risks are highest in women with early syphilis.

Other means of transmission are very rare, but include transfusion and accidental direct inoculation. Indirect evidence suggests that needle sharing by intravenous drug users may contribute some cases *(9)*.

ETIOLOGY

Syphilis is caused by an anaerobic spirochete, *T. pallidum*, a member of the family Spirochaetaceae, which also includes Borrelia and Leptospira. The treponemes are subdivided by their ability to cause disease in humans. *T. pallidum* subspecies endemicum causes epidemic syphilis (nonvenereal); *T. pallidum* subspecies pertenue causes yaws and *T. carateum* causes pinta. The treponemes tend to have similar morphology, share antigens, and have a relatively high degree of DNA homologies *(1)*. This can cause difficulty in interpreting the results of serological tests, especially in patients who come from or have traveled to areas where the other treponemes are common. Other nonpathogenic treponemes colonize the human gastrointestinal tract or can be found in soil, water, or other animals.

T. pallidum is a thin, elongated organism with characteristic regularly round coils, with corkscrew mobility and the ability to flex at a 90° angle *(1)*. It measures 7–14 μm in length and 0.25 μm in width. *T. pallidum* replicates every 30–33 hours. Although infections have been established in other animal models (rabbits and guinea pigs), spontaneous clinical infections are confined to humans.

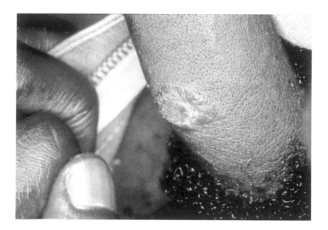

Penile syphilis chancre.

CLINICAL MANIFESTATIONS
Initial Infection

T. pallidum penetrates through the skin or mucosal tissue, especially through defects caused by microtrauma associated with sexual activity. The spirochete then enters the blood stream and spreads throughout the body. Spirochetemia occurs even before skin lesions develop or blood tests can detect infection. The incubation period for syphilis ranges from 10 to 90 days, with an average of 3 weeks. The incubation period depends on the size of the inoculum, as was demonstrated in a 1936 study, which would not be permitted under today's ethical standards. In this study, when prisoners were transdermally inoculated with 10 spirochetes, chancres developed 28.7 days later on average. The incubation period was reduced to 18.6 days when the inoculum was increased to 100,000 organisms *(6)*.

Primary Stage

Primary syphilis, the earliest clinical stage of the disease, is defined by the lesion at the site of inoculation—the chancre. In three quarters of cases, the chancre is a solitary nodule, most commonly found on the penis, rectum, vagina, anus, cervix, or vulva. In some instances, chancres may be found at extragenital sites, such as the lips, tongue, oral mucosa, tonsils, fingers, or breasts. In men, most oral chancres develop on the upper lip, whereas women tend to have lower lip involvement. Chancres can also develop peripherally on the tongue or in the tonsillar area *(10)*. The lesion begins as a small red papule that enlarges and erodes into a round or slightly elongated, ulcerated lesion. The margins are raised, sharply defined, indurated, and firm. The base is dry, clean, and measures 1–2 cm across.

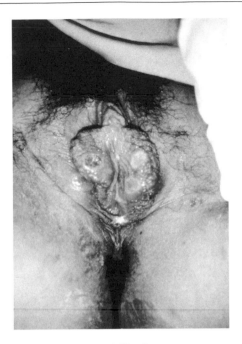

Libia syphilis chancre.

The chancre is painless and highly infectious. There are no exudates, unless the lesion became secondarily infected *(11)*. The chancre is often accompanied by nontender and bilateral enlargement of the inguinal nodes.

Without intervention, the chancre will dry up and heal spontaneously in 3–6 weeks. Chancres often are not noticed, particularly if they are located in the vagina or the anus. In that situation, the patient will remain asymptomatic for months.

The differential diagnosis of primary syphilis includes other genital ulcerative diseases, such as genital herpes, chancroid, aphthous ulcers, primary HIV ulcers, lymphogranuloma venereum and granuloma inguinale, trauma, neoplasm, autoimmune diseases such as Behçet syndrome, Crohn's disease, Reiter syndrome, and fixed drug eruptions *(12)*.

Secondary Stage

The secondary stage represents greater hematogenous dissemination of *T. pallidum* and involves more widespread physical findings as well as constitutional signs and symptoms. Syphilis has been called the great imitator because of its varied manifestations at every stage. Onset of secondary syphilis follows an average of 3 weeks after the appearance of the chancre, or 6–8 weeks after initial exposure. However, it may overlap with the chancres or be delayed for

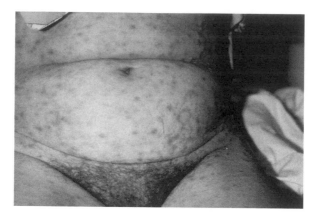

Secondary syphilis abdominal lesions.

months *(12)*. In this stage, the patient is highly infectious. The secondary stage of syphilis is characterized by one or more of the following clinical findings:

- Constitutional signs: low-grade fever, headache, sore throat, malaise, loss of appetite, severe weight loss, muscle aches, and nasal discharge.
- Generalized skin rashes.
- Alopecia (hair loss).
- Mucous patches (painless silvery ulcerations of mucous membranes of the oral cavity or genital tract).
- Condylomata lata.
- Generalized, nontender lymphadenopathy or enlarged liver or spleen.
- Secondary anemia, leukocytosis.

The rashes associated with secondary syphilis are characteristically variable. Rash is the presenting complaint in more than 70% of patients with secondary syphilis and can be found on exam in all but 10% of patients. The first eruptions are macular or erythematous. They start on the flanks, back, shoulder, upper extremities, and flexor surfaces of the arms or forearm. The non-blanching, light red-colored rash is more intensely colored in the center and fades at the edge. After the initial rash resolves in about 2 weeks, it is replaced with hyperpigmentation that resembles a variety of other dermopathies.

This is followed in 50–80% of cases by generalized copper-red, maculopapular or papulosquamous eruptions involving the central portion of the face, trunk, and flexor surface of the upper extremities. These lesions may appear on the palms of the hands and soles of the feet. Mucous patches may also be present on the mucosa of the lips, tongue, gums, pharynx, palate, and buccal surfaces as well as on the moist surfaces of the genitals. These oval-shaped patches have a slightly raised border surrounding a shallow ulcer that is covered by a gray-white membrane. Ulceration of these patches can be seen on the tip and sides of the tongue.

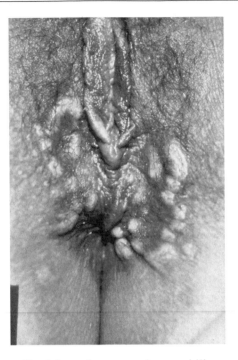

Condyloma lata secondary syphilis.

The next generation of lesions is papular. They are larger than the macular eruptions but fewer in number. The papular lesions are deep-seated, flat, and scaly, uniformly involving the soles and palms. These lesions resemble lichen planus or psoriasis. In the hair-bearing areas of the body, they are more follicular and can cause alopecia of the scalp and beard as well as patchy alopecia of the eyebrows. When the papular lesions develop along the scalp hairline on the forehead, it is called the "Crown of Venus." Lesions along the anterior neck and chest are called the "Collar of Venus." Resolution of these lesions occurs more slowly than the other rashes and almost invariably leaves postinflammatory hyperpigmentation.

Condyloma lata develop on the moist surfaces, especially in the genital areas. They result from coalescence of papular lesions. They appear hypertrophic, red-brown or grey, flat-topped, and moist. Pustular lesions are less common but result when papules soften, ulcerate, and crust. They can involve the fingernails and toenails. When more generalized, they may be due to immunosuppression or be a prelude to fatal malignant syphilis, the original "Great Pox."

Recurrent secondary syphilis may be marked by larger, more discrete and darker lesions often characterized as annular syphilitic lesions. They occur in the midline facial structures (mouth corners, nasolabial folds, chin), as well as the

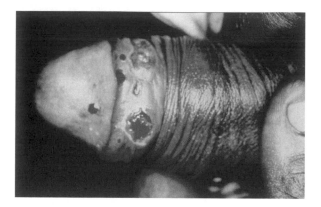

Syphilis chancre of the penis.

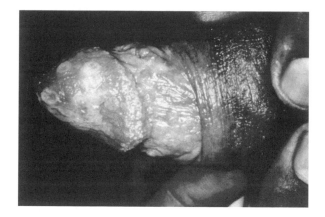

Penile syphilis chancre.

genital areas. Recurrent large condyloma lata may also be a manifestation of recurrent secondary syphilis. The rashes, mucous patches, and moist lesions (condyloma lata) in the anogenital areas are all highly infectious.

Because secondary syphilis is a systemic process, it can cause neurological, meningeal, renal, gastrointestinal, hepatic, bone, or ophthalmological diseases *(12)*. It has been suggested that patients with primary or secondary syphilis who are incompletely treated may be more likely to develop meningeal or meningovascular as well as ocular syphilis (uveitis) than are untreated patients. The hypothesis is that when partial therapy clears the spirochetes from the peripheral sites, the normal immune response to infection becomes muted so that the pathogens in the eye and central nervous system (CNS) are able to multiply and cause neurological and ocular diseases *(1)*. Early neurosyphilis, in particular, with ocular involvement, may present at any time after initial infections.

Table 1
Manifestations of Tertiary Syphilis

- Neurosyphilis.
    - Most often associated with the tertiary stage but can occur at any time. Late neurosyphilis occurs when the spirochetes attack the brain or the meninges (lining that covers it).
    - May produce dementia, tremors, loss of muscle coordination, paralysis, and/or blindness.
- Gummatous syphilis.
    - Localized areas of granulomatous inflammation found on the liver
- Cardiovascular syphilis.
    - Inflammatory lesions of the cardiovascular system.
    - Causes aortic aneurism, thickening of cardiac valves or angina pectora.

Untreated, symptoms of secondary syphilis will spontaneously disappear in 3–12 weeks. The differential diagnosis of the symptoms associated with secondary syphilis includes primary HIV, pityriasis rosea, and condylomata acuminata.

Latent Stage

Following resolution of secondary syphilis, the organism persists in the body, but there are no clinical manifestations of syphilis in the latent stage. The latent stage is subdivided into early and late latent phases. The CDC defines early latent phases as occuring within the year of initial infection. When the diagnosis is made more than 1 year after the initial infection or when the duration of infection is unknown, the CDC classifies it as late latent. The World Health Organization uses a 2-year watershed as the dividing line between early and late latent. The distinction between early and late latent stages is clinically important because people are infectious during recurrences, which occur during early latent phase. Those with late latency syphilis generally are noninfectious.

Tertiary Stage

Approximately one-third of untreated latent stage syphilis cases will develop signs of the devastating and even fatal complications of tertiary syphilis (*see* Table 1). The tertiary stage may begin as early as 1 year after infection or at any time during an infected person's lifetime. Today, however, the clinical manifestations of tertiary syphilis are rarely seen. When present, the clinical expression of tertiary stage syphilis depends on which of the specific complications develop. Damage that occurs during the tertiary syphilis is irreversible.

NEUROSYPHILIS

Neurosyphilis is divided into early and late forms. *T. pallidum* invades the CNS early in the course of the infection. Spontaneous clearance of the spirochete occurs in 75% of cases; with adequate antibiotic treatment of early infection, few immunocompetent individuals do not clear. However, those who have persistent spirochetes in the CNS are at risk for symptomatic neurosyphilis. Overall, in untreated populations, 4–9% of cases developed into early neurosyphilis. Early neurosyphilis co-exists with primary or secondary infections and may be symptomatic (5%), but usually is not (95%). The cerebrospinal fluid, cerebral blood vessels, and meninges are often involved, but the brain and spinal cord are usually spared. Meningeal syphilis presents with headache, stiff neck, nausea, and vomiting with or without cranial nerve involvement. Meningovascular syphilis causes focal ischemia or stroke.

On the other hand, late neurosyphilis affects the meninges and brain or spinal cord; it develops in 4–14% of cases of untreated early neurosyphilis. There are two major manifestations of late neurosyphilis: general paresis (2–5%) and tabes dorsales (2–9%). General paresis (paretic neurosyphilis) is a chronic, progressive dementia, which can have some psychotic features (this was the condition that filled American mental institutions between World Wars I and II). Tabes dorsales (locomotor ataxia) is a spinal cord disorder with sensory ataxia (including blindness because of optic atrophy), lightening pains, and bladder and bowel dysfunction. Adolph Hitler was affected by this.

GUMMATOUS DISEASE

Gummatous disease is particularly disfiguring manifestation of tertiary syphilis. It affects 15% of untreated cases and develops 1–46 years after initial infection. Most experts believe that the appearance of a gumma represents a delayed hypersensitivity or allergic response to *T. pallidum*. The gummatous lesion is most often nodular and characterized by granulomatous inflammation and necrosis. The size of these benign but highly tissue destructive lesions ranges from microscopic to many centimeters in diameter and may be found in any tissue or organ. They are, however, most commonly found in soft tissue and bone. Once healed, deep scarring occurs at the site of the gumma. Although spirochetes may not be detectable in biopsy specimens, the treponemal serological tests will be reactive in the presence of gummatous disease.

CARDIOVASCULAR DISEASE

After the introduction of antibiotics, cardiovascular syphilis became extremely rare. Today it is estimated that only 10% of the untreated cases of syphilis will develop serious cardiac involvement. Because syphilis affecting the cardiovascular system only manifests clinically in the tertiary stage of the disease, the onset of symptoms may be delayed for 20–30 years after the initial infection. Cardiovascular syphilis may lead to aortic aneurysms, aortic insufficiency, coronary stenosis, and myocarditis.

TESTING TECHNIQUES

T. pallidum cannot be cultured. In initial disease, dark-field microscopy of exudate from the lesion is a reliable diagnostic method used to confirm the presence of spirochetes. Incident light through a microscope fitted with polarizing lenses allows the viewer to identify the corkscrew morphology of treponemes as white against a black background. Exudate for dark-field microscopy can be collected from the base of the chancre that has been cleaned with saline. Microscopic examination must be performed promptly because drying of the specimen can reduce the sensitivity of the test. In the absence of darkfield microscopy, direct fluorescent antibody stains of the exudates can also be used to identify *T. pallidum*. Each of these tests suffers from a low sensitivity. Most clinicians do not have the equipment (dark-field microscope) or laboratory support to perform these tests.

Serological testing for antibodies to *T. pallidum* forms the basis of diagnostic testing in the United States. The initial test used is the one that tests quantitatively for the presence of nontreponemal antibodies, using either the Venereal Disease Research Laboratory (VDRL) or the reactive plasma reagin (RPR) tests. Nontreponemal tests are used to test patients for the presence of nonspecific reagin antibodies, which develop and rise in titer following infection.

It must be remembered that the test requires that the patient has had time and ability to mount an antibody response to the infection. In early primary syphilis, antibody levels may be too low to detect and nontreponemal tests may be nonreactive. Only 30% of individuals infected with primary stage syphilis will become serologically positive 1 week after appearance of the chancre, but 90% will be positive after 3 weeks *(16)*. Nontreponemal tests are 78–89% sensitive in primary syphilis, but are almost 100% sensitive in secondary syphilis *(2)*. Later in the infection, when the antibody titer again may fall, sensitivity again drops to 95–98% *(2)*. In late syphilis, titers decline and previously reactive results revert to nonreactive in 25% of cases, and test sensitivity averages only 70%. Therefore, nontreponemal tests cannot establish a definitive diagnosis of syphilis, especially in the early or latent stages of the disease.

False-positive results for nontreponemal tests occur in 1–2% of Americans *(2)*. These are associated with auto-immune disease, intravenous drug use, vaccination, pregnancy, HIV, pneumonia, hepatitis, hepatic disease (mononucleosis), tuberculosis, bacterial endocarditis, and other spirochetal malarial or rickettsial infections *(13)* *(see* Table 2). In 90% of cases of false-positive results, the titers were 1:8 or lower.

Because nontreponemal tests are associated with false-positive test results, specific treponemal tests, such as fluorescent treponemal antibody absorption

Table 2
Potential Causes of False-Positive Serological Tests for Syphilis

Bacterial reaginic or nontreponemal tests (RPR, VDRL)

Infectious causes	Noninfectious causes
• Pneumococcal pneumonia	• Pregnancy
• Scarlet fever	• Chronic liver disease
• Leprosy	• Advanced cancer
• Lymphogranuloma venereum	• Intravenous drug use
• Relapsing fever	• Multiple myeloma
• Bacterial endocarditis	• Advancing age
• Malaria	• Connective tissue disease
• Rickettsial disease	• Multiple blood transfusions
• Psittacosis	
• Leptospirosis	
• Chancroid	
• Tuberculosis	
• Mycoplasmal pneumonia	
• Trypanosomiasis	

Viral reaginic or nontreponemal tests (RPR, VDRL)

Infectious causes

- Vaccinia (vaccination)
- Chickenpox
- HIV
- Measles
- Infectious mononucleosis
- Mumps
- Viral hepatitis

Treponemal tests (FTA-ABS, MHA-TP, TP-PA)

Infectious causes	Noninfectious causes
• Lyme disease	• Systemic lupus erythematosus
• Leprosy	
• Malaria	
• Infectious mononucleosis	
• Relapsing fever	
• Leptospirosis	

RPR, reactive plasma reagin; VDRL, Venereal Disease Research Laboratory; HIV, human immunodeficiency virus; FTA-ABS, fluorescent treponemal antibody absorption; MHA-TP, microhemagglutination assay-*T. pallidum*; TP-PA, *T. pallidum* particle agglutination.
Source: From ref. *1*.

(FTA-ABS) test or *T. pallidum* passive particle agglutination (TP-PA) test are used to confirm the diagnosis of syphilis in patients with a reactive nontreponemal tests. These treponemal tests also are subject to some false-positive results, but the causes are different. Therefore, when used sequentially, the positive predictive value of the combined tests is high and reactive results are likely to represent true infection with syphilis *(14)*. Treponemal tests become reactive before nontreponemal tests do. For this reason, the FTA-ABS or *T. pallidum* passive particle agglutination may be useful in diagnosing primary syphilis (in the absence of a history of prior infection). However, these antibodies remain positive in 75–85% of individuals, even after the infection has cleared.

The potential for polymerase chain reaction tests to detect *T. pallidum* has been demonstrated. However, these tests are expensive and require sophisticated laboratory processing, so they are not expected to be in widespread use in the near future.

As a demonstration of what can be done to respond to local problems with syphilis, the San Francisco Department of Public Health has developed an Internet-based, confidential online syphilis testing service (STDTest.org), which allows people to print out a laboratory request slip, have blood drawn, and receive the test results online *(15)*. It also has launched a Web site (www.inspot.org) for partner notification.

DIAGNOSIS

In early infection, a presumptive diagnosis of syphilis can be made based on the patient's history and findings on physical examination. Specific tests, such as dark-field microscopy, are more secure, but often not available. A positive treponemal-specific test (in the absence of prior infection) can be confirmatory even if the nontreponemal test is negative.

After the initial infection, however, diagnosis requires that both the nontreponemal and treponemal tests be reactive. Occasionally, a low titer reactive result may be obtained, indicating either new infection or a false-positive. Recent infection can be confirmed by documenting increase in titer of the nontreponemal test over time. Because the accuracy of the test may vary by a dilution, the increase must be two dilutions or a fourfold increase on titers (such as 1:8 to 1:32) to demonstrate a clinically significant difference between tests. The CDC cautions that when serially monitoring patients for diagnosis, the same nontreponemal test (RPR or VDRL) should be used and preferably, the tests should be processed by the same laboratory. Some HIV-infected patients may have unusual serological tests results over time, so other modalities, including biopsy or direct microscopy may be needed.

Neurosyphilis may occur at any stage of infection with *T. pallidum*. Therefore, any syphilitic person presenting with neurological complaints, such as stiff neck, severe persistent headache, or hearing compromise should undergo lumbar puncture and cerebrospinal fluid evaluation using a combination of tests including cell count, protein, and VDRL-CSF with or without FTA-ABS testing. Those with visual complaints should be evaluated for uveitis using a slit-lamp examination.

In the tertiary stage of syphilis, the sensitivity of nontreponemal tests ranges from 71 to 73%. Treponemal-specific tests are positive in this stage with a sensitivity of 94–96%.

All patients diagnosed with syphilis should be tested for HIV and for other STIs. In areas of high HIV prevalence, HIV tests should be repeated in 3 months.

TREATMENT

Table 3 summarizes the CDC-recommended treatments for syphilis in non-pregnant and non-HIV-infected individuals. Intramuscular administration of penicillin G is the preferred drug for treatment of all stages of syphilis. The preparation(s) used (i.e., benzathine, aqueous procaine, or aqueous crystalline), the dosage, and the length of treatment depend on the stage and clinical manifestations of disease (12). The most important property is that bacteriocidal levels of the medication are maintained for several weeks to kill the slowly metabolizing T. pallidum. Careful attention must be paid to the type of penicillin administration. One clinic inadvertently used bicillin C-R instead of bicillin L-A to treat 429 patients with confirmed syphilis infections and an additional 234 patients who were sexual contacts. About one in five cases required retreatment once the mistake was identified (16).

Doxycycline and tetracycline may be used in non-pregnant patients with penicillin allergy, or if there is concern with compliance and follow-up, these individuals can be desensitized and treated with penicillin (see Table 4). Penicillin alternative therapies, used for the treatment of late latent or latent syphilis of unknown duration, should be used only in conjunction with close serological and clinical follow-up (12). Some investigators have suggested that macrolides (e.g., azithromycin) should be considered in the treatment of syphilis, because they share the property of long tissue half-life. However, cases of macrolide resistance and treatment failures have now been reported (17).

No alternatives to penicillin have been proved effective for treatment of syphilis during pregnancy (see Syphilis in Pregnancy section).

Within 24 hours of treatment, up to 60% of cases have a Jarisch-Herxheimer reaction, which includes fever, myalgia, headache, malaise, sore throat, and vasodilatation with mild hypotension and tachycardia (18). The reaction results from an antigen overload, which is more likely to occur in early syphilis. It may result from prostaglandin release or as an immune response. This reaction can induce early labor or fetal distress.

Table 3
Syphilis—CDC STD Treatment Guidelines 2006

Recommended regimens	Alternative regimens
Primary, secondary, or early latent syphilis Benzathine penicillin G[a] For adults: 2.4 million units IM in a single dose[b] For children: 50,000 units/kg IM, up to the adult dose or 2.4 million units in a single dose	***For non-pregnant adult patients with penicillin allergy*** *Select one of the following:* Doxycycline[c] 100 mg orally twice daily for 14 days Tetracycline[c] 500 mg orally four times daily for 14 days Desensitizing protocols for treatment with benzathine penicillin G
Late latent, latent of unknown duration, or tertiary syphilis Benzathine penicillin G[a] For adults: 7.2 million units total, administered as three doses of 2.4 million units IM each at 1-week intervals For children: 50,000 units/kg IM, up to the adult dose of 2.4 million units, administered as three doses at 1-week intervals (total 150,000 units/kg up to the adult total dose of 7.2 million units)	***For non-pregnant adult patients with penicillin allergy*** *Select one of the following:* Doxycycline[c] 100 mg orally twice daily for 28 days Tetracycline[c] 500 mg orally four times daily for 28 days *WITH* close serological and clinical follow-up.
Neurosyphilis Aqueous crystalline penicillin G[a] 18–24 million units per day, administered as 3–4 million units iv every 4 hours or continuous infusion, for 10–14 days	***For non-pregnant adult patients with penicillin allergy:*** Procaine penicillin 2.4 million units IM once daily for 10–14 days *PLUS* Probenecid 500 mg orally four times a day for 10–14 days

Source: From ref. 23.

[a] Patients with penicillin allergy who are pregnant or whose compliance with therapy or follow-up cannot be ensured should desensitized and treated with penicillin.

[b] Some experts recommend repeating this regimen after 7 days.

[c] Contraindicated for pregnant and lactating women and for children under 8 years old.

Table 4
Oral Desensitization Protocol for Patients With a Positive Skin Test

Penicillin V suspension dose [a]	Amount [b] (units/mL)	mL	Units	Cumulative dose (units)
1	1000	0.1	100	100
2	1000	0.2	200	300
3	1000	0.4	400	700
4	1000	0.8	800	1500
5	1000	1.6	1600	3100
6	1000	3.2	3200	6300
7	1000	6.4	6400	12,700
8	10,000	1.2	12,000	24,700
9	10,000	2.4	24,000	48,700
10	10,000	4.8	48,000	96,700
11	80,000	1.0	80,000	176,700
12	80,000	2.0	160,000	336,700
13	80,000	4.0	320,000	656,700
14	80,000	8.0	640,000	1,296,700

Observation period: 30 minutes before parenteral administration of penicillin.

[a] Interval between doses, 15 minutes; elapsed time, 3 hours and 45 minutes; cumulative dose, 1.3 million units.
[b] The specific amount of drug was diluted in approximately 30 mL of water and then administered orally.
Reprinted from ref. 29 with permission.

FOLLOW-UP

Treatment failure is possible with any regimen. The CDC recommends that patients should be re-examined clinically and serologically 6 and 12 months following treatment. More frequent evaluations may be prudent if follow-up is uncertain. HIV-infected patients require more frequent and prolonged follow-up intervals (3, 6, 9, 12, and 24 months). Patients with latent syphilis should have quantitative nontreponemal tests repeated at 6, 12, and 24 months. Those with neurosyphilis need CSF tests done every 6 months until their cell count normalizes.

It is expected that titers of nontreponemal tests will decline by at least two titers (fourfold) to demonstrate initial response. Over time, most successfully treated patients will revert to undetectable levels of nontreponemal titers. The treponemal-specific antibodies generally remain positive throughout life. There are exceptions to these observations. One study found that 25% of treated primary syphilis and 44% of those treated for secondary syphilis had persistence of nontreponemal tests 36 months after treatment and 24% of primary syphilis cases had disappearance of the FTA (19).

Patients with persistent or recurrent signs or symptoms or who sustain a four-fold increase in nontreponemal test titer over the baseline titer should be considered to be treatment failures or re-infected. They need to be retreated and re-evaluated for HIV infection.

PARTNER NOTIFICATION AND REPORTING REQUIREMENTS

It is important to identify and treat any possible sexual contacts of patients with syphilis. In patients with primary syphilis, all contacts for 3 months before the appearance of the chancre should be evaluated clinically and with serological tests. In patients with secondary syphilis, contacts for 6 months before the onset of the signs associated with secondary syphilis should be evaluated clinically and serologically. In patients with early latent syphilis and no history or signs suggestive of primary or secondary stage disease, contacts for 12 months prior should be evaluated clinically and serologically. Persons with known exposure to a patient with early syphilis within the previous 3 months can be infected and seronegative and should, therefore, be treated presumptively. Syphilis is a reportable disease in all states and territories.

PREGNANCY-RELATED ISSUES

Antepartum syphilis produces serious adverse outcomes for the pregnant woman and her fetus. Maternal syphilis has been associated with obstetric complications, such as hydramnios, abortion, and preterm delivery, and fetal complications such as fetal syphilis, hydrops, prematurity, fetal distress, and stillbirth (20). The frequency of congenital syphilis varies with both the stage and duration of maternal infection; the highest incidence occurs in neonates born to mothers with early syphilis and the lowest incidence occurs with late latent disease (21). If the maternal infection is acquired within 4 years of the pregnancy, infection of the fetus occurs in more than 70% of cases (22).

Fortunately, as the national rates of primary and secondary syphilis have decreased among reproductive aged women, so have the rates of pregnancy complications associated with syphilis. In 2002, 80% of congenital syphilis cases occurred in mothers who had no documented treatment or had received inadequate treatment of syphilis before or during pregnancy (4). Lack of prenatal care, late or limited prenatal care, and maternal use of illicit drugs, including methamphetamine and crack cocaine, are associated with congenital syphilis (5).

Syphilis screening is recommended for all women at the first prenatal visit, again at 32 weeks gestation for high-risk patients, and at delivery. In addition, any woman who delivers a stillborn after 20 weeks gestation should be tested for syphilis (23). No infant should be discharged from the hospital without maternal serological test results determined at least once during the pregnancy.

Only penicillin should be used to treat pregnant women. Other agents may eradicate the maternal infection, but they do not reliably treat the fetus. Therefore, a pregnant woman who is allergic to penicillin should undergo desensitization in a hospital setting and then be treated with the penicillin regimen that is appropriate to the stage of her infection with syphilis *(12)* *(see* Table 4).

Another important feature of treatment in pregnant women is the impact Jarisch-Herxheimer reaction may have on the pregnancy. About 40% of pregnant women treated have uterine contractions and recurrent variable decelerations in the fetal heart tracing within 48 hours of treatment, although the risk persists for several weeks after therapy *(18)*. Rarely, is it associated with fetal demise. As a result, it seems prudent to warn patients about possible side effects and urge them to seek care if they have fever, change in fetal activity, or uterine contractions. Some experts have suggested a routine nonstress test be performed for all viable pregnancies in the 24- to 48-hour period after treatment.

In addition, because congenital syphilis may result in polyhydramnios and enlarged placentas, it is generally recommended that women with syphilis have detailed fetal ultrasounds studies to rule out intrauterine growth retardation that may not be detected by comparing fundal height to gestational age. In addition, ultrasound of the fetus may detect signs of fetal infection, such as hepatosplenomegaly, hydrops or ascites. Placental infection with syphilis may increase maternal–fetal transmission of HIV infection.

HIV AND SYPHILIS

Epidemiological studies demonstrate that a history of sexually transmitted diseases, including syphilis, is associated with an increased risk for HIV infection, and that genital ulcers caused by sexually transmitted diseases are cofactors for acquiring HIV infection *(24,25)*. Isolated case reports have suggested that co-existent HIV infection may alter the natural history of syphilis and the dosage or duration of treatment required to cure syphilis *(26,27)*. Numerous case reports have documented the rapid progression of early syphilis to neurosyphilis manifested as meningitis or cranial nerve defects such as optic neuritis or deafness *(12)*. It is suggested that impairment of both cell-mediated and humeral immunity by HIV limits the host's defenses against *T. pallidum*, thereby altering the clinical manifestations or natural course of the disease *(28)*.

Standard serological tests appear to be accurate and reliable for the diagnosis of syphilis and the evaluation of treatment response in HIV-infected individuals, although additional testing may be needed to rule out some of the complications of advanced disease, such as neurosyphilis. More frequent and prolonged follow-ups are also necessary.

HIV-infected patients with primary, secondary, or early latent syphilis should be treated with the same regimens as a non-infected individual, but it is recommended that those with late latent or syphilis of unknown durations have a analysis of the cerebrospinal fluid before initiation of therapy *(12)*. These patients should be managed by an expert in HIV infection.

CASE STUDY

Martin, age 34, was recently released from the county jail where he served a 9-month sentence. He is here today for his pre-employment physical. He has a history of generalized non-pruritic rash, which resolved without treatment after about 2 weeks. His RPR serological test was 1:128 with FTA-ABS testing being done to confirm the diagnosis. He has no history of treatment for syphilis. Titers done at the time of his incarceration were normal.

Questions

1. What is his diagnosis?
2. What other tests need to be performed?
3. What therapies would you offer?
4. Are there any reporting requirements?
5. What do you do about his sexual partners?

Answers

1. From his history and early laboratory findings, it appears that Martin has early latent syphilis. His tests are high enough (>1:32) to be outside range of biologically false-positive results. His symptoms of the rash confirms secondary syphilis.
2. He needs to be tested for other STIs. Particular attention should be paid to obtaining rectal and pharyngeal specimens.
3. He should be treated for early latent syphilis with single-dose therapy according to the CDC guidelines. He will need to be vaccinated for hepatitis B virus if his tests confirm he has not been previously infected. If any other STIs are diagnosed, they will also be treated.
4. Syphilis is a reportable disease.
5. Case tracking will inevitably lead to the jail, but all of his other sexual partners also need to be contacted.

   - All partners exposed in the last 90 days might be infected, even if their tests were negative. They should be treated presumptively.
   - Sex partners exposed more than 90 days ago should also be treated presumptively if serological tests are not available immediately and follow-up is not certain.
   - Long-term sex partners should be evaluated serologically and treated on the basis of those findings.

REFERENCES

1. Hook EW 3rd, Marra CM. Acquired syphilis in adults. N Engl J Med 1992; 326:1060–1069.
2. Golden MR, Marra CM, Holmes KK. Update on syphilis: resurgence of an old problem. JAMA 2003; 290:1510–1514.
3. Centers for Disease Control and Prevention. Sexually transmitted disease surveillance, 2004. Atlanta, GA: US Department of Health and Human Services, 2005. Available from: http://www.cdc.gov/std/stats/. Accessed Nov 24, 2006.
4. Centers for Disease Control and Prevention. Congenital syphilis—United States, 2002. MMWR Morb Mortal Wkly Rep 2004; 53:716–719.
4a. Bernstein KT, Curriero FC, Jennings JM, Olthoff G, Erbelding EJ, Zenilman J. Defining core gonorrhea transmission utilizing spatial data. Am J Epidemiol 2004; 160(1):51–58.
4b. Rosenberg D, Moseley K, Kahn R, et al. Networks of persons with syphilis and at risk for syphilis in Louisiana: evidence of core transmitters. Sex Transm Dis 1999; 26(2):108–114.
5. McFarlin BL, Bottoms SF, Dock BS, Isada NB. Epidemic syphilis: maternal factors associated with congenital infection. Am J Obstet Gynecol 1994; 170:535–540.
5a. Kahn RH, Peterman TA, Arno J, Coursey EJ, Berman SM. Identifying likely syphilis transmitters: implications for control and evaluation. Sex Transm Dis 2006; 33(10):630–635.
6. Magnuson HJ, Thomas EW, Olansky S, Kaplan BI, De Mello L, Cutler JC. Inoculation syphilis in human volunteers. Medicine (Baltimore) 1956; 35:33–82.
7. Garnett GP, Aral SO, Hoyle DV, Cates W Jr, Anderson RM. The natural history of syphilis. Implications for the transmission dynamics and control of infection. Sex Transm Dis 1997; 24:185–200.
8. Cunningham G, MacDonald P, Gant N, et al. Sexually transmitted diseases. In: *Williams Obstetrics*, 21st Ed. Stamford, CT: Appleton & Lange, 2001.
9. Nelson KE, Vlahov D, Cohn S, Odunmbaku M, Lindsay A, Antohony JC, Hook EW 3rd. Sexually transmitted diseases in a population of intravenous drug users: association with seropositivity to the human immunodeficiency virus (HIV). J Infect Dis 1991; 164:457–463.
10. Fiumara NJ, Walker EA. Primary syphilis of the tonsil. Arch Otolaryngol 1982; 108:43–44.
11. DiCarlo RP, Martin DH. The clinical diagnosis of genital ulcer disease in men. Clin Infect Dis 1997; 25:292–298.
12. Musher DM. Early syphilis. In: Holmes KK, Sparling PF, Mardh PA, Lemon SM, Stamm WE, Piot P, Wasserheit JW, eds., *Sexually Transmitted Diseases*, 3rd Ed. New York, NY: McGraw Hill, 1999, pp. 479–485.
13. Hook EW 3rd, Marra CM. Acquired syphilis in adults. N Engl J Med 1992; 326:1060–1069.
14. United States Preventive Services Task Force. Screening for syphilis infection: recommendation statement. Ann Fam Med 2004; 2:362–365.
15. Levine DK, Scott KC, Klausner JD. Online syphilis testing—confidential and convenient. Sex Transm Dis 2005; 32:139–141.
16. Centers for Disease Control and Prevention. Inadvertent use of Bicillin C-R to treat syphilis infection—Los Angeles, California, 1999–2004. MMWR Morb Mortal Wkly Rep 2005; 54:217–219.
17. Lukehart SA, Godornes C, Molini BJ, et al. Macrolide resistance in Treponema pallidum in the United States and Ireland. N Engl J Med 2004; 351:154–158.
18. Myles TD, Elam G, Park-Hwang E, Nguyen T. The Jarisch-Herxheimer reaction and fetal monitoring changes in pregnant women treated for syphilis. Obstet Gynecol 1998; 92:859–864.
19. Romanowski B, Sutherland R, Fick GH, Mooney D, Love EJ. Serologic response to treatment of infectious syphilis. Ann Intern Med 1991; 114:1005–1009.

20. Wendel GD Jr, Sheffield JS, Hollier LM, Hill JB, Ramsey PS, Sanchez PJ. Treatment of syphilis in pregnancy and prevention of congenital syphilis. Clin Infect Dis 2002; 35:S200–S209.
21. Centers for Disease Control and Prevention. Primary and secondary syphilis—United States, 1998. MMWR Morb Mortal Wkly Rep 1999; 48:873–878.
22. Ingraham NR. The value of penicillin alone in the prevention and treatment. Acta Derm Venereol (Stockh) 1951; 31:60–88.
23. Centers for Disease Control and Prevention. Sexually transmitted diseases treatment guidelines 2002. MMWR Recomm Rep 2002; 51:1–78.
24. Darrow WW, Echenberg DF, Jaffe HW, O'Malley PM, Byers RH, Getchell JP, Curran JW. Risk factors for human immunodeficiency virus (HIV) infections in homosexual men. Am J Public Health 1987; 77:479–483.
25. Greenblatt RM, Lukehart SA, Plummer FA, et al. Genital ulceration as a risk factor for human immunodeficiency virus infection. AIDS 1988; 2:47–50.
26. Johns DR, Tierney M, Felsenstein D. Alteration in the natural history of neurosyphilis by concurrent infection with the human immunodeficiency virus. N Engl J Med 1987; 316:1569–1572.
27. O'Mahony C, Rodgers CA, Mendelsohn SS, et al. Rapidly progressive syphilis in early HIV infection. Int J STD AIDS 1997; 8:275–277.
28. Bowen DL, Lane HC, Fauci AS. Immunopathogenesis of the acquired immunodeficiency syndrome. Ann Intern Med 1985; 103:704–709.
29. Wendel GO, Jr, Stark BJ, Jamison RB, Melina RD, Sullivan TJ. Penicillin allergy and desensitization in serious infections during pregnancy. N Engl J Med 1985; 312:1229–1232.
30. Pearlman MD, Yashar C, Ernst S, Solomon W. An incremental dosing protocol for women with severe vaginal trichomoniasis and adverse reaction to metronidazole. Am J Obstet Gynecol 1996; 174:934–936.

10 Trichomoniasis

Anne Moore

INTRODUCTION

Trichomonas vaginalis was first discovered by Donné in 1836. Today, it is responsible for 25% of all cases of clinically diagnosed vaginitis. More than half of infected women and nearly 90% of infected men are asymptomatic, which increases the reservoir of people spreading the infection. Trichomoniasis increases the risks of human immunodeficiency virus (HIV) transmission and HIV acquisition.

FAST FACTS

- There are 5 million new infections with *T. vaginalis* in the United States each year.
- The routine diagnostic test—microscopic evaluation of a vaginal specimen—detects only 50–60% of infections.
- Treatment of the non-pregnant woman and her partner is necessary even if they had no symptoms.
- Some strains of *T. vaginalis* are now resistant to metronidazole and require higher dose therapy with metronidazole or treatment with tinidazole.

PREVALENCE AND INCIDENCE

Trichomoniasis is the second most common sexually transmitted infection (STI) after human papillomavirus. Because this STI is not a reportable disease, data regarding actual numbers of cases remain elusive. However, it has been estimated that there are 5 million new cases in the United States each year, which is more than the sum of all cases of chlamydia and gonococcal infections *(1,2)*. The World Health Organization estimates that there are 173 million new infections worldwide per year *(3)*.

Prevalence rates for trichomoniasis infections with *T. vaginalis* vary with different types of clinical settings. For example, Soper reported that studies in

From: *Current Clinical Practice: Sexually Transmitted Diseases:*
A Practical Guide for Primary Care
Edited by: A. L. Nelson and J. A. Woodward © Humana Press, Totowa, NJ

sexually transmitted disease clinics found that between 15 and 54% of women in those sites had culture or polymerase chain reaction (PCR) evidence of trichomonal infection, 43% of patients in substance abuse facilities, 47% of prison inmates, 10–13% of women in student health, and 11–22% of HIV-infected or at-risk women were found to have trichomonal infections *(4)*.

Earlier studies suggested that 6–15% of asymptomatic women undergoing annual Pap smears had *T. vaginalis (5)*. In contrast to other STIs, such as chlamydia and gonorrhea, peak years of prevalence for trichomoniasis occur later in life—among 20- to 46-year-olds. There is generally a longer duration of infectiousness and a high level of asymptomatic infections, especially in men.

RISK FACTORS

Risk factors for trichomoniasis include all the risks generally associated with STI acquisition—multiple or new partners, non-use of barrier method of contraception, young age, minority member, lower socioeconomic status, and other STIs. Chlamydial infection is a particularly high risk factor; up to 30% of women with chlamydial cervicitis also have trichomoniasis.

INFECTIVITY AND TRANSMISSION

The primary mode of transmission of *T. vaginalis* is through sexual contact. Transmission by fomites is possible, but is rarely the cause of a symptomatic infection. An inoculum of at least 10,000 organisms is needed to establish a clinically significant infection; fomites are usually not able to deliver that large a deposit of organisms. Male-to-female transmission rates are higher than female-to-male rates; about 85% of exposed women will contract the infection. Female-to-male transmission rates are more variable, but may be as high as 70% within 48 hours of exposure *(4)*. Incubation period varies from 4 to 28 days *(6)*.

ETIOLOGY

T. vaginalis is a unicellular, anaerobic, flagellated protozoan. The organism was the first described in 1836 by Donné. The usual size range of this parasite is 5–15 μ long, but it can grow to 30 μ. It has a short undulating membrane, which extends only half way to the end of the body. The organism relies heavily on the host to obtain all nutrients as preformed molecules; it has little or no biosynthetic capability of its own. It even lacks mitochondria. *T. vaginalis* resembles anaerobic bacteria more than eukaryotic behavior in that it ferments large amounts of carbohydrates into carbon dioxide and hydrogen gases, causing bubbles. Its presence in the vaginal vault changes the vaginal microbiology—the lactobacilli disappear and anaerobic bacteria predominant. *T. vaginalis* swims freely in the vaginal discharge but can also attach to the vaginal wall. The cell membranes of

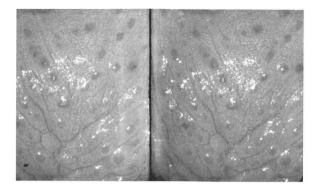

Trichomoniasis: strawberry spots on the vaginal wall.

the parasite and those of the host interdigitate. Trichomonads adhere to vaginal and cervical epithelial cells. *T. vaginalis* also infects the urethra, Skene's glands, and Bartholin glands. The organism does not invade into the underlying tissues but precipitates an intense inflammatory response locally *(7)*.

This inflammatory response is responsible not only for the characteristic clinical and laboratory findings of leukocytosis, but it also explains the increased vulnerability people infected with *T. vaginalis* have to acquiring HIV. HIV can gain ready access through disruptions in the epithelium to HIV target cells, such as CD4-bearing lymphocytes and macrophages concentrated in the area in response to the *T. vaginalis* infection. Trichomoniasis also increases the infectivity of HIV-infected individuals *(8,9)*. Treatment of *T. vaginalis* in HIV-infected women decreases cell-free HIV-1 virus by 4.2-fold in the vagina. Similarly, trichomoniasis-infected men with HIV have a sixfold higher concentration of HIV RNA in their seminal plasma than those without trichomonal infections *(10)*.

CLINICAL MANIFESTATIONS

Half of women infected with *T. vaginalis* are asymptomatic, but about 30% of these women will develop symptoms when they are followed for 6 months *(11)*. Women who develop symptoms may complain of increased vaginal discharge, which has a green hue, frothy appearance, and foul odor. The odor may not be because of the original trichomonal infection, but may result from concomitant bacterial vaginosis. Women may also have complaints of urinary frequency, dysuria, dyspareunia, and/or postcoital spotting. Dysuria and frequency may be caused by a urethral infection; dyspareunia and postcoital spotting generally result from the inflamed and friable cervix. Some women may note vulvar irritation, pruritus, or edema.

Only about 10% of men infected with *T. vaginalis* develop symptoms. Latif et al. suggested that men may be more resistant to infection or may be able to clear the infection without developing symptoms or treatment *(12)*. It is unlikely that men are resistant to infection, because a serological survey found that men and women were as likely to have antibodies to *T. vaginalis (13)*. This high level of asymptomatic infection in men is important to emphasize when counseling women who are diagnosed with trichomoniasis; they should expect that their sex partners will deny having symptoms. Symptoms in men are nonspecific. They may have urethral discharge and/or dysuria. More severe symptoms are more likely to be reported in cases in which the infection involves the prostate or seminal vesicles. One study found trichomoniasis in 5.5% of men with nongonococcal urethritis. Interestingly, the men with *T. vaginalis* as a cause of nongonococcal urethritis had experienced symptoms for nearly twice as long than men with other etiologies *(12)*. The discharge these men experienced was also different from other STI-related urethral discharges; it was characterized as a white, watery discharge with tiny clumps of material. When these clumps were examined microscopically, large numbers of epithelial cells with some white cells were seen. Interestingly, the diagnosis of *T. vaginalis* also occurred in men who were treated for laboratory-confirmed cases of gonococcal urethritis, suggesting that initially the men had dual infections. Prostatitis with or without epididymitis is an uncommon complication. Therefore, other STIs should be ruled out before attributing these complications to trichomonal infection.

On physical examination, an infected woman may have copious amounts of frothy discharge at her introitus with erythema and some edema in the vestibule and surrounding labia. The vaginal vault may be coated with gray or yellow-green-colored frothy discharge, which often pools in the upper vault. The bubbles in the discharge, which are characteristic of this infection, result from the metabolism of carbohydrates into carbon dioxide and hydrogen gases. However, frothiness was found in only 12–34% of cases in Gardener and Duke's series *(14)*. Wiping away the discharge from the cervix, the portio may seem to have an injected, edematous appearance speckled with clusters of petechia (punctate mucosal hemorrhages), which has classically been described as a "strawberry" or "flea-bitten" cervix. These petechiae are best seen with colposcopic magnification. The cervix may be quite friable, but in the absence of other STIs, there should not be cervical motion tenderness.

TESTING AND DIAGNOSIS

T. vaginalis can be isolated in urine, semen, and vaginal discharge. The standard diagnostic test is microscopic examination of vaginal discharge. Collecting and handling of the specimen are critically important in improving the sensitivity of the wet-mount test. The classic technique of placing a drop of the vaginal

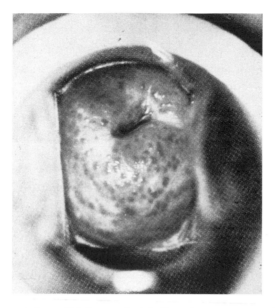

Trichomonas (a.k.a., Trichomoniasis). Strawberry spots on the cervix.

secretions directly onto a slide and mixing in some normal saline, then trapping the specimen under a cover slide is most effective when the specimen is promptly examined. Any substantial delay in examining the specimen (e.g., when other specimens are collected, bimanual exam is performed, and the patient is counseled about physical findings) allows the specimen to dry out. After drying, the protozoan loses its characteristic pear shape and becomes rounded. In this shape, it is easy to overlook it in sheets of similar shaped (but smaller) leukocytes, which are present in abundance. Twenty percent of wet mounts initially positive for *T. vaginalis* become negative within 10 minutes, and 87% disappear within 2 hours. In order to retain the pear-shape morphology of *T. vaginalis*, the clinician should suspend the vaginal specimen in a test tube with normal saline that has no preservatives. When it is time to do microscopy, a drop of the dilute specimen can be placed onto the slide for examination. At room temperature, *T. vaginalis* may lose its rapid motion, but if the pear-shaped organism is observed, a slow undulation will be seen. This dilution of the specimen also allows separation of the epithelial cells so that their borders are easier to examine to rule out concomitant bacterial vaginosis.

The sensitivity of the microscopic examination of the vaginal discharge varies from 42 to 92% *(15)*, with most studies reporting sensitivities of 50–60% *(16)*. The variation seen is a function not only of the technique used, but also the time spent searching for *T. vaginalis* in the microscopic sample. Sweet reported that experienced technicians can detect 80% of cases, but that the sensitivity drops to 50% when the test is performed by busy clinicians *(15)*. Ledger reports even lower accuracy. He found considerable errors in diagnoses; only 51.2% of patients with culture proven infection were detected on microscopy and 25% of women diagnosed with trichomoniasis microscopically did not have the infection on culture *(17)*.

There are two FDA-cleared tests for trichomonas in women: the OSOM Trichomonas Rapid test (Genzyme Diagnostics, Cambridge, MA), which uses an immunochromatographic capillary flow dipstick technology and a nucleic acid probe test called the Affirm VP II System (Becton Dickinson), which uses synthetic probes for detection of *T. vaginalis*, bacterial vaginosis, and *Candida* from a single vaginal swab. These tests have greater than 83% sensitivity and specificity greater than 97%, compared to culture.

Other techniques that have been tested for diagnosis of *T. vaginalis* infection include monoclonal antibody staining of direct specimens *(18)*. This technology has been shown to have a 92% sensitivity overall and a 77% sensitivity in women with negative microscopy. Monoclonal antibody staining provides rapid answers; however, the need for specific reagents and high-quality microscopy rules this out as an office-based procedure *(19)*. PCR tests have been developed that are more sensitive than cultures and can distinguish *T. vaginalis* from other trichomonal species. The test is too expensive for routine use at this time. Lobo et al. reported that the sensitivity of traditional testing modalities, when compared with PCR, are lower than generally recognized. For example, when compared with PCR, culture is only 79% as sensitive, wet mounts are 66% as sensitive, and Pap smear sensitivity was 61% *(20)*.

The gold standard technique for diagnosis has been culture, the sensitivities of other tests are measured against it. Culture is straightforward, but special culture media are needed. The two most commonly used media are Diamond or Kupferberg media, but laboratory support for processing cultures is frequently not available. Products such as InPouch™ TV (Biomed Diagnostics, San Jose, CA) have been developed to combine culture and microscopy *(21)*. Generally, only 1000–10,000 organisms are necessary for an infection to be detected on culture. Negative results will not be available for up to 7 days, but positive results may be available earlier. The best specimen to culture in women is material from the vaginal vault. In men, urethral pus or a spun-down urine specimen (urine sediment) may be cultured.

In general, the conventional Pap smear has been found to be a poor diagnostic test of trichomoniasis. It has low sensitivity (52–67%) and a low specificity (83–99%), even when the smear is prepared with a vital strain, such as acridine orange *(15)*. Although it is acknowledged that conventional Pap smears are not useful in screening women for this infection, clinicians are often left with the challenge of how best to manage women whose Pap smear reports the presence of *T. vaginalis*. Today it is recognized that asymptomatic infections in non-pregnant women warrant treatment, but the accuracy of the Pap smear must be questioned. In one study comparing various test procedures, cytological smear were interpreted as positive in 56% of the women who actually had infection detected by other methods, but another 1% of the population tested were read as positive and 3% were read as "suspicious" when they had negative cultures. The authors found a positive predictive value of only 69% *(18)*. For many women the issue of having an infection, which is probably sexually transmitted, is important to their relationships. Therefore, the correct management of an asymptomatic woman with an isolated Pap smear reporting *T. vaginalis* is controversial. Some argue that because trichomoniasis is an important STI and treatment is not associated with much cost or side effects, women should be offered treatment based on the Pap smear results alone. This automatic treatment is a reasonable approach for women who are in high-prevalence populations or who are at higher personal risk for having the infection. One example would be the woman who has been recently diagnosed with chlamydia and her Pap smear reported *T. vaginalis*. For lower risk women, there is more conflict. This is because the traditional diagnostic test used—the wet mount—is very insensitive. The argument is that if a woman really had trichomoniasis (suggested by her Pap smear), there would be a 40–50% of missing it with a microscopic evaluation of her vaginal discharge. One solution would be to seek the woman's counsel about her willingness to be treated with no further work-up. If she prefers to have more information, perform a wet mount and treat the positive results. If her wet mount is negative, perform more sensitive testing (such as a culture).

Liquid-based Papanicolaou cervical cytology testing may improve the detection of *T. vaginalis* compared with conventional Pap smear. One study found that compared to culture, liquid-based Pap testing had a sensitivity of 61.4% (virtually the same as conventional tests) but an improved specificity of 99.4%. This improved the positive predictive value to 96.4% *(16)*.

In men, diagnosis is even more challenging. It is difficult to identify *T. vaginalis* in either a centrifuged deposit of urine or urethral discharge suspended in normal saline. In one study, only 50% of men with the infection had it detected on first microscopic examination. Wet-mount microscopic studies of urethral samples had only 30% sensitivity and urethral cultures detected only 60% of infections *(22)*. PCR has the ability to detect four times more infections than combined cultures of urethra and urethral swabs. Culture testing of ureteral swabs, urine, and semen is required for optimal sensitivity. The intrinsic insensitivity of tests of men is another reason that male sex partners of infected women need to be treated on an epidemiological basis—even if they have no evidence of personal infection. Patients with trichomoniasis should be evaluated for other STIs.

Table 1
Trichomoniasis CDC STD Treatment Guidelines 2006

Recommended regimens— Select one of the following:	Alternative regimen
Metronidazole [a] 2 g orally in a single dose Tinidazole [a] 2 g orally in a single dose	Metronidazole [a] 500 mg orally twice a day for 7 days

[a] Patients should be advised to avoid consuming alcohol during treatment with metronidazole or tinidazole and for 24 hours after metronidazole and 72 hours after completion of tinidazole.

TREATMENT

Metronidazole has been the drug of choice for the treatment of infections with *T. vaginalis* since 1960 *(23)*. The Center for Disease Control and Prevention recommendations for treatment of uncomplicated trichomoniasis have remained constant for the last several years *(see* Table 1). The recommended regimen is metronidazole 2 g or tinidazole 2 g orally in a single dose. Metronidazole single-dose therapy has a cure rate of 90–95% *(24)*. Tinidazole's cure rate is 86–100%. Tinidazole has more complete tissue penetration and lower minimum lethal concentrations than metronidazole *(24a)*. Lower doses of metronidazole have been studied in an attempt to decrease gastrointestinal side effects. The 1.5-mg dose was roughly equivalent to the 2 mg dose, and had fewer side effects, but even lower doses were associated with unacceptably high failure rates *(25)*. The alternative recommendation of metronidazole 500 mg orally twice a day for 7 days is thought to be equivalent and to have similar side effect rates as single dose therapy *(26)*, but is associated with lower compliance rates. Incomplete use of 7-day treatments has resulted in the emergence of strains of *T. vaginalis* that are more resistant to metronidazole. Oral systemic therapies are needed because *T. vaginalis* can be sequestered in the Bartholin glands or Skein's glands, not treatable by topical therapies. A trial of single 2 mg intravaginal metronidazole cream resulted in a 50% cure rate compared to an 88% cure rate with systemic therapy *(27)*.

Use of metronidazole or tinidazole is associated with potential side effects, including a metallic taste, headache, and a 12% incidence of nausea *(28)*. Ingestion of alcohol should be avoided for 24 hours preceding and up to 72 hours following drug administration. Prolonged therapies of these agents can potentiate the effects of warfarin and impact phenytoin and lithium levels *(29)*.

For patients with metronidazole allergy, Pearlman et al. have reported successful use of an "incremental" protocol for desensitization used in two patients

Table 2
Metronidazole Desensitization Protocol

- Verify immediate hypersensitivity reaction (wheal to MetroGel on skin).
- Pretreat with antihistamines or corticosteroids.
- Monitor with frequent measurements of blood pressure and EKGs with continuous oxygen saturation monitoring.
- Crash cart and intubation tray.
- Provide doses every 15–20 minutes.
- Monitor for minimum of 4 hours after desensitization.

Dose	Metronidazole	Volume
5 µg	5 µg/mL	1 mL
15 µg	5 µg/mL	3 mL
50 µg	50 µg/mL	1 mL
150 µg	50 µg/mL	3 mL
500 µg	500 µg/mL	1 mL
1.5 mg	500 µg/mL	3 mL
5 mg	5 mg/mL	1 mL
15 mg	5 mg/mL	3 mL
30 mg	5 mg/mL	6 mL
60 mg	5 mg/mL	12 mL
125 mg	5 mg/mL	25 mL
250 mg	250 mg tablet	—

Source: From ref. 20.

(30). The first step is to verify an immediate hypersensitivity reaction by placing a small amount of MetroGel-Vaginal® gel on the skin and observing for the development of a wheal. If the patient has a demonstrated reaction, desensitizing therapy may be performed in a setting able to handle anaphylactic shock (generally a hospital). Patients should be pretreated with antihistamine or corticosteroids. They should be monitored with blood pressure, electrocardiogram, and continuous measurement of O_2 saturation. A crash cart and intubation tray should be available with trained personnel ready. Metronidazole is given intravenously starting at a 5-µg dose and increasing increments every 15–20 minutes as outlined in Table 2.

No routine test of cure is needed for patients who are treated unless the patient remains symptomatic. In this case, the most likely cause of symptoms is re-infection. Inquire about sexual exposures since treatment and their timing in relation to partner's treatments. Re-infections can be treated as initial infections. Routine doses of metronidazole may be subtherapeutic in patients taking drugs such as phenytoin, which increase hepatic microsomal enzyme activity.

Resistance to metronidazole is emerging. Current estimates are that 2.5–5% of infections are resistant to recommended or alternative treatments *(31)*. Because clusters of patients with highly resistant *T. vaginalis* have not been reported, Pattman suggested that the mechanisms of metronidazole resistance are likely to be idiosyncratic and unstable *(32)*. In resistant infections, the patient and partner should be treated with a 7-day course of metronidazole 500 mg twice a day. Both should undergo immediate tests of cure following completion of treatment. If the infection persists, use metronidazole 500 mg orally four times a day for 3–5 days. Side effects and complication rates (including irreversible neurological problems) increase at doses greater than 3 g daily. It should be noted that there are seven cases reported in the literature of metronidazole-induced acute pancreatitis *(33)*. Various combinations of tinidazole orally and vaginally have been reported to be effective in the treatment of metronidazole-resistant trichomonal infections. Sobel reported an 89% cure rate with 1 g orally three times a day combined with 500 mg per vagina three times a day for 14 days *(24a)*.

Some infections require culture and sensitivity testing to determine metronidazole dosing and the appropriate route of administration (oral or intravenous). Technical assistance and consultation are available at the Centers for Disease Control and Prevention (telephone: [770] 488-4115, Web site: http://www.cdc. gov/std/).

PARTNER NOTIFICATION
AND REPORTING REQUIREMENTS

Although trichomonas is not reportable disease, it is important to have partners treated before resuming sexual contract. If this does not take place, re-infection of the treated patient is almost a certainty. Caution patients that most men will deny any symptoms and may resist treatment, but they should be treated presumptively for trichomonas and related STIs even in the absence if any clinical finding of *T. vaginalis* infection.

PREGNANCY-RELATED ISSUES

Pregnancy complications include an increased incidence of premature rupture of membranes and increased preterm delivery rates and low-birthweight infants *(34)*. Treatment with metronidazole (Pregnancy Category B) does not appear to reduce this prenatal morbidity. The safety of tinidazole in pregnancy has not been established. Pregnant women with symptomatic infections should be treated with metronidazole 2 mg orally all at once at any trimester. This therapy minimizes fetal exposure. Reports have found no teratogenicity associated with *in utero* exposure even if administered in the first trimester *(35,36)*. Treatment of asymptomatic pregnant women is more controversial. Metronidazole has been associated with higher risk of preterm delivery in women with prior history of preterm delivery compared with untreated asymptomatic controls in one doubled-blinded, placebo-controlled trial *(36)*. However, treatment might reduce the spread of this STI and might prevent respiratory or genital infection of the newborn. The CDC does not recommend treatment of asymptomatic pregnant women. Breastfeeding women should discard their breast milk during treatment and for 12–24 hours after their last dose of metronidazole. If using tinidazole, breast milk should be discarded for 3 days after the last dose.

PREVENTION

The National Institutes of Health expert panel cited a study that reports a 30% reduction in risk of infection of *T. vaginalis* in women using condoms, but concludes that the paucity of epidemiological studies of condom effectiveness for trichomonas does not allow an accurate assessment of the reduction in risk of trichomonas infection by condom use *(37)*.

Education regarding transmission of *T. vaginalis* and the signs and symptoms of trichomoniasis is needed by patients and providers. The health risks associated with trichomonal infection must be more respected, especially its connection with transmission of HIV. Health care professionals should adopt effective techniques for detection of this infection to reduce its prevalence. Patients need instruction in safer sex practices to avoid this infection.

CASE STUDY

Angela, age 19, had a routine Pap smear, which indicated that she had an infection with T. vaginalis. Angela did not have a wet mount at the time of the Pap smear because she was asymptomatic. You treated her for chlamydia 4 months ago.

Questions

1. What should you do with the results?

Possible Answers

a. Perform a wet mount and treat only if the infection was confirmed.
b. Perform a wet mount and treat regardless of the outcome.
c. Culture her for *T. vaginalis*.
d. Decide that no follow-up is needed because she is asymptomatic.

Correct Answers

1. b. Try to find the infection on microscopy, but given that she is high risk, treat.

Teaching Points

- Sensitivity of the wet mount for detecting trichomonas is only 60%; therefore, in an asymptomatic low-risk patient, confirmatory testing would be advisable.
- However, this patient, by virtue of her recent chlamydia diagnosis is a high-risk patient.
- Women and their partners need to be treated.
- A repeat chlamydia test should be done at the first visit. (It has been 4 months since her chlamydial cervicitis was treated.)
- A more comprehensive sexual history is indicated. This offers an opportunity for safer sex counseling.

REFERENCES

1. Cates W Jr. Estimates of the incidence and prevalence of sexually transmitted diseases in the United States. American Social Health Association Panel. Sex Transm Dis 1999; 26:S2–S7.
2. Gerbase AC, Rowley JT, Heymann DH, Berkley SF, Piot P. Global prevalence and incidence estimates of selected curable STDs. Sex Transm Infect 1998; 74:S12–S16.
3. World Health Organization. Sexually Transmitted Infections Fact Sheet. Geneva, Switzerland: World Health Organization. 2004. Available from: www.who.int/reproductive-health/rtis/docs/sti_factsheet_2004.pdf. Accessed April 18, 2005.
4. Soper D. Trichomoniasis: under control or undercontrolled? Am J Obstet Gynecol 2004; 190:281–290.
5. Spence MR, Hollander DH, Smith J, McCaig L, Sewell D, Brockman M. The clinical and laboratory diagnosis of *Trichomonas vaginalis* infection. Sex Transm Dis 1980; 7:168–171.
6. Petrin D, Delgaty K, Bhatt R, Garber G. Clinical and microbiological aspects of *Trichomonas vaginalis*. Clin Microbiol Rev 1998; 11:300–317.
7. Horowitz BJ, Mårdh P-A, eds. *Vaginitis and Vaginosis*. New York, NY: Wiley-Liss, 1999.
8. Hook EW III. *Trichomonas vaginalis*—no longer a minor STD. Sex Transm Dis 1999; 26:388–389.
9. Laga M, Manoka A, Kivuvu M, et al. Non-ulcerative sexually transmitted diseases as risk factors for HIV-1 transmission in women: results from a cohort study. AIDS 1993; 7:95–102.
10. Hobbs MM, Kazembe P, Reed AW, et al. Trichomonas vaginalis as a cause of urethritis in Malawian men. Sex Transm Dis 1999; 26:381–387.
11. Thomason JL, Gelbart SM. *Trichomonas vaginalis*. Obstet Gynecol 1989; 74:536–541.
12. Latif AS, Mason PR, Marowa E. Urethral trichomoniasis in men. Sex Transm Dis 1987; 14:9–11.
13. Mason PR, Forman L. Serological survey of trichomoniasis in Zimbabwe Rhodesia. Cent Afr J Med 1980; 26:6–8.
14. Gardner HL, Dukes CD. Haemophilus vaginalis vaginitis: a newly defined specific infection previously classified non-specific vaginitis. Am J Obstet Gynecol 1955; 69:962–976.
15. Sweet RL, Gibbs RS. *Infectious Diseases of the Female Genital Tract*, 4th Ed. Philadelphia, PA: Lippincott Williams & Wilkins, 2002, pp. 339–340.
16. Lara-Torre E, Pinkerton JS. Accuracy of detection of *Trichomonas vaginalis* organisms on a liquid-based Papanicolaou smear. Am J Obstet Gynecol 2003; 188:354–356.
17. Ledger WJ, Monif GR. A growing concern: inability to diagnose vulvovaginal infections correctly. Obstet Gynecol 2004; 103:782–784.

18. Krieger JN, Tam MR, Stevens CE, et al. Diagnosis of trichomoniasis. Comparison of conventional wet-mount examination with cytologic studies, cultures, and monoclonal antibody staining of direct specimens. JAMA 1988; 259:1223–1227.
19. van Der Schee C, van Belkum A, Zwijgers L, et al. Improved diagnosis of *Trichomonas vaginalis* infection by PCR using vaginal swabs and urine specimens compared to diagnosis by wet mount microscopy, culture, and fluorescent staining. J Clin Microbiol 1999; 37:4127–4130.
20. Lobo TT, Feijo G, Carvalho SE, et al. A comparative evaluation of the Papanicolaou test for the diagnosis of trichomoniasis. Sex Transm Dis 2003; 30:694–699.
21. Borchardt KA, Li Z, Zhang MZ, Shing H. An in vitro metronidazole susceptibility test for trichomoniasis using the InPouch TV test. Genitourin Med 1996; 72:132–135.
22. Weston TE, Nicol CS. Natural history of trichomonal infection in males. Br J Vener Dis 1963; 39:251–257.
23. Durel P, Roiron V, Siboulet A, Borel LJ. Systemic treatment of human trichomoniasis with a derivative of nitro-imidazole, 8823 RP. Br J Vener Dis 1960; 36:21–26.
24. Centers for Disease Control and Prevention. Sexually transmitted diseases treatment guidelines, 2006. MMWR 2006; 55(RR-11):52–54. Available from: http://www.cdc.gov/std/treatment/. Accessed Nov. 24, 2006.
24a. Sobel JD, Nyirjesy P, Brown W. Tinidazole therapy for metronidazole-resistant vaginal trichomoniasis. Clin Infect Dis 2001; 33:1341–1346.
25. Spence MR, Harwell TS, Davies MC, Smith JL, The minimum single oral metronidazole dose for treating trichomoniasis: a randomized, blinded study. Obstet Gynecol 1997; 89:699–703.
26. Hager WD, Brown ST, Kraus SJ, Kleris GS, Perkins GJ, Henderson M. Metronidazole for vaginal trichomoniasis. Seven-day vs single-dose regimens. JAMA 1980; 244:1219–1220.
27. Tidwell BH, Lushbaugh WB, Laughlin MD, Cleary JD, Finley RW. A double-blind placebo-controlled trial of single-dose intravaginal versus single-dose oral metronidazole in the treatment of trichomonal vaginitis. J Infect Dis 1994; 170:242–246.
28. Smilack JD, Wilson WR, Cockerill FR III. Tetracyclines, chloramphenicol, erythromycin, clindamycin, and metronidazole. Mayo Clin Proc 1991; 66:1270–1280.
29. Flagyl. Prescribing Information. Chicago, IL: Pfizer Inc., 2004.
30. Pearlman MD, Yashar C, Ernst S, Solomon W. An incremental dosing protocol for women with severe vaginal trichomoniasis and adverse reaction to metronidazole. Am J Obstet Gynecol 1996; 174:934–936.
31. Schmid G, Narcisi E, Mosure D, Secor WE, Higgins J, Moreno H. Prevalence of metronidazole-resistant *Trichomonas vaginalis* in a gynecology clinic. J Reprod Med 2001; 46:545–549.
32. Pattman RS. Recalcitrant vaginal trichomoniasis. Sex Transm Infect 1999; 75:127–128.
33. Feola DJ, Thornton AC. Metronidazole-induced pancreatitis in a patient with recurrent vaginal trichomoniasis. Pharmacotherapy 2002; 22:1508–1510.
34. Cotch MF, Pastorek JG II, Nugent RP, et al. *Trichomonas vaginalis* associated with low birth weight and preterm delivery. The Vaginal Infections and Prematurity Study Group. Sex Transm Dis 1997; 24:353–360.
35. Burtin P, Taddio A, Ariburnu O, Einarson TR, Koren G. Safety of metronidazole in pregnancy: a meta-analysis. Am J Obstet Gynecol 1995; 172:525–529.
36. Piper JM, Mitchel EF, Ray WA. Prenatal use of metronidazole and birth defects: no association. Obstet Gynecol 1993; 82:348–352.
37. National Institute of Allergy and Infectious Diseases. Workshop summary: scientific evidence on condom effectiveness for sexually transmitted disease (STD) prevention. Washington, DC: National Institutes of Health, Department of Health Services, 2001. Available from: http://www.niaid.nih.gov/dmid/stds/condomreport.pdf. Accessed Nov. 24, 2006.

11

Lymphogranuloma Venereum, Chancroid, Granuloma Inguinale, and Molluscum Contagiosum

JoAnn Woodward

INTRODUCTION

Genital infections with lymphogranuloma venereum (LGV), chancroid, granuloma inguinale, and molluscum contagiosum are sexually transmitted infections (STIs) that are generally more frequently found in tropical areas, but do present in the United States. Each is more common in human immunodeficiency virus (HIV)-infected individuals than in the general population. Ulcerative infections increase the risks of transmission and acquisition of HIV. Diagnosis of each of these infections is usually done clinically; the availability of laboratory testing to support the diagnosis is limited.

FAST FACTS

- Chancroid lesions are very painful and often spread by auto-inoculation, especially in women.
- LGV initially presents as a painless lesion that may go unnoticed, but the subsequent adenopathy can be very painful. In the third stage of the disease, fibrosis causes significant genital distortion, including elephantiasis.
- Granuloma inguinale is also a chronic, ulcerative, progressively destructive STI. In the advanced stages, the lesions swell, become superinfected, and induce irreversible genital deformity. Social isolation is common because of the characteristic aroma of this infection.
- Molluscum contagiosum in the genital area is an STI. The characteristic lesion is a raised, centrally umbilicated papule or nodule.

LYMPHOGRANULOMA VENEREUM
Introduction

LGV was not identified as a separate pathological entity until 1913. Before that time, it was confused with chancroid, syphilis, or herpes. It has also been called

From: *Current Clinical Practice: Sexually Transmitted Diseases:*
A Practical Guide for Primary Care
Edited by: A. L. Nelson and J. A. Woodward © Humana Press, Totowa, NJ

tropical, strumous, climatic bubo, lymphogranuloma inguinale, poradenitis inguinalis, and Durand-Nicolas-Favre disease *(1)*. LGV is a chronic STI caused by *Chlamydia trachomatis*. LGV has three stages of clinical manifestations—a small, short-lived, relatively asymptomatic primary lesion; a secondary stage character-ized by inguinal adenopathy or acute hemorrhagic proctitis and systemic symp-toms; and a third stage marked by ulceration, fistula formation, rectal strictures, and genital elephantiasis. Because of the ulcerative nature of LGV, patients are at increased risk of transmitting or acquiring HIV and other STIs.

Prevalence and Incidence

Although LGV is found worldwide, it most commonly occurs in tropical areas. LGV is endemic in East and West Africa, India, part of Southeast Asia, Central American, South American, and the Caribbean. For example, a surveyed clinic in Ethiopia reported several thousand cases each year *(1)*. By contrast, LGV is rela-tively rare in the United States and occurs sporadically. In 2004, there was a slight increase in cases reported among men who have sex with men (MSM) on the west coast. Most cases in the United States are found in men and in urban areas. Peak years of infection are in the 30s. Although LGV infections are five times more likely to occur in men than in women, the long-term complications are more common in women because the infection is more asymptomatic in women and, therefore, more frequently goes undetected until a more advanced stage.

Risk Factors

As an STI, the risk of the infection is increased by a history of multiple sexual partners and young age. However, in the most recent outbreaks in the United States, most cases were found among MSM practicing anal receptive sex who have had contact with MSM from Europe. Travel to endemic countries is another risk factor in those engaging in high-risk sexual practices.

Infectivity and Transmission

LGV is spread by sexual contact. It is not known if LGV can be transmitted as a fomite on shared sex toys or by fisting, which would be important to know when counseling MSM *(2)*. The infectivity is not known, but is generally thought to be less than gonorrhea.

Etiology

LGV is an STI caused by *C. trachomatis*, serotypes L_1, L_2, and L_3. *C. tracho-matis* cannot penetrate intact skin or mucous membranes. It enters the body through microabrasions in the skin. The life cycle of *C. trachomatis* is discussed in Chapter 6. These strains are more invasive in tissue culture than the strains that cause chlamydial cervicitis and urethritis. It is believed that most of the extensive tissue damage seen with LGV is caused by a cell-mediated "hypersensitivity" to chlamydia antigen *(3)*.

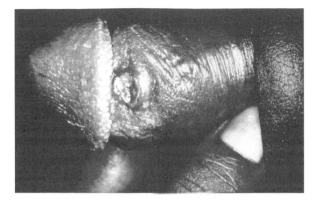

Penile lymphogranuloma venereum.

Clinical Manifestation

The incubation period for LGV is 3–30 days. The disease has both systemic manifestations and a wide spectrum of anogenital lesions, lymphadenopathy with destruction, and distortion of the genital areas. Subclinical infections are also possible, especially in women. The clinical manifestations progress through three stages. The primary lesion is generally self-limited and painless except in primary rectal LGV, which may present with proctitis and diarrhea, discharge, and ulcerations (4). The primary lesion, which develops at the site of inoculation, is typically small (2–10 mm in diameter). This primary lesion can take one of four forms: a small, nonpainful papule; a shallow ulcer or erosion; a small herpetiform lesion; or nonspecific urethritis (1). The primary lesion usually bursts quickly and forms an ulcer that oozes pus, but heals rapidly thereafter. In women, the lesion typically forms in the posterior vaginal wall, the fourchette, cervix, or vulva. In men, the primary lesion occurs in the coronal sulcus, but may develop on the frenulum, prepuce, penis, urethral glans, or scrotum. It may be associated with a cordlike lymphangitis of the dorsal penis and form large painful lymphangial nodule called a "bubonulus" (1). If the bubonulus ruptures, both draining sinuses of the urethra and deforming scars on the penis can develop. In women, LGV cervicitis can spread into the parametrium or salpinges. Alternatively, the lesion may remain undetected in the urethra, vaginal vault or rectum as it ulcerates.

Most people first seek care during the second stage of the infection because the first stage goes unnoticed by them. The secondary stage of LGV represents the spread of the infection into lymphatic tissue. The secondary stage develops days to months (average 10–30 days) after the primary lesion. The first symptoms of the second stage may be systemic—such as fever, malaise, headache,

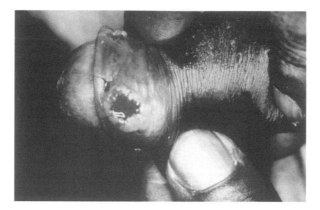

Penile lymphogranuloma venereum.

anorexia, myalgia, and arthralgia. In the inguinal syndrome, these symptoms are followed rapidly by the development of adenopathy. The inguinal syndrome is the most frequent clinical manifestation of LGV. The superficial inguinal nodes are most often involved, but femoral nodes may also be affected. Adenopathy is unilateral in two-thirds of cases in women. Initially firm, discrete, multiple, slightly tender nodes develop. As the inflammation of the lymph nodes becomes more intense in the following few weeks, the nodes enlarge, necrose, and form fluctuant abscesses or buboes. These become adherent to the subcutaneous tissue and the overlying skin. If both the inguinal and femoral nodes are involved, Poupart's ligament creates a groove between the nodes and the patient develops the classic "groove sign;" this occurs in 10–20% of cases *(3)*. If untreated, the bubo ruptures in one-third of cases. Rupture relives the pain and fever, but multiple sinus tracts form in the base of the ulcer and drain thick pus for months. Even after rupture, buboes recur in 20% of untreated patients *(1)*. Buboes that do not rupture undergo slow involution and form chronic inguinal masses.

Another second stage manifestation of LGV is the anogenitorectal syndrome, in which perianal or perirectal lymphatic tissue (usually of the distal left side of the large intestine) becomes inflamed, resulting in hemorrhagic proctocolitis, perirectal abscesses, ischiorectal or rectovaginal fistulas, or anal fistulas. Ultimately, anal or rectal strictures result. The clinical and histological presentations of LGV proctocolitis may mimic the initial manifestations of inflammatory bowel disease *(5)*. The rectal strictures of LGV must be distinguished from carcinoma, tuberculosis, actinomycosis, and schistosomiasis.

A minority of patients infected with LGV will progress to the third stage of the infection, which involves the external genitalia and the rectal area. Because healing from LGV infection is by fibrosis, the normal structure of the lymph nodes is altered, which causes obstruction of the lymphatics of the scrotum,

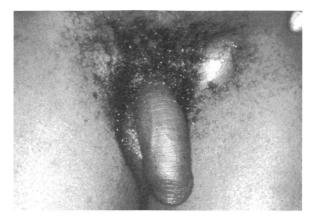

Male inguinal node lymphogranuloma venereum.

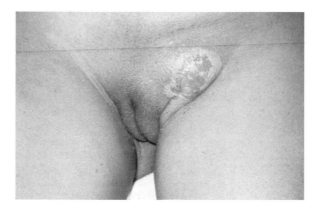

Female inguinal node lymphogranuloma venereum.

penis, or vulva. The chronic infection of the lymphatics, and the resulting edema and sclerosing fibrosis of the subcutaneous tissue cause induration and enlargement. This presents clinically as elephantiasis. In men, elephantiasis occurs within the penoscrotal area.

It is believed that much of the tissue damage in LGV is caused by a cell-mediated hypersensitivity to chlamydia antigens *(3)*. The term *esthiomene*, which is derived from the Greek word for "eating away," is used to describe the findings of LGV of the lymphatic system of the vulva, penis, and scrotum *(1)*. Ulceration of the lesion starts superficially, but later becomes destructive. In women, the areas of the labia major, genitocrural folds, and lateral areas of the perineum are most frequently involved.

Other clinical presentations include papillary growths in the urethral meatus of women, smooth pedunculated perianal lesions ("lymphorrhoids"), and follicular conjunctivitis. Rarely, the infecting organism enters the blood stream and involves unusual sites, such as the gallbladder, liver, or pericardium. Primary infections of the oral cavity or pharynx have also been reported.

Diagnosis

Diagnosis is based primarily on clinical findings; routine laboratory confirmation may not be possible (6). However, given the wide variety of clinical manifestations, clinical diagnosis may be difficult. This difficulty is compounded by the relative rarity of this infection, which means that many clinicians may not recognize the clinical findings.

Serological tests such as microimmunofluorescent or complement fixation tests are most commonly used to support the clinical diagnosis. Titers of complement fixation tests more than 1:64, or a fourfold increase in titer, are considered diagnostic (3) as are titers more than 1:128 on the microimmunofluorescent test (7). A list of laboratories that perform serologic tests for C. trachomatis and might provide titered results is available from http://www.cdc.gov/std/lgv-labs.htm.

The most accurate tests used to diagnose LGV today are those using polymerase chain reaction (PCR) and other amplification techniques, although nonculture nucleic acid testing is not specific for LGV. The Food and Drug Administration has not approved the use of rectal swabs for nucleic acid testing (6). In research settings and specialized laboratories, the genotype can be determined by performing restriction endonuclease pattern analysis of the amplified outer membrane protein A gene. Cultures of aspirates from the buboes or lesions are often performed, but are positive in only 30–50% of suspected lesions (1,8).

Evaluation of gastrointestinal syndromes that may have been sexually transmitted requires either anoscopy or sigmoidoscopy and testing for C. trachomatis, syphilis, herpes, N. gonorrhoeae, and common enteric pathogens that can be sexually transmitted (6). In order to evaluate rectal strictures, mucosal biopsy may be needed to rule out carcinoma or other chronic infections.

Treatment

The treatment of LGV is displayed in Table 1. Treatment should be started empirically pending return of laboratory test results. If the laboratory test results all return negative, therapy can be discontinued, if appropriate. The goal is to cure the infection and prevent ongoing tissue damage. Antibiotics are needed for 3 weeks. In addition, buboes may require aspiration through intact, uninfected tissue or incision and drainage to prevent inguinal/femoral ulcerations. Patients should be followed clinically until all signs and symptoms have resolved.

Table 1
Lymphogranuloma Venereum
CDC STD Treatment Guidelines 2006

Recommended regimen	Alternative regimen
Doxycycline [a] 100 mg orally twice a day for 21 days	Erythromycin base [b] 500 mg orally four times a day for 21 days

Source: ref. 6.

[a] Contraindicated for pregnant and lactating women and for children under 8 years old.

Partner Notification and Reporting Requirements

All partners who have had sexual contact with the patient within 60 days of the onset of symptoms should be examined (6,7). In the absence of symptoms, sexual contacts should be treated for a chlamydia cervicitis or urethritis (see Table 3 in Chapter 6). Symptomatic partners should be treated according to LGV treatment guidelines outlined in Table 1. If the patient is in the second stage of the infection, earlier partners may benefit from therapy. LGV is a reportable infection in many large metropolitan cities (Los Angeles, New York, and so on), but case reporting is not mandatory in all public health jurisdictions (9).

Pregnancy-Related Issues

Transplacental congenital infection can occur, but most neonatal infection occurs because of exposure during passage through an infected birth canal. For infected pregnant and lactating women, the Centers for Disease Control and Prevention (CDC) recommends only the use of erythromycins. Doxycycline is contraindicated in pregnancy.

CHANCROID

Introduction

Chancroid is commonly referred to as "soft chancre." It is a highly contagious STI caused by *Haemophilus ducreyi*. *H. ducreyi* was first identified as the causative organism for chancroid in 1889 when August Ducrey inoculated the forearms of infected patients with pus from their genital lesions (10). Causation was made even clearer later when Bezancon et al. inoculated the forearms of healthy volunteers with culture-purified organisms (*H. ducreyi*) and produced characteristic soft chancres from which the organisms were re-isolated (11).

The infection causes genital ulceration, regional lymphatitis, and bubo formation. It is a major cause of genital ulcer disease in many resource-poor countries in Africa, Asia, and Latin America (12). The genital ulceration caused by chancroid causes significant distress and increases the transmission and acquisition

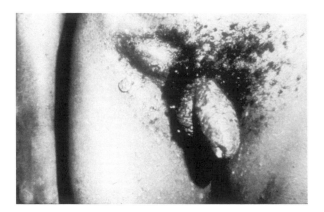

Male bubo chancroid.

of HIV infection *(13)*. The relative risk of acquiring HIV if a genital ulcer is present ranges from 3 to 18, with a per act increase in transmission of 10- to 100-fold *(14)*. About 10% of US patients with chancroids are co-infected with HIV or *T. pallidum*; this rate is higher than found in infected individuals in other countries.

Prevalence/Incidence

In 1997, the World Health Organization estimated that 6 million cases of chancroid occurred worldwide each year *(15)*. In developing countries, chancroid is the cause of most genital ulcerative disease and accounts for 10–30% of all STIs in Africa. In tropical countries, such as Kenya and Thailand, chancroid is one of the most common STIs *(16)*. The infection is common in Africa, Southeast Asia, and the Caribbean *(17)*. In developed countries, chancroid occurs sporadically, and most frequently among those individuals who have traveled to endemic areas. In the United States, 80% of infections occur in heterosexual men. The male to female ratio of infection in the United States is between 5:1 and 10:1.

Risk Factors

Commercial sex workers are felt to have been reservoirs of infection in the outbreaks that have occurred in the United States in the last decade. This is because chancroid is most commonly diagnosed in men who have recent exposure. Uncircumcised men are more susceptible to infection *(18)*.

Infectivity and Transmissibility

Chancroid is a relatively contagious infection. Estimates are that 70% of women who are sex partners of chancroid-infected men are infected *(19)*. The probability of sexual transmission with a single exposure has been estimated to be 0.35 *(20)*. An estimated delivery dose of approximately 30 colony-forming units of *H. ducreyi* organisms has been reported to form a papule formation rate of 95% and a pustule formation rate of 69% in a human experimental challenge model *(21)*.

Etiology

Chancroid is caused by a small, nonmobile facultative anaerobic, Gram-negative rod bacterium, *H. ducreyi*. The organism is only remotely related to *Haemophilus* influenza and has been reclassified in the *Actinobacillus* cluster of the Pasteurellae *(14)*. *H. ducreyi* only infects humans. It is believed that the organism gains entry into the skin and mucosal surfaces only through microabrasions and other trauma; it is not able to penetrate normal skin.

Clinical Manifestations

The lesions of chancroid are generally limited to the genital areas. In women, they are found on the labia, clitoris, vestibule, and fourchette. In men, the lesions are most commonly sited in the inner surface of the prepuce and frenulum.

The incubation period of chancroid is 3 to 11 days, with the most common frequency being 4 to 7 days. A small papule develops at the site of entry. The papule is haloed by erythema. In 2 to 3 days, the lesion becomes pustular or vesiculopustular, and ulcerates. The base of the ulcer is soft, shallow and necrotic-appearing; the edges are irregular, ragged, and undermined and are surrounded by deep red-colored halos. The ulcers are covered by a grey-colored, foul-smelling exudate. There is no induration around the lesion. The lesion is exquisitely painful and tender. In men, the most common initial presentation is a single ulcer. In women, multiple ulcers form and often become interconnected in serpentine streaks measuring up to 2 cm. Many times, they are bilateral (so-called "kissing lesions") created by auto-inoculation. Mixed infections with syphilis and herpes simplex can complicate the diagnosis of chancroid.

In 7 to 10 days, a bubo develops in about half the cases. The bubo is unilateral (same side as lesion) and unilocular in up to two-thirds of the time. It is an acute, painful, tender inflammatory inguinal adenopathy. Untreated buboes may rupture and form large weeping ulcers in the inguinal area. Phimosis may develop in men. Extragenital infections are possible but rare.

Symptoms in men relate to the lesions themselves; the pain of the lesion of the adenopathy will prompt men to seek professional care. In women, the symptoms generally are more nonspecific; infected women complain of dysuria, dyspareunia, vaginal discharge, or rectal bleeding depending on the location of infection.

Relapses after antibiotic therapy occur in up to 5% of patients.

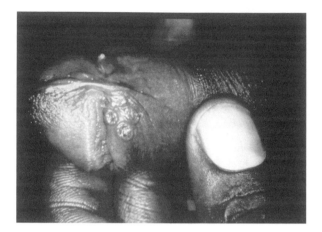

Chancroid: male.

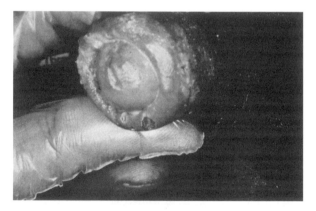

Chancroid: male.

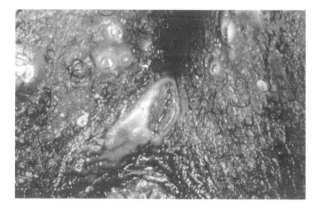

Ulcerate chancroid.

Diagnostic Testing

The classical presentation of a painful ulcer and tender suppurative inguinal adenopathy is almost pathognomonic for chancroid. However, this complex occurs in only abut one-third of cases. Therefore, the diagnosis of chancroid generally relies on other tests. The exudates from the lesion or from aspiration of the lesion may reveal the Gram-negative rods extracellularly located in chains with clustering. The Gram stain patterns of *H. ducreyi* have been described as "schools of fish," "railroad tracks," and "fingerprints." However, the sensitivity of the Gram stain is only 50%, and should not be used to rule out chancroid *(22)*. Definitive laboratory diagnosis depends on culture and isolation of *H. ducreyi*; but those tests are rarely available in standard labs. Even in the best of situations, the sensitivity of cultures is only about 80%. Because *H. ducreyi* is so fastidious, it must be plated directly onto the culture media or plated on Stuart's, Amies', and thioglycolate hemin based transport media and transported at 4°C.

PCR and multiplex PCR tests have been described for *H. ducreyi*, but none has received Food and Drug Administration approval. The PCR tests lose sensitivity when used to test genital ulcer specimens but are still superior to culture tests *(12)*. Multiplex PCR is particularly useful in the face of co-infection, because it can detect the presence of *H. ducreyi* as well as herpes simplex virus, and *T. pallidum (23)*.

Studies have shown that the accuracy of clinical diagnosis of *H. ducreyi* infection is related to the prevalence of chancroid in the population, as well as the experience of the clinician *(12)*. Overall, the accuracy ranges from 33 to 80% *(24,25)*. Also complicating this situation is the fact that co-infection of HIV and *H. ducreyi* is common. HIV can modify the appearance of chancroid *(12)*.

Despite these limitations, the diagnosis is often made on clinical grounds, and testing is used to rule out other infections that cause genital ulceration, such as syphilis or herpes. The CDC recommends that the probable diagnosis of chancroid be made if:

- The individual has one or more painful genital ulcers.
- There is no evidence of syphilis by darkfield examination of the lesions, or by serology performed at least 7 days after onset of the ulcers.
- Either the clinical presentation of the genital ulcers and regional adenopathy are typical for chancroid or test results for herpes simplex virus are negative.

Patients diagnosed with chancroid should be tested for HIV, not only because of the high concordance, but also because HIV-infected patients do not respond to therapy as well.

Treatment

The CDC treatment guidelines are for chancroid outlined on Table 2. The agents currently used are more expensive than the traditional treatments based on

Table 2
Chancroid CDC STD Treatment Guidelines 2006

Recommended regimens—select one of the following:

Azithromycin [a]	1 g orally in a single dose
Ceftriaxone	250 mg intramuscularly in a single dose
Ciprofloxacin [b]	500 mg orally twice a day for 3 days
Erythromycin base	500 mg orally three times a day for 7 days

Source: Centers for Disease Control and Prevention. Sexually transmitted diseases treatment guidelines 2002. MMWR Recomm Rep 2002; 51:11–12.
[a] Safety and efficacy among pregnant and lactating women have not been established (pregnancy category B).
[b] Contraindicated for pregnant and lactating women.
CDC, Centers for Disease Control and Prevention; STD, sexually transmitted disease.

tetracycline or penicillin. Resistance to chloramiphene, sulfonamide, and aminoglycosides has emerged *(26)*. Azithromycin and ceftriaxone have the advantage of being single-dose therapies.

Patients should be re-examined within 3 to 7 days of initiation of therapy. If treatment is successful, the patient should improve symptomatically within 3 days. The clinical appearance should improve within 7 days. If the patient does not improve adequately within 7 days, there are several possibilities:

- The diagnosis was incorrect
- The diagnosis was incomplete and the patient was co-infected with another STI.
- The strain of *H. ducreyi* is resistant to the antibiotic given.
- The treatment was not correctly taken.
- The patient is immunocompromised, as with HIV infection.

The time to complete healing depends on the size of the ulcer. Larger ulcers may require more than 14 days to heal. Ulcers located under the foreskin of uncircumcised men are also slower to heal; uncircumcised men also have higher treatment failure rates.

The bubo (fluctuant adenopathy) may require aspiration through uninfected adjacent tissue. Bubos larger than 5 cm may need incision and drainage. After aspiration, fluid may re-accumulate; repeated aspirations may be required until healing is complete.

HIV-infected patients require closer and more prolonged monitoring because they are more likely to respond slowly or inadequately to conventional therapy. They may also require longer courses of antibiotics.

In developing countries with little or no ability to preform diagnostic testing, the World Health Organization recommends the use of a syndromic management

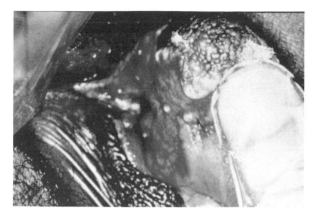

Chancroid.

approach for genital ulcer disease. Syndromic management calls for patients to be treated at the first visit with a combination of antibiotics that treat the sexually transmitted diseases (STDs) commonly found locally *(27)*. This means that neither clinical experience nor laboratory support is needed. It has been shown to be more successful that traditional targeted and therapies in management of genital ulcers in Rwanda *(28)*.

Patients should avoid sexual contact until the ulcers are completely healed.

Partner Notification and Reporting Requirements

Sex partners of patients who had contact with the infected patient in the 10 days preceding the onset of the patient's symptoms should be examined. Treatment should be given even if the contact is asymptomatic. Chancroid is a reportable disease.

Pregnancy-Related Issues

No direct adverse effects of chancroid infection have been demonstrated on the pregnancy or on the neonate. Ciprofloxacin is contraindicated in pregnancy and lactation. The CDC 2006 guidelines also state that the safety and efficacy of azithromycin for pregnant or lactating women have not been established and recommend in favor of other agents. However, other expert panels have not limited the use of azithromycin in those patients *(29)*.

GRANULOMA INGUINALE

Introduction

Granuloma inguinale, also known as Donovanosis, is a chronic, ulcerative, progressively destructive bacterial infection of the genital and anal skin and subcutaneous tissue caused by the bacterium *Klebsiella granulomatis* (formerly known as *Calymmatobacterium granulomatis*). It is classified as an STI because it is spread predominantly by sexual contact, but it can be spread by other means.

The differential includes other causes of genital ulceration (syphilis, LGV, herpes, chancroid), other granulomatous conditions and carcinomas. When a biopsy from a large necrotic lesion that appears neoplastic shows only inflammatory changes, consider granuloma inguinale and order special stains to reveal *K. granulomatis*.

Prevalence/Incidence

This infection rarely occurs in the United States but granuloma inguinale is endemic in some tropical and developing areas, including India, southern Africa, Papua New Guinea, central Australia, and the Caribbean islands. In the United States, fewer than 100 cases are reported each year. Infection is more common in men; the male-to-female ratio is about 2.5:1 *(30)*. Infection rates peak among 20- to 30-year olds.

Infectivity/Transmissibility

The infection can be spread as an STI, but can also be spread by close, personal, nonsexual contact. It is not highly contagious; usually repeated or chronic exposure is needed to contract the infection. The infection is found in 1–52% of sexual partners of women with the infection *(31)*. It is also found is sexually abstinent children and very old adults without sexual contact, which suggests that nonsexual transmission is possible. Indirect contact through vaginal contamination by fecal organisms may be an important contributor, as auto-inoculation may be *(30)*.

Etiology

Granuloma inguinale is caused by an intracellular Gram-negative bacterium *K. granulomatis*. This organism is a small (0.1 μm), nonmotile, non-sporing, encapsulated coccobacillus that shares common antigens with Klebsiella and *Escherichia coli*. It may be part of the intestinal flora, which is made pathogenic by a bacteriophage *(30)*. *K. granulomatous* is pathogenic only for humans and chick embryos.

Clinical Presentation

Granuloma inguinale is an acute or chronic infection characterized by ulcerating, necrosing, superinfected lesions of the skin and subcutaneous tissues in the anogenital area. The incubation period varies from 1 to 2 weeks. The initial lesion of granuloma inguinale can be single or multiple papules. In women, the usual sites of infection are the inner aspect of labia and fourchette. In men, the lesions are generally found on the penis. In 10% of cases, the initial lesion develops in the inguinal area. The lesion is friable and bleeds easily on contact. The skin over each nodule ulcerates. The characteristic lesion is an area of coalesced beefy-red ulcers with fresh granular tissue. As the adjacent areas of ulceration grow together, the normal vulvar/penile architecture is destroyed. The lesion is generally not painful and there is minimal adenopathy. Four different types of granuloma inguinale have been described *(32)*:

- Ulcerogranulomatosis (the most common type) marked by beefy-red, non-tender ulcers that bleed easily if touched and may become quite extensive if not treated.
- Hypertrophic or verrucous ulcer, which presents as a growth with an irregular edge.
- Necrotic type with a foul-smelling, deep ulcer causing tissue destruction.
- Dry, sclerotic or cicatricial lesion.

Massive swelling of the labia is common. Inguinal swelling may occur, but not because of enlarged or obstructed lymph nodes. Instead, "pseudo buboes" form because of subcutaneous granulation. The pseudo buboes break down and are replaced by ulcers. Adenopathy may develop in response to bacterial infection of the ulcerated lesions. Social isolation is common because of the smell of the infected tissue.

As the infection progresses, scarring and lymphatic obstruction produce marked enlargement of the vulvar area. Although correct treatment can eradicate the infection, long-standing infection can cause irreversible genital deformities such as skin depigmentation; stenosis of the urethral, vaginal, and anal orifices; and massive edema *(30)*. Loss of sexual function often follows because of destruction of genital tissue, scarring, and deformities *(33)*.

Relapse of granuloma inguinale is relatively frequent and may occur 6 to 18 months after apparently effective treatment *(34)*.

Extragenital lesions have been reported up to 6% of cases. Involvement on the face, neck, mouth, larynx, pharynx, and chest have all been reported. Metastatic lesions involving bones, joints, and liver have been reported *(30)*. The patients affected with these distant lesions often had cervical or uterine disease.

Diagnosis

In endemic areas, the infection is usually diagnosed by its clinical presentation. Identification of Donovan bodies using special stains in either smears or crushed specimens taken from the depth of the ulcer and the fresh edge confirms the clinical diagnosis. Biopsies should be taken with punch biopsy or small curettes. Air-dry the specimen then fix in 95% ethanol for 5 minutes. The specimen should then be stained. Donovan bodies are seen on Giemsa stain or Wright stain as clusters of dark-staining bacteria that appear as small, straight, or curved dumbbell-shaped "safety pin" (bipolar) appearance in the cytoplasm of macrophages. They stain purple with a surrounding pink capsule. In patients who have taken even small amounts of small antibiotics, however, the Donovan bodies may not be present. Biopsy may be necessary to rule out carcinoma.

Standard laboratory approaches are not fruitful. *K. granulomatosis* is difficult to culture; it has been cultured successfully only in chick embryonic yoke sac *(35)*. A PCR test has been developed using swabs rather than biopsy or tissue samples, but this is not readily available *(36,37)*. In vitro antibiotic sensitivity testing is unavailable *(38)*. Serological tests are nonspecific.

Treatment

The granuloma inguinale treatment guidelines recommended by the CDC are outlined in Table 3. In general, at least 3 weeks of broad-spectrum antibiotics are necessary. Therapy should be continued until there is healing of all ulcers. This requires prolonged self-administration, which raises the possibility of poor compliance. Poor compliance increases the likelihood of antibiotic resistance, reducing the observed cure rates, and raising community and patient dissatisfaction. This in turn increases the likelihood of poor compliance *(39)*.

Initial response should be recognizable within 7 days, although maximal effect may take 3 to 5 weeks to see. Tetracycline resistance is widespread. Gentamicin should be added if the lesions fail to respond after the first few days of therapy. The advanced lesions seen in endemic areas respond poorly to conventional treatment regimens.

Partner Notification and Reporting Requirements

Individuals who had sexual contact with a patient in the 60 days before the onset of the patient's symptoms should be contacted and offered testing. Empiric therapy in asymptomatic partners has not been studied, but given the low infectivity of this organism, it is not recommended at this time. Reporting to the local health departments is necessary.

Pregnancy-Related Issues

There have been no reports of congenital transmission of this infection, but transmission may occur during vaginal delivery. Otitis media and mastoiditis have been reported in exposed children, so careful cleansing of the heads of newborns born to infected mothers is recommended *(40)*. In pregnancy, women tend to have less genital tract bleeding and fewer sites of infection. Erythromycin is the recommended treatment agent, but the addition of gentamicin is highly advisable. Azithromycin might prove useful for treating a granuloma in pregnancy, but data is lacking.

Table 3
Granuloma Inguinale (Donovanosis) CDC STD Treatment Guidelines 2006

Recommended regimen	*Alternative regimens—select one of the following:*	
Doxycycline [a] 100 mg orally twice a day for at least 3 weeks	Azithromycin	1 g orally once per week for at least 3 weeks
	Ciprofloxacin [c]	750 mg orally twice a day for at least 3 weeks
	Erythromycin base	500 mg orally four times a day for at least 3 weeks
	Trimethoprim	One double-strength tablet
	Sulfamethoxazole [b]	One (800 mg/160 mg) tablet orally twice a day for at least 3 weeks

Therapy should be continued at least 3 weeks or until all lesions have completely healed. Some specialists recommend the addition of an aminoglycoside to the above regimens if improvement is not evident within the first few days of therapy (e.g., Gentamicin, 1 mg/kg IV every 8 hours)

Source: ref. 6.
[a] Contraindicated for pregnant and lactating women and for children under 8 years old.
[b] Pregnancy is a relative contraindication to the use of sulfonamides.
[c] Contraindicated for pregnant and lactating women.
CDC, Centers for Disease Control and Prevention; STD, sexually transmitted disease.

MOLLUSCUM CONTAGIOSUM
Introduction

Molluscum contagiosum is a viral infection that is an increasingly common prevalence, especially in those infected with HIV. The characteristic lesion is a raised, umbilicated papule or nodule. The lesions are self-limited, but may persist for up to 5 years. Molluscum is often sexually transmitted in adults, but it may be asexually transmitted in children.

Prevalence/Incidence

Molluscum contagiosum is found worldwide, but has higher prevalence in tropical areas. Its incidence is estimated to be between 2 and 8% (41). Statistics in the United States are not available; indirect evidence suggests that it is increasing in frequency of diagnosis. Molluscum contagiosum accounts for 1% of all diagnosed dermatological conditions (42). In the last 30 years, the number of molluscum-related office visits increased dramatically (43). The infection is most frequently found in patients in the 15- to 29-year-old age range. Estimates are that 5 to 18% of HIV-infected patients are also infected with molluscum contagiosum (44). The disease is endemic with a higher incidence within institutions and communities where overcrowding, poor hygiene, and poverty enable its spread (43).

Infectivity/Transmissibility

The virus is spread by direct skin contact with an infected individual, and is often spread sexually in adolescents and adults. It develops more frequently in patients who have deficient cell-mediated immunity. The communicability of molluscum contagiosum is not known, but the condition is known to be only mildly contagious (45). Transmission of the virus is also possible by fomites (e.g., bath towels, tattooing instruments, equipment in beauty parlors and Turkish baths, as well as underwear) as well as by auto-inoculation (43).

Etiology

Molluscum contagiosum is a member of the pox virus (Poxviridae) family, to which small pox and variola also belong. Pox viruses are complex, double-stranded DNA viruses that contain an envelope. The virus infects only squamous skin, not mucous membranes.

Pox viruses enter cells by endocytosis or by cell fusion. They then uncoat, and transcription of the viral DNA takes place to produce infective virions. These intracytoplasmic virions can be seen microscopically. Intact virus is shed through the epidermis and spread over the skin. Infection with the virus causes hyperplasia and hypertrophy of the epidermis (46). The molluscum bodies contain large numbers of maturing virions within a collagen-lipid-rich sac-like structure that evades host immunological detection (47).

Clinical Presentations

Incubation time averages 14–50 days *(48)*, but can be as long as 6 months. Infections are usually self-limited, but can persist for up to 5 years *(45)*. Molluscum contagiosum causes lesions in adults and adolescents in the groin, genitalia, and lower abdomen. Younger children may develop asexually transmitted lesions on the face, truck, extremities, axilla, and crural folds. The lesions are generally discrete, smooth, firm, skin-colored (opalescent), raised (domed) lesions with central umbilication. "Water wart" is a descriptive term for the lesion. The central depression contains a white, waxy, or curd-like core. The lesions are either papules measuring 1–5 mm in diameter or larger nodules measuring 6–10 mm in diameter. They may appear as solitary lesions or clusters generally of less than 30 lesions.

Infections rarely cause inflammatory changes. However, trauma may rupture the lesions and cause acute inflammation *(49)*. Deep infections may have one or more shallow cysts filled with molluscum bodies.

The lesions are generally asymptomatic but may cause pruritus or tenderness. Lesions spread by sexual contact may appear in the perianal or perioral areas. In some cases, there may be eczema around the lesion, which resolves after the resolution of the lesion *(45)*. Bacterial superinfection of the lesion is a concern *(31)*. The appearance of the infection in immunocompromised patients may be atypical. HIV-infected patients also tend to grow giant lesions (>1 cm) or may have clusters of hundreds of small lesions. These lesions last longer and tend to spread to other locations (especially the face) and are more resistant to common treatments *(45)*. For the smaller lesions, the differential diagnosis includes condyloma acuminata or vulvar syringoma. For the larger, solitary lesions, carcinoma must be ruled out.

Diagnosis

Diagnosis of genital molluscum contagiosum is generally made based on the clinical appearance of the lesions. If there is any question, biopsy of the lesion with Gram, Wright, or Giemsa staining can be helpful. The most common histological feature of molluscum contagiosum is the intracytoplasmic purplish-to-red inclusion known as the molluscum body (Henderson-Patterson body) *(50)*.

The virus cannot be grown in culture other than human skin as its host. On the vulva, molluscum contagiosum can co-exist with condyloma acuminata, which can make identification of the lesions more challenging.

Treatment

A debate remains over the need to treat molluscum contagiosum, because it is a self-limited infection in most cases. The CDC does not discuss this entity in its 2006 treatment guidelines. Many clinicians recommend therapy to reduce the

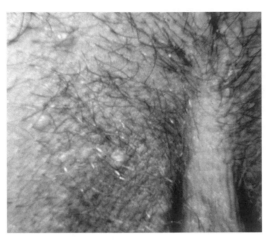

Molluscum contagiosum.

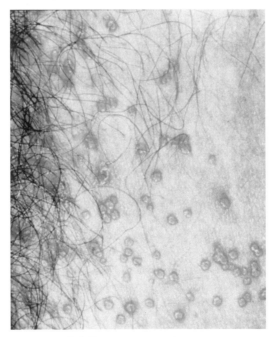

Molluscum contagiosum.

risk of transmission to sex partners and auto-inoculation, and for quality-of-life reasons *(45)*.

Physician-administered ablative procedures are commonly used to treat molluscum. Cryotherapy is one of the most common, quick, and efficient methods of treatment. Liquid nitrogen, dry ice, or Frigiderm may be applied to each lesion for a few seconds. Repeat treatments may be needed in 2- to 3-week intervals *(51)*. Hyperpigmentation, hypopigmentation, or scaring may be created by this treatment.

Enucleation of the molluscum body by needle or by curettage is also commonly used. The area is cleansed with an antiseptic agent, and the core of each lesion is removed. Silver nitrate, ferric subsulfate, or 85% trichloroacetic acid is applied to the center for hemostasis. General curettage of the area to unroof lesions with a sharp dermal curette is more practical when there are numerous lesions present. Pulsed dye laser has also demonstrated excellent results in single treatment without scarring or pigment abnormalities *(52)*. Cost makes this approach less desirable *(53)*. Cantharidin (0.9% solution of collodion and acetone) has been used with success in the treatment of molluscum contagiosum. This is a blister-inducing agent. It should be carefully applied to the dome of the lesion and left in place for 4 hours before being washed off. If tolerated on a single test lesion, it may be applied to other lesions every week until clearance occurs. It should not be used on the face *(54)*. Use of chemocauterizing agents, such as trichloroacetic acid or podophyllin, are no longer used in most practices because of their lack of efficacy.

Patient-provided therapies can be used off-label to treat the lesions caused by molluscum contagiosum. Imiquimod 5% cream has been shown to be an effective and safe therapy when applied once daily, 5 days a week for 4–16 weeks *(55)* to people with lesions that are resistant to standard therapies. In another study with imiquimod 5% cream, given only 3 days a week (every other day) for a maximum of 16 weeks, lesions in 78% of study completers cleared completely *(56)*. Potassium hydroxide 5–10% can be applied twice a day to each of the lesions with a swab. Resolution occurs in a mean of 30 days *(57)*. Other agents that have been reported to have efficacy include cidofovir topically applied, cimetidine orally, iodine solution and salicylic acid plaster, and tape stripping *(58)*.

Partner Notification and Reporting Requirements

Sexual partners should be examined and treated if lesions are present. There are no reporting requirements.

Pregnancy-Related Issues

Molluscum contagiosum is not known to have any adverse impact on pregnancy.

CASE STUDY

Molly is a 24-year-old woman who comes to your office for her annual exam. As she is preparing for her pelvic exam, she mentions that she has recently developed some "bumps on her vagina." They do not irritate her but her new boyfriend told her they looked "funny." On exam, you find about six small clear, fluid-filled vesicles along the outer aspect of her intertriginous area. Closer inspection reveals another four lesions in the adjacent hair-bearing area. The exam is complicated by a mild folliculitis that has resulted from her bikini wax treatments. You test her for chlamydia and HIV, and tell her she has:

- An STI and needs antibiotics applied to the lesions.
- A common infection, but that it will go away in a few years.
- She has lesions that can be treated with cream at home or treated in the office as a small procedure.

Molly needs to be tested for chlamydia because she is under age 26 and for HIV because she has a new sex partner. Molluscum is an STD, which can be conservatively managed. However, because Molly's partner has already commented in the lesions, she is seeking treatment. The preferred therapy is self-applied imiquimod (off label) or provider-performed enucleation of the central core of each of the lesions.

REFERENCES

1. Schwartz DA. Lymphogranuloma venereum. In: Connor DH, Chandler FW, Schwartz DA, Mantz HJ, Lack EE, eds., *Pathology of Infectious Diseases*. Stamford, CT: Appleton & Lange, 1997, pp. 491–497.
2. Blank S, Schillinger JA, Harbatkin D. Lymphogranuloma venereum in the industrialised world. Lancet 2005; 365:1607–1608.
3. Sweet RL, Gibbs RS. Sexually transmitted diseases. In: *Infectious Diseases of the Female Genital Tract*. Philadelphia, PA: Lippincott Williams & Wilkins, 2002, pp. 118–175.
4. Bolan RK, Sands M, Schachter J, Miner RC, Drew WL. Lymphogranuloma venereum and acute ulcerative proctitis. Am J Med 1982; 72:703–706.
5. Bauwens JE, Lampe MF, Suchland RJ, Wong K, Stamm WE. Infection with Chlamydia trachomatis lymphogranuloma venereum serovar L1 in homosexual men with proctitis: molecular analysis of an unusual case cluster. Clin Infect Dis 1995; 20:576–581.
6. Centers for Disease Control and Prevention. Sexually transmitted diseases treatment guidelines, 2006. MMWR Recomm Rep 2006; 55(RR-11):15,16,20–22. Available from: http://www.cdc.gov/std/treatment/. Accessed Nov. 24, 2006.
7. County of Los Angeles Department of Health Services. Provider alert: lymphogranuloma venereum infections in California. Public's Health 2005; 5(3):1–2. Available from: http://www.ladhs.org/media/tph/TPHMarch2005.pdf. Accessed Nov. 24, 2006.
8. Schachter J, Smith DE, Dawson CR, et al. Lymphogranuloma venereum. I. Comparison of the Frei test, complement fixation test, and isolation of the agent. J Infect Dis 1969; 120:372–375.
9. Koo D, Wetterhall SF. History and current status of the National Notifiable Diseases Surveillance System. J Public Health Manag Pract 1996; 2:4–10.
10. Ducrey A. Experimentelle Untersuchungen uber den Ansteckungsstof des weichen Schankers und uber die Bubonen. Monatsh Prakt Dermatol 1889; 9:387–405.
11. Bezancon F, Griffin V, LeSourd L. Culture du bacille du chancre mou. C R Seances Soc Biol Fil 1900; 52:1048–1051.
12. Lewis DA. Diagnostic tests for chancroid. Sex Transm Infect 2000; 76:137–141.

13. Fleming DT, Wasserheit JN. From epidemiological synergy to public health policy and practice: the contribution of other sexually transmitted diseases to sexual transmission of HIV infection. Sex Transm Infect 1999; 75:3–17.
14. Spinola SM, Bauer ME, Munson RS Jr. Immunopathogenesis of Haemophilus ducreyi infection (chancroid). Infect Immun 2002; 70:1667–1676.
15. World Health Organization (WHO). Sexually transmitted infections fact sheet. Geneva, Switzerland: WHO, 2004. Available from: www.who.int/reproductive-health/rtis/docs/sti_factsheet_2004.pdf. Accessed April 18, 2005.
16. Nikolaidis G, Rosen T. Chancroid. In: Connor DH, Chandler FW, Schwartz DA, Mantz HJ, Lack EE, eds., Pathology of Infectious Diseases. Stamford, CT: Appleton & Lange, 1997, pp. 469–471.
17. Crowe MA, Hall MA. Chancroid. Updated 2005. Available from: www.emedicine.com/derm/topic71.htm. Accessed Nov. 24, 2006.
18. Ronald AR, Albritton W. Chancroid and Haemophilus ducreyi. In: Holmes KK, Mardh P-A, Sparling PF, et al., eds., Sexually Transmitted Diseases. New York, NY: McGraw-Hill, 1999, pp. 515–523.
19. Plummer FA, D'Costa LJ, Nsanze H, Dylewski J, Karasira P, Ronald AR. Epidemiology of chancroid and Haemophilus ducreyi in Nairobi, Kenya. Lancet 1983; 2:1293–1295.
20. Brunham RC. Epidermiology of sexually transmitted diseases in developing countries. In: Wasserheit J, Aral S, Holmes KK, eds., Research Issues in Human Behavior and STDs in the AIDS Era. Washington: American Society of Microbiology, 1991, pp. 61–80.
21. Al-Tawfiq JA, Thornton AC, Katz BP, et al. Standardization of the experimental model of Haemophilus ducreyi infection in human subjects. J Infect Dis 1998; 178:1684–1687.
22. Lockett AE. Serum-free media for the isolation of Haemophilus ducreyi. Lancet 1991; 338:326.
23. Orle KA, Gates CA, Martin DH, Body BA, Weiss JB. Simultaneous PCR detection of Haemophilus ducreyi, Treponema pallidum, and herpes simplex virus types 1 and 2 from genital ulcers. J Clin Microbiol 1996; 34:49–54.
24. Chapel TA, Brown WJ, Jeffres C, Stewart JA. How reliable is the morphological diagnosis of penile ulcerations? Sex Transm Dis 1977; 4:150–152.
25. Dangor Y, Ballard RC, da L Exposto F, Fehler G, Miller SD, Koornhof HJ. Accuracy of clinical diagnosis of genital ulcer disease. Sex Transm Dis 1990; 17:184–189.
26. Lewis DA. Chancroid: clinical manifestations, diagnosis, and management. Sex Transm Infect 2003; 79:68–71.
27. World Health Organization (WHO). Program for sexually transmitted diseases, global program on AIDS. Recommendations for the management of sexually transmitted diseases. WHO/GPA/TEM/94. Geneva: WHO, 1994.
28. Bogaerts J, Vuylsteke B, Martinez Tello W, et al. Simple algorithms for the management of genital ulcers: evaluation in a primary health care centre in Kigali, Rwanda. Bull World Health Organ 1995; 73:761–767.
29. California STD/HIV Prevention Training Center. California STD treatment guidelines for adults and adolescents, 2004. Revised January 2005. Available from: http://www.dhs.ca.gov/dcdc/STD/docs/CA%20Tx%20Guide%20Jan%202005.pdf. Accessed Nov. 24, 2006.
30. Majmudar B. Granuloma inguinale. In: Connor DH, Chandler FW, Schwartz DA, Mantz HJ, Lack EE, eds., Pathology of Infectious Diseases. Stamford, CT: Appleton & Lange, 1997, pp. 1:565–570.
31. Droegemueller W. Infections of the lower genital tract. In: Stenchever MA, Droegemueller W, Herbst AL, Mishell DR, eds., Comprehensive Gynecology, 4th Ed. St. Louis, MO: Mosby Inc., 2001, pp. 641–706.
32. O'Farrell N. Donovanosis. Sex Transm Infect 2002; 78:452–457.

33. Merianos A, Gilles M, Chuah J. Ceftriaxone in the treatment of chronic donovanosis in central Australia. Genitourin Med 1994; 70:84–89.
34. Richens J. The diagnosis and treatment of donovanosis (granuloma inguinale). Genitourin Med 1991; 67:441–452.
35. Kuberski T. Granuloma inguinale (donovanosis). Sex Transm Dis 1980; 7:29–36.
36. Carter J, Bowden FJ, Sriprakash KS, Bastian I, Kemp DJ. Diagnostic polymerase chain reaction for donovanosis. Clin Infect Dis 1999; 28:1168–1169.
37. Carter JS, Kemp DJ. A colorimetric detection system for Calymmatobacterium granulomatis. Sex Transm Infect 2000; 76:134–136.
38. Sehgal VN, Prasad AL. Donovanosis. Current concepts. Int J Dermatol 1986; 25:8–16.
39. Merianos A, Gilles M, Chuah J. Ceftriaxone in the treatment of chronic donovanosis in central Australia. Genitourin Med 1994; 70:84–89.
40. Govender D, Naidoo K, Chetty R. Granuloma inguinale (donovanosis): an unusual cause of otitis media and mastoiditis in children. Am J Clin Pathol 1997; 108:510–514.
41. Brown ST, Nalley JF, Kraus SJ. Molluscum contagiosum. Sex Transm Dis 1981; 8:227–234.
42. Taillac PP, Bretz S. Molluscum contagiosum. Available from: http://www.emedicine.com/emerg/topic317.htm. Accessed Nov. 24, 2006.
43. Postlethwaite R. Molluscum contagiosum. Arch Environ Health 1970; 21:432–452.
44. Gottlieb SL, Myskowski PL. Molluscum contagiosum. Int J Dermatol 1994; 33:453–461.
45. Tyring SK. Molluscum contagiosum: the importance of early diagnosis and treatment. Am J Obstet Gynecol 2003; 189:S12–S16.
46. Billstein SA, Mattaliano VJ Jr. The "nuisance" sexually transmitted diseases: molluscum contagiosum, scabies, and crab lice. Med Clin North Am 1990; 74:1487–1505.
47. Bugert JJ, Darai G. Recent advances in molluscum contagiosum virus research. Arch Virol Suppl 1997; 13:35–47.
48. Fenner F. Poxviruses. In: Fields BN, Knipe DM, eds., Virology, 2nd Ed. New York, NY: New York Press, 1990.
49. Henao, Freeman RG. Inflammatory molluscum contagiosum. Clinicopathological study of seven cases. Arch Dermatol 1964; 90:479–482.
50. Cockerell CJ. Poxvirus infections. In Connor DH, Chandler FW, Schwartz DA, Mantz HJ, Lack EE, eds., Pathology of Infectious Diseases. Stamford, CT: Appleton & Lange, 1997, pp. 273–279.
51. Janniger CK, Schwartz RA. Molluscum contagiosum in children. Cutis 1993; 52:194–196.
52. Hughes PS. Treatment of molluscum contagiosum with the 585-nm pulsed dye laser. Dermatol Surg 1998; 24:229–230.
53. Becker TM, Blout JH, Douglas J, Judson FM. Trends in molluscum contagiosum. Dermatol Ther 2000; 13:285–289.
54. Silverberg NB, Sidbury R, Mancini AJ. Childhood molluscum contagiosum: experience with cantharidin therapy in 300 patients. J Am Acad Dermatol 2000; 43:503–507.
55. Hengge UR, Esser S, Schultewolter T, et al. Self-administered topical 5% imiquimod for the treatment of common warts and molluscum contagiosum. Br J Dermatol 2000; 143:1026–1031.
56. Liota E, Smith KJ, Buckley R, Menon P, Skelton H. Imiquimod therapy for molluscum contagiosum. J Cutan Med Surg 2000; 4:76–82.
57. Romiti R, Ribeiro AP, Grinblat BM, Rivitti EA, Romiti N. Treatment of molluscum contagiosum with potassium hydroxide: a clinical approach in 35 children. Pediatr Dermatol 1999; 16:228–231.
58. Hanson D, Diven DG. Molluscum contagiosum. Dermatol Online J 2003; 9:2.

12 Ectoparasites
Scabies and Pediculosis Pubis

JoAnn Woodward

INTRODUCTION

Scabies has existed for more than 2500 years. It was described in ancient texts from the Middle East, China, and India *(1)*. The word "scabies" is believed to have originated from *scabere*, the Latin term meaning "to scratch." It was not until 1687 that Bonomo and Cestoni described the casual relationship between the mite and the disease *(2)*. More than 300 million cases of scabies are diagnosed each year. It is a sexually transmitted infection (STI), but it can be spread by other activities that involve close personal skin contact. The pruritus caused by the infestation is very distressing in itself, but the burrows directly caused by the mite and the excoriations caused by the scratch also make the host susceptible to secondary skin infection and systemic sepsis.

Infestation with lice is referred to as pediculosis. About 4000 species of lice exist; only about 560 species suck blood and feed only on mammals; 3 species infest humans. Phthiriasis (pediculosis pubis) is a lice infestation usually located in the pubic region, commonly called "crabs." *Pthirus pubis* is a blood-sucking louse that is a very successful obligate parasite of humans. Infestations are found in all socioeconomic strata.

FAST FACTS

- Scabies is highly contagious and is spread by close personal contact, including sexual contact.
- Lesions from scabies are intensely pruritic but may not be visible.
- Diagnosis of scabies is clinical and can be confirmed by microscopic examination of a skin scraping.
- Treatment for scabies must include treatment of the entire body as well as treatment of clothing and bedding.

From: *Current Clinical Practice: Sexually Transmitted Diseases:*
A Practical Guide for Primary Care
Edited by: A. L. Nelson and J. A. Woodward © Humana Press, Totowa, NJ

- Crusted or Norwegian scabies, which can involve infestation with hundreds of thousands or millions of mites, are more common in immunocompromised hosts.
- Scabies complicated by superinfection can be fatal.
- Pediculosis pubis is more contagious than any other STI.
- *P. pubis* (crab louse) is visible with the naked eye.
- Diagnosis is made if the louse and the nits (eggs) are seen on body hair.
- Thirty percent of patients with pediculosis pubis have another STI.
- Children with crab lice in their eyelashes should be evaluated as potential victims of sexual abuse.
- Pediculosis pubis can involve all hairy parts of the body except the scalp, so treatment should not be restricted to the genital area.
- The louse contains host DNA, which may be helpful in identifying rapists.

SCABIES
Prevalence/Incidence

Prevalence of scabies worldwide is not known but it has been estimated that more than 300 million people are infested *(3)*. Historically, epidemics of scabies occur in times of war, famine, and overcrowding *(4)*. In the United States and Europe, scabies occurs in cycles every three decades. Prevalence is 0–6% *(5)*. Individuals under age 20 are more commonly infected, but gender and ethnicity are not risk factors. In developing countries, the infestation is chronic and affects up to 30% of the population *(6)*. The disease spreads rapidly in institutions such as correctional facilities, health care facilities, and nursing homes, but is not commonly found in schools. The current epidemic has disproportionately affected people infected with human immunodeficiency virus (HIV).

Transmission/Infection

Scabies is a highly contagious condition. Spread of the scabetic mite ("itch mite") requires direct skin-to-skin contact with an infested person. Occasionally, cases are transmitted by contaminated clothing or bedding. Human and canine scabies mites remain infective at room temperature off the host for only 3 days *(7)*. Fomites, therefore, are possible, but inefficient, vectors. Mites are attracted by heat and odor to seek out hosts. The mites are motionless at room temperature. They cannot fly or jump, but they can crawl as fast as 1 inch per minute on warm skin *(4)*. Unlike most STIs, which can spread by brief sexual contact, scabies is more likely to be transmitted by sharing a bed for a night *(8)*.

Etiology

Scabies is caused by an eight-legged blind mite, *Sarcoptes scabiei*. In the female, the front two legs have suckers and the rear two ones are tipped with bristles, but the male has pods on his last pair of legs to hold the female during mating *(9)*. *S. scabiei* is an obligate parasite, requiring an appropriate host for survival. It subsists on dissolved human tissue but does not feed on blood *(4)*. The female mite is shield-shaped and measures in 0.3–0.4 mm; the male mite is half as large. The mites mate on the skin surface. The male mite dies. The female mite burrows beneath the epidermis secreting enzymes that dissolve the skin, which she then ingests. It takes the mite 30 minutes to enter the skin as she burrows head first using her jaws and cutting claws on her forelegs to create the burrow. The female lays one to three eggs each day for the rest of her 4- 6-week life span. The egg hatches in 2–4 days as six-legged larvae, which cuts through the burrow roof to reach the skin surface. The larvae hides in the hair follicles and skin folds and progresses through two more developmental phases before then it molts into adults. The adult moves to the skin surface to mate. Less than 1% of the eggs laid complete this life cycle *(10)*.

Canine mites, which cause mange in dogs, may also attach to humans. The infestation occurs in areas of the body that come in contact with the dog (arms and trunk). The canine mite cannot live on humans, so there are no burrows.

Clinical Manifestation

Scabies presents with intensely pruritic papular rash. The pruritus worsens at night. The initial symptom starts 2–6 weeks after initial infestation and often has a gradual onset. Typically, the patient is infested with 10–15 mites (range 3–50). The pruritus results from a delayed type IV hypersensitivity reaction to the mites, their eggs, saliva and scybala (pockets of feces) *(7)*. Patients who are re-infested are already sensitized and develop symptoms in only 1–4 days.

On exam, the mite burrows can be found on the patient's hands, interphalangeal finger webs, wrists, peri-umbilical skin, waistline, and axillary folds. The mites prefer the keratinized skin with a few pilosebaceous follies *(9)*. The sexually transmitted infestations often involve the penis, scrotum, labia, areola, nipples, and buttocks. In adults, the face and scalp are spared, as are the palms and soles. The back is also usually spared except in bedridden individuals. The burrows are short, thin, elevated, serpiginous, gray-colored tracks. The burrows are often destroyed by scratching and may be difficult to see. At the end of the burrow, a small papule may be found. There is often widespread secondary excoriation, pustules, or crusting.

There are different scabies lesions. The most common is erythematous papular or vesicular lesions that are associated with burrows. They may be bullous or urticarial due to an intense immune response *(11,12)*. Other forms include nodular, bullous, and keratotic variations. Nodular scabies, which comprises 10% of cases, presents with dark pruritic nodules that are 5–20 mm in diameter. The nodules are smooth and red, pink, tan, or brown in color. The nodules spontaneously resolve in weeks or months, but may leave postinflammatory hyperpigmentation. Keratotic, crusting, or "Norwegian" scabies are variants that most commonly afflict immunocompromised hosts. The lesions are generally more widespread and represent infestation with hundreds of thousands to millions of mites. The lesions are large, hyperkeratotic, warty crusts that are filled with burrows, which can last for years. The areas under the fingernails are filled with debris; the palms and soles show deep fissuring of the crusts. Because these hosts are not able to mount an inflammatory reaction, there is less pruritus associated with keratotic scabies. A second type of lesion seen in scabies is a generalized papular eruptions not located in the area of the mite. The papules are formed on the trunk and thighs. They appear erythematous and are thought to be an allergic response to the mite (13).

The classical presentations are not always seen. It takes 4–6 weeks to demonstrate a primary infestation. Early infestations are difficult to detect because the lesions are scarce; the burrows are only 5 mm long and may be difficult to visualize. Wide and sparse lesions may also be seen in patients using systemic or topical lesions. Elderly patients may have intense itching without a visible inflammatory response. Often the excoriation can reduce the number of mites and either obscure or destroy the burrows. In long-standing scabies infections, the skin has a more eczematous appearance. If the secondary infection develops, the lesions look pustular.

Scabies is generally self-limiting in humans. However, untreated scabies can become superinfected, which can lead to cellulitis, abscesses, sepsis, and glomerulonephritis (14). Because the mites and the mite fecal pellets contain streptococcus and staphlyococci, it is possible that the mite also contributes to the infection. Secondary infection of scabies with group A streptococcus pyogenes is a major precursor to acute poststreptococcal glomerulonephritis (15,16).

Diagnosis

Diagnosis can be made empirically based on the history of intense pruritus, which worsens at night, and the presence of characteristic lesions located in areas typically affected by the infestation. If other family members are affected, the diagnosis is even more secure. The lesions can be better visualized with a hand lens. If there is difficulty identifying the burrow, the best method to find them is by staining. The Burrows Ink Test is performed by flooding an area of skin with fountain pen ink, wiping it clean with alcohol and identifying the wavy burrows that retain the ink (17). Liquid tetracycline can be substituted for the ink and Wood's light and magnifying lens are used to visualize the tetracycline-filled burrows.

Microscopic analysis of the infestation may be prudent, particularly when the lesions have atypical appearances. In order to obtain a specimen, gently scrape the roof off five or six burrows with an oil-covered blunt scalpel blade; the oil will help the material adhere to the blade. The best sites to examine are new, nonexcoriated burrows in the skin webs between the fingers. Place the material on a glass slide. Add a drop of mineral oil or 10% potassium hydroxide and study the

Table 1
Scabies—CDC Treatment Guidelines 2006

Recommended regimens— *select one of the following:*	*Alternative regimen*

Permethrin cream (5%) [a]
   Applied to all areas of the body
   from the neck down and washed
   off after 8–14 hours
Ivermectin
   200 µg/kg orally, repeated in 2 weeks
	Lindane (1%) [b]
	   1 oz. of lotion or 30 g of cream applied
	   in a thin layer to all areas of the body
	   from the neck down and thoroughly
	   washed off after 8 hours

Source: From ref. *22.*
[a] Permethrin is effective and safe but costs more than lindane.
[b] Lindane should not be used immediately after a bath or shower, and it should not be used by persons who have extensive dermatitis, pregnant or lactating women, or children aged under 2 years.
CDC, Centers for Disease Control and Prevention.

specimen under low power. Visualizing the mite, eggs, or egg shells confirms the diagnosis. Video dermatoscopy is an effective and sensitive diagnostic tool, which allows in vivo visualization of the skin with magnification up to 600 times *(4).*

Treatment

The Centers for Disease Control and Prevention (CDC) treatment guidelines are outlined in Table 1. Careful selection of the correct topical agent depends on the patient's age, pregnancy status, and skin condition. Permethrin cream 5% is a widely used synthetic pyrethroid insecticide whose parent compound was derived from chrysanthemums *(18).* It is poorly absorbed through the skin and well-tolerated. It should be applied from the neck down and washed off after 8–14 hours. Ivermectin is a macrocyclic lactone antibiotic that is given orally in two doses 1 week apart. Lindane is not recommended as first-line therapy because of toxicity. Lindane is an organochloride insecticide to which the mites have shown some resistance. In addition, it can be absorbed through the skin (especially directly after bathing or through damaged skin) and cause severe neurotoxicity and aplastic anemia. It should be washed off 8 hours after application. Bedding and clothing require attention. Because the mites cannot survive more than 3 days without a host, isolating the materials for 72 hours will kill all the mites. However, machine washing or drying on a hot cycle will also kill any mites on clothing or bedding immediately. Trimming fingernails helps reduce the potential injury from scratching. The pruritus and inflammation in scabies can be treated with antihistamines or steroids *(7).* Additional dosing is needed to treat keratotic (crusting or "Norwegian") scabies because the magnitude of infestations is so impressive. Combined therapies with topical and oral agents or repeated treatment with oral agents has been suggested by experts.

It should be noted that the pruritus might persist for up to 2 weeks after effective eradication of the infestation. However, if symptoms persist beyond 14 days, the diagnosis should be re-evaluated. It is also possible that the treatment was applied incorrectly or that re-infestation has occurred *(19)*. Resistance, particularly to lindane, has been well-documented *(20)*.

Partner Notification and Reporting Requirements

Both sexual and close personal and household contacts within the preceding month should be examined and treated for scabies. Scabies is not a reportable disease.

Special Pregnancy-Related Issues

The CDC recommended treatment in pregnant and breastfeeding women is permethrin. Permethrin has been rated (BM) compatible in pregnancy and breastfeeding by other experts *(21)*. Those same experts rate lindane a category BM drug (limited human data but animal suggest low-risk manufacturer rating), but because of lindane's potentially serious neurotoxicity, the CDC states that it should not be used for pregnant or lactating women *(22)*. The CDC recommends that Ivermectin not be used in lactating women, but the American Academy of Pediatrics classifies Ivermectin as compatible with breastfeeding *(23)*.

PEDICULOSIS PUBIS

Prevalence and Incidence

It has been estimated that 3 million cases of pediculosis pubis are treated each year in the United States *(8)*. Pediculosis pubis most commonly infests adults and young adults. In the 15- to 19-year-old age group, women are more likely to be infested than men are. Over age 20, men are more likely to be infested *(24)*.

Transmission and Infectivity

Pubic lice infestation is generally classified as an STI. Transmission occurs most commonly by close physical contact, such as sexual intercourse or sleeping in the same bed. The infection is more contagious than any other STI, with a 95% chance of contacting the infestation after only one single sexual encounter *(25)*. However, fomite transmission is also possible by sharing towels or underwear.

Etiology

P. pubis (the crab louse) is one of three types of lice that uniquely infest humans and are generally site-specific. The crab louse measures 0.8–1.2 mm in length and width. It is tough skinned and gray-brown in color (but turns rusty color after feeding). It is a wingless, dorsoventrally flattened louse. The louse has

Pediculosis pubis.

six-paired clawed legs, the last two pairs that are adapted to grasp widely spaced pubic hair. The front pair of legs is shortened. Lice pierce the skin every few hours to obtain a blood meal. The louse inserts its mouth parts into the skin and injects saliva that has vasodilating properties to facilitate access to the blood. Crab lice move 10 cm per day *(26)*. Within 24 hours after mating, the female starts to lay about four eggs per day. The eggs are laid on hair near the root and cemented in a characteristic angle from that strand. The nits incubate for 7 days, after which time a nymph hatches. The nymph proceeds through three moltings in the next 8–9 days and enters into the adult phase. The life span of the female adult crab louse is about 17 days; for the male, it is 22 days *(7)*. *P. pubis* can live away from the host for about 2 days *(27)*.

Clinical Presentation

The incubation time of pediculosis pubis is 30 days. People generally will present with pruritus, irritation, and/or rash. The pruritus is owing to allergic sensitivity *(25)*. Patients may also have papular urticaria and excoriation. Occasionally, patients will seek care because they see the louse moving over the skin or along the hair follicle. If the patient suffers large numbers of bites in a short time of period, he or she may have low-grade fevers, malaise, or irritability.

The lice, nits, and excoriation are hallmarks of infestations. For longer-standing infestations, another characteristic finding is maculae ceruleau, which are bluish-gray macules found on the skin of the lower abdomen and thighs from the bites of the *P. pubis*. The color of the macules is assumed to be related to hemosiderin deposits in the deep dermis. Patients may also note some spots of blood or crusting in their underwear.

Pubic lice are not limited to the pubic region. They may be found in other short hairs of the body, such as facial, back, chest, or thigh hairs; eyebrows; eyelashes; and hair at the scalp line. Infestation in the eyelashes is called pediculosis ciliaris. Atypical locations are more common if the pubic region was already locally treated (17).

Diagnosis

The diagnosis of pediculosis pubis can be made if the louse or the nits (lice egg cases) are seen with the naked eye. Identification of the nits may be facilitated with the use of a hand-held magnifying lens. Pluck suspicious-looking hairs and examine in mineral oil under the microscope. It may be possible to differentiate the pubic lice nits from the hair louse nit. The pubic lice nits are attached to the hair shaft at a relatively more acute angle (26). Nits on the pubic hairs may be confused with white piedra or trichomycosis pubis. Excoriation may result from concurrent infestation with scabies or contact dermatitis.

The diagnosis of pediculosis pubis should prompt testing for other STIs. Thirty percent of individuals with pubic lice have another concurrent STI and, therefore, should undergo screening for HIV, syphilis, gonorrhea, Chlamydia, herpes, warts, and trichomoniasis (26). Children with *P. pubis* in the eyelashes should be evaluated for sexual abuse.

Treatment

The pubic louse is totally encased in a proteinaceous sheath (except for the orifice through which it feeds). As a result, it is more resistant to topical therapies than are other lice. The CDC treatment recommendations are displayed in Table 2 (22). Each is a rinse or shampoo, which must be applied to the pubic areas and all other affected areas and later rinsed off as directed. Infestation in the eyelashes should not be treated with any of the recommended regimens. Pediculosis of the eyelids should be treated by applying occlusive ophthalmic ointment (such as Vaseline petroleum jelly) twice a day for 10 days. Patients with pediculosis pedis should be evaluated for other STIs.

Bedding and clothing should be decontaminated. Decontamination can be done actively with machine washing and drying using hot cycles or dry cleaning, or passively by removing it from body contact for 72 hours, during which time all the pubic lice will die. Fumigation of living areas is not necessary.

If symptoms persist, the patient should be re-evaluated after 1 week. Retreatment may be necessary if lice are found or if eggs are observed at the hair–skin junction. Patients who do not respond to a recommended therapy should be retreated with an alternative regimen.

Treatment must include the patient's sex partner(s) within the last month. Sexual and other close contact with partner(s) should be avoided until both partners have been treated and re-evaluated after 1 week to rule out persistent disease.

Table 2
Pediculosis Pubis—CDC Treatment Guidelines 2006

Recommended regimens— select one of the following:	Alternative regimen— select one of the following:

Permethrin 1%
    Creme rinse applied to affected
    areas and washed off after 10 minutes
	Malathion 0.5%
	    Lotion applied for 8–12 hours and
	    then washed off

Pyrethrins with piperonyl butoxide
    Applied to the affected area and
    washed off after 10 minutes
	Ivermectin 250 µg/kg orally
	    Taken orally and repeated in 2 weeks

Note: The recommended regimens should not be applied to the eyes. Pediculosis of the eyelashes should be treated by applying occlusive ophthalmic ointment to the eyelid margins twice a day for 10 days.

Source: From ref. 22.

If pubic lice infestation is diagnosed in a sexual assault investigation, there may enough blood in a single louse to identify a rapist's DNA by polymerase chain reaction. Mechanical removal of as many lice as possible may be important to obtain evidence (26).

Partner Notification and Reporting Requirements

Partners in the last month should be contacted and treated. Partners should also be tested for other STIs. There is no uniform requirement to report *P. pubis* to the local public health department.

Pregnancy-Related Issues

Pregnant and lactating women should be treated with either permethrin or pyrethrin with piperonyl butoxide. The CDC says that lindane is contraindicated for use by pregnant or breastfeeding women.

CASE STUDY

Pat is a 23-year-old graduate student who presents with intense pruritus in her pelvic area. She had initially thought that she had a yeast infection; she treated herself with an over-the-counter antifungal cream, but the itching got worse. Her last menstrual period started 5 weeks ago. She received her first injection of depo-medroxyprogesterone acetate 3 days later. She is in a fairly stable relationship with her boyfriend except one episode just before her last period, when she and her boyfriend had a fight. She slept with a former partner and thinks they used condoms. On exam, she has an impressive infestation of P. pubis.

Questions

1. Would you require her to have a pregnancy test before administering drug therapy?
2. Does she need any other tests?
3. Who should be tested and treated? For which infection(s)?
4. What other measures does she need to take?
5. What if she is still symptomatic in a week?

Answers

1. It is highly unlikely that she is pregnant, given that she had a timely injection of depo-medroxyprogesterone acetate. Because the first-line treatment is permethrin, there is no need to do pregnancy testing.
2. She needs testing for at least chlamydia and a microscopic assessment to rule out vaginal infections. HIV testing in a month might also be prudent. Other STI tests may also be indicated once more history about the infecting partner is obtained.
3. All of her sexual contacts in the last month should be examined and treated for *P. pubis* and tested for other STIs.
4. Her bedding and clothing must be decontaminated. She must not have intimate contact until 1 week after she and her partner have both been treated.
5. If she is symptomatic 1 week after therapy, consider re-exposure. If she has a resistant infection, she may need to be treated with lindane. A pregnancy test would be needed before this therapy. All of her sexual contacts who were treated would also have to be re-evaluated for their response to therapy.

REFERENCES

1. Alexander JO'D. Scabies. In: *Arthropods and Human Skin*. Berlin, Germany: Springer-Verlag, 1984, pp. 227–292.
2. Parish LC. History of scabies. In: Orkin M, Maibach HI, Parish LC, Schwartzman RM, eds., *Scabies and Pediculosis*. Philadelphia, PA: Lippincott, 1977, pp. 1–6.
3. Taplin D, Meinking TL, Chen JA, Sanchez R. Comparison of crotamiton 10% cream (Eurax) and permethrin 5% cream (Elimite) for the treatment of scabies in children. Pediatr Dermatol 1990; 7:67–73.
4. Steen CJ, Carbonaro PA, Schwartz RA. Arthropods in dermatology. J Am Acad Dermatol 2004; 50:819–842.
5. Epstein E, Orkin M. Scabies: clinical aspects. In: Orkin M, Maibach HI, eds., *Cutaneous Infestations and Insect Bites*. New York, NY: Marcel Decker, 1985, pp. 19–24.
6. Burkhart CG. Scabies: an epidemiologic reassessment. Ann Intern Med 1983; 98:498–503.
7. Huynh TH, Norman RA. Scabies and pediculosis. Dermatol Clin 2004; 22:7–11.
8. Sweet RL, Gibbs RS. Sexually transmitted diseases. In: Sweet RL, Gibbs RS, eds., *Infectious Diseases of the Female Genital Tract*, 4th Ed. Philadelphia, PA: Lippincott Williams & Wilkins, 2001, pp. 118–175.
9. Conner DH. Scabies. In: Conner DH, Chandler FW, Schwartz DA, Manz HJ, Lack EE, eds., *Pathology of Infectious Diseases*. Stamford, CT: Appleton and Lange, 1997, pp. 1695–1698.

10. Mellanby K. Scabies in 1976. R Soc Health J 1977; 97:32–36, 40.
11. Witkowski JA, Parish LC. Scabies. Subungual areas harbor mites. JAMA 1984; 252:1318–1319.
12. Chapel TA, Krugel L, Chapel J, Segal A. Scabies presenting as urticaria. JAMA 1981; 246:1440–1441.
13. Mellanby K. *Scabies*, 2nd Ed. Hampton, UK: EW Classey, 1972.
14. Burgess I. *Sarcoptes scabiei* and scabies. Adv Parasitol 1994; 33:235–292.
15. Svartman M, Finklea JF, Earle DP, Potter EV, Poon-King T. Epidemic scabies and acute glomerulonephritis in Trinidad. Lancet 1972; 1:249–251.
16. Hersch C. Acute glomerulonephritis due to skin disease, with special reference to scabies. S Afr Med J 1967; 41:29–34.
17. Woodley D, Saurat JH. The Burrow Ink Test and the scabies mite. J Am Acad Dermatol 1981; 4:715–722.
18. McCarthy JS, Kemp DJ, Walton SF, Currie BJ. Scabies: more than just an irritation. Postgrad Med J 2004; 80:382–387.
19. Karthikeyan K. Treatment of scabies: newer perspectives. Postgrad Med J 2005; 81:7–11.
20. Boix V, Sanchez-Paya J, Portilla J, Merino E. Nosocomial outbreak of scabies clinically resistant to lindane. Infect Control Hosp Epidemiol 1997; 18:677.
21. Briggs GG, Freeman RK, Yaffe SJ, eds. *Drugs in Pregnancy and Lactation: A Reference Guide to Fetal and Neonatal Risk*, 7th Ed. Baltimore, MD: Williams & Wilkins, 2005.
22. Centers for Disease Control and Prevention. Sexually transmitted diseases treatment guidelines, 2006. MMWR Recomm Rep 2006; 55(RR-11):79–80. Available from: http://www.cdc.gov/std/treatment/. Accessed Nov. 24, 2006.
23. American Academy of Pediatrics Committee on Drugs. Transfer of drugs and other chemicals into human milk. Pediatrics 2001; 108:776–789.
24. Fisher I, Morton RS. *Phthirus pubis* infestation. Br J Vener Dis 1970; 46:326–329.
25. Felman YM, Nikitas JA. Pediculosis pubis. Cutis 1980; 25:482, 487–489, 559.
26. Ko CJ, Elston DM. Pediculosis. J Am Acad Dermatol 2004; 50:1–12.
27. Steen CJ, Carbonaro PA, Schwartz RA. Arthropods in dermatology. J Am Acad Dermatol 2004; 50:819–842, quiz 842–844.

13

Patient–Clinician Communication and STI Care

Assessing Risk, Conveying a Diagnosis, and Supporting Behavior Change

Felicia Guest

STI HISTORY:
ASSESSING RISK BEHAVIOR

Primary care patients who are sexual with another person—or who have ever in the past been sexual with another person—deserve a thorough history to review sexual patterns and events and to assess present risk of sexually transmitted infections (STIs) and illnesses. The STI history is a key part of the new patient work-up, and those initial findings help set the interval for future assessments. For celibate patients, ask at least annually, "Has anything changed since you last told me you are not sexual with anyone?" For patients with one or more sex partners, repeat the STI history anytime you ask history questions of any kind. For patients with a history of risky behavior or an STI diagnosis, assess risk taking at every encounter, look for opportunities to praise and support safer sex steps, and intervene promptly when you discover behavioral risk taking or clinical evidence of infection.

Getting Started

Whether the STI history is brief or extensive, it merits a good setting and a good beginning. Provide privacy, and conduct the history when the patient is fully clothed. Be sure to begin with a rationale for why you are about to ask intimate questions: "I'm going to ask you some personal sexual questions that we routinely ask all our patients, is that all right with you?" This type of opening reassures the patient that you have not singled her or him out for some reason, and reinforces the importance of sex in the overall health picture.

From: *Current Clinical Practice: Sexually Transmitted Diseases:
A Practical Guide for Primary Care*
Edited by: A. L. Nelson and J. A. Woodward © Humana Press, Totowa, NJ

When do you first include sexual risk assessment questions in history taking with a young patient? Most clinicians follow cues about physical maturity, dress style, behavior, and the responses to such questions as, "Tell me about your friends. What do you and your friends do? Do you have a boyfriend or girlfriend? What do the two of you like to do?" With some cues that your patient might be beginning sexual exploration, it is appropriate to ask, "What do you do to protect yourself from acquired immune deficiency syndrome (AIDS) and pregnancy?" as a positive way to probe about sex behaviors. Whatever the response, you have a clue about where to go next in your discussion with your young patient. (For more on using this query with patients, *see* the following section.)

Should older teens and adult patients record their own answers to STI history questions on a questionnaire form or computer screen, or should the clinician ask the questions aloud and write down the answers? Three factors determine which methodology might work better in your setting:

- Literacy of the patient population.
- Sexual openness of the patient population (often influenced by culture).
- Waiting time available for completing questionnaires.

Print or electronic questionnaires may work well with patients who are literate (in the language of your questionnaire) and who are comfortable with sexual topics. College health services might use questionnaires successfully, for example. In other settings, taking an oral history might be more effective.

One Question

If you can budget only scant moments for the STI risk history, ask something like, "What are you doing to protect yourself from AIDS?" From the patient's answer to this one question, you can get some sense of STI awareness and safer sex practices, and you can respond with praise for clear thinking and positive steps, and with at least one focused and personalized suggestion to build on knowledge and/or skill. (You may choose to frame the question in different ways, such as, "What are you doing to protect yourself from a sexual infection?" or, "Thinking about AIDS and other sexual infections, what do you think is the riskiest thing you do?" Use whatever form of the question that suits your personal style.)

When you ask, "What are you doing to protect yourself from AIDS?" you may hear some of these typical responses:

- "I don't have sex!" You can reply, "Thanks for telling me. If that situation changes for you, remember I'm someone you can talk to about protecting your health as a sexual person."
- "My boyfriend is very healthy, he doesn't have AIDS!" You can reply, "I'm glad to hear that. Remember some serious infections do not show at all for years, such

as AIDS. The only way to be sure is to get a test. Would you like me to tell you some places the two of you could go for a test if you decide to have one?"

- "I use condoms sometimes." You can reply, "Good for you! Use them every time if you possibly can because that is what it takes to protect the two of you from infections. Would you like to pick up some condoms while you are here today? There's no charge." (If you have a minute more, ask, "What do you think it would take for you to use condoms each and every time?" This question helps your patient develop insight about barriers to condom use and about possible steps to conquer these barriers. This motivational interviewing technique is discussed in more detail in the section, "Supporting Behavior Change".)

- "Who me? I'm married!" "I know. We ask everyone this question, as I said before, because it is such an important issue. I hope you never have any worries about your spouse's faithfulness, but if you should, I urge you to listen to your inner voice! If you are feeling worried it may be for a good reason. I'm someone you can talk to if this ever comes up."

Brief Assessment

If you can budget 2 or 3 minutes for a fuller assessment, add a few questions that elucidate history of infection, risk taking, and relationships in more detail. Possible questions to ask are discussed below, and they appear in Table 1 in checklist form.

- "Have you ever had an STI, a sexually transmitted infection?" (Some clinicians frame this as, "Have you ever worried that you had a sexually transmitted infection?")
- "Have you ever felt that alcohol or drugs was a problem for you?"
- "What do you do to protect yourself (or your partner) from an unplanned pregnancy?"
- "Are you in a relationship now? Tell me how it's going."
- "Have you ever had a sexual experience against your will?"

These questions introduce a discussion about patterns of relationships, sexual risk taking, and safer sex practices. It would be extremely useful to follow up with additional in-depth questions when time permits, even if it is at a later visit. The next section suggests some questions to expand on each of the categories covered in these brief questions above.

Fuller Assessment

SEXUAL RISK BEHAVIORS

These questions can appropriately follow "What are you doing to protect yourself from AIDS?" if needed, to expand your understanding of sexual risk exposure.

- "Have you ever had a sexual experience of any kind with another person?" Avoid asking, "Have you ever had sex?" or "Have you ever had intercourse?"

Table 1
STI Risk Assessment Questions

One question	*What are you doing to protect yourself from AIDS?*

Note: *Brief assessment questions are in bold italic*,
with additional in-depth questions if time permits.

What are you doing to protect yourself from AIDS?

- Have you ever in your life had a sexual experience with another person?
- Can you tell me with about how many people? One? Two or three? Four to ten? More than ten?
- Have your sexual partners been men? Women? Men sometimes and women sometimes?
- What about this past year? About how many sex partners have you had? One? Two or three? Four to ten? More than ten?

Have you ever had an STI, a sexually transmitted infection?

- Have you ever had a test for HIV or AIDS? What prompted you to have the test?
- In the past year, have you had vaginal intercourse? Anal intercourse? Oral sex? (for STI examination and testing)

Have you ever felt that alcohol or drugs were a problem for you?

- In the past 7 days, how many times have you used alcohol? Recreational drugs?
- Have you ever, even once, shared needles and injection equipment with another person for any reason? (Drugs, tattoo, skin piercing, steroids) Have you ever had a sexual partner who used injection drugs?
- When you are sexual with a partner, are you usually sober? Using alcohol? High?

What do you do to protect yourself (or your partner) from an unplanned pregnancy?

- Do you have pain or discomfort with intercourse or any other sexual activity?
- Have you ever had an injury or illness involving your internal or external reproductive organs?

Are you in a sexual relationship now? Tell me how it is going.

- How would you describe your marriage these days?
- Is there anything about your sexual life that you would like to be different?

Have you ever had a sexual experience against your will?

- Have you ever had sex when you did not want to?
- Have you ever traded sex for money, drugs, shelter, or food?
- Have you ever been hurt by a sex partner, or been afraid you might be hurt?

STI, sexually transmitted infection; AIDS, acquired immune deficiency syndrome; HIV, human immunodeficiency virus.

"Sex" is defined differently by different people, and "intercourse" leaves out some forms of sexual expression that are important to include, such as oral sex.

- For patients who answer "yes," ask, "Can you tell me with about how many people in your lifetime? One? Two or three? Four to ten? More than ten?" Asking the question with these options cues your patient that any answer is acceptable, and she/he does have to guess at what you want to hear.

- Follow this question with "Have your sexual partners been men? Women? Men sometimes and women sometimes?" (This question might be omitted if the answer to the previous question is completely unambiguous, such as, "I've never made love with anyone but my husband." Otherwise, ask and do not guess.)

- Next, probe about your patient's partner(s). "Has your partner ever had a same-sex partner to your knowledge?" Although bisexuality is often a hidden behavior, it makes sense to ask, especially in an STI context, and some federal programs require this question as a component of sexual risk assessment.

- Next, ask about the most recent 12-month period to assess current patterns. "What about this past year? About how many sex partners have you had? One? Two or three? Four to ten? More than ten?" Follow this query with a probe about partner practices, as described in the paragraph above.

- Next, ask about current safer sex practices. "In this past year, did you or your partner(s) use condoms? Tell me how you use them." It is normal for patients to want you to think well of them, so someone might answer "yes" to condom use when a better answer might be "sometimes," "when I'm worried," or "until I get to know my partner." Asking, "Tell me how you use them" gives you a chance to listen for correct and consistent use and to remind patients that only correct and consistent use assures good STI protection *(1,2)*.

Sexually Transmitted Infections

Once you have a basic understanding of sexual patterns in the patient's life, move to an STI assessment: "Have you ever been told you had an STI, a sexually transmitted infection of any kind?" Explore any positive responses. You might add, "Have your ever had a human immunodeficiency virus (HIV) test?" (If yes), "What prompted you to have the test?"

Especially when a physical exam will follow, make an assessment of body structures that should be checked for signs of sexual infection or injury, and sites that should be sampled for STI testing. "Have you had vaginal intercourse? Anal intercourse? Oral sex?"

Substance Use

Disinhibiting substances such as alcohol and drugs can promote unsafe sexual decision making, and addiction can promote sex-for-drugs and sex-for-money-for-drugs risk behaviors. No sexual or STI history is complete without an understanding of the role these substances play in the patient's sexual life. Asking, "Have you ever felt that alcohol or drugs was a problem for you?" is a good one-question assessment not only for alcohol and drug use patterns, but also for the patient's perception of use patterns. If time permits, ask additional questions:

- "In the past 7 days, how many times have you used alcohol? Drugs?" Quantifying questions can be helpful as long as you take into account the human tendency to minimize reports of these behaviors. Also, avoid potentially confusing terminology. "Week" means Monday through Friday, as opposed to "weekend" to some people. "Seven days" is a clearer term. Asking how many "drinks" can be confusing, because for some people "drinks" are hard liquor beverages only. You could ask instead, "In the last 7 days, about how many total alcoholic beverages have you had, including hard liquor, beer, wine, and spritzers?"
- "Have you ever, even once, shared needles or other injection equipment with another person for any reason? Drugs? Tattooing? Skin piercing? Steroids?" You can explain that sharing unsanitary injection equipment is extremely risky for transmitting such blood-borne infections as HIV and hepatitis. Also, be sure to include, "Have you ever had a sexual partner who used injection drugs?"
- "When you are sexual with another person, are you usually sober? Using alcohol? High?" Disinhibition may improve sex for some people, but may impair judgment about safer sex practice.

REPRODUCTIVE MEDICAL EVENTS

Once you have assessed current contraceptive practice with, "What do you do to protect yourself from an unplanned pregnancy?" you can follow with these questions to pinpoint any STI-related events.

- "Do you ever have pain or discomfort with intercourse or with any other sexual activity?" Listen to your patient's answer to sort out physical pain from illness or injury, physical pain related to sexual technique, and emotional pain as clearly as you can.
- "Have you ever had any injury or illness involving your internal or external reproductive organs?" This question, framed in medical, genitourinary terms, may undercover STI-related issues that the patient defines in more medical terms.

RELATIONSHIP CONCERNS

Assess whether the patient is in a primary relationship: "Are you in a relationship now? How is it going?" or for married patients, "How would you describe your marriage these days?" Always be prepared to make referral recommendations to qualified mental health professionals who do marriage or couples counseling, in case you learn about relationship troubles.

For patients who are married or in another type of stable relationship, consider asking about sexual satisfaction and sexual compatibility. This gives patients an opportunity to express any common sexual concerns such as lack of desire, differences between the two partners about how often they want sex, or differences between the two partners about what specific sexual activities are and are not enjoyable. "Patients sometimes have concerns about sex. Is there anything about your sexual life that you would like to be different?" Ask your colleagues who specialize in marriage and couples counseling for advice about useful sexual therapy books and Web sites, and have referral recommendations ready for patients who need more extensive support than you are able to offer in the primary care setting.

ABUSE AND VIOLENCE

It is vitally important to ask about the presence of sexual coercion and intimate partner violence in a patient's life, past or present, because of the lasting impact of these experiences on self-esteem and well-being. Your patient may or may not want to disclose anything to you, but it is helpful for you to ask, so she/he is reassured that you are a willing and concerned listener should she/he feel ready to talk. In the words of one woman who experienced childhood sexual abuse, "I bet at least 10 health care providers asked me about abuse before I was ready to talk about it. And I don't think I could have told the eleventh one if the first 10 hadn't asked!" Some alternative or additional questions are:

- "Have you ever had sex when you didn't want to?"
- "Have you ever traded sex for money, drugs, shelter, or food?"
- "Have you ever been hurt by a sex partner, or been afraid you might be hurt?"

Shaping a Risk Assessment History

Only you know how to consider your time pressures, the cultural and social contexts of your patients' lives, and the prevalence of various STIs in your area. From your understanding of these issues, you (and your colleagues) can craft a set of STI risk-assessment questions that will make sense in your setting, using the questions suggested in this chapter as a starting place. You are free to add, subtract, and modify these questions in ways that make the history work best for you.

CONVEYING AN STI DIAGNOSIS

With every patient comes the potential for breaking the news that she/he has an STI. If the STI is curable, the news will be temporarily dismaying, and may unsettle a sexual relationship. Alternatively, it may not seem to faze the patient. If the STI is incurable and serious, such as HIV or hepatitis C, it is likely to be extremely upsetting, perhaps even marking life with a milestone for "before I knew" and "after I knew." It is never easy to tell a patient about an STI diagnosis, and we can never anticipate how seriously the patient will take the news. The conversation requires all your skill and compassion as an advocate and teacher. Excellent books and articles on the topic of breaking bad news are available for further study (3–5). The following section distills ideas from these sources and from a series of workshops conducted by the author. Although many of these concepts are gleaned from settings in which patients learned about diagnoses such as HIV or cancer, they can be applied to an STI diagnosis as well.

Break bad health news in a private place, when the patient is dressed, and both of you are seated. Have tissues handy. Use a preparatory remark such as, "I'm afraid I have bad news," and convey the diagnosis in simple, plain language. Use two or three straightforward sentences to explain the situation, then say, "I'm sorry" or something similar in your own speaking style, and then stop talking for a moment to give you patient time to absorb what you have said.

One of the eternal pitfalls of telling a patient that she or he has an STI is that in medical language, bad news is a "positive" test result. Be careful not to say, "I'm sorry to say your test was positive." For some patients, "positive" always means "good," and they will be bewildered that you are sorry.

If possible, avoid giving an STI diagnosis by telephone. If you must use the telephone, say something like, "I'm sorry to tell you this on the telephone," and check to see if the patient can speak privately. Because you will not be able to assess body language, ask frequently, "How are you doing?" and "Is it still okay to talk?"

How Patients Respond

The emotional response to bad health news is varied and unpredictable. Be careful not to assume how your patient feels. When clinicians and counselors in workshops were asked to recall their own experience of hearing bad news, their emotional responses, roughly in order of frequency, included: numb or dazed, frightened, angry, resentful, disbelief, guilty, and helpless.

When it is not apparent to you what your patient's immediate emotional response is, ask: "Can you tell me how you're feeling right now?" Allow time to regain composure before you move on with the discussion.

Clinician Goals and Patient Goals

Most care providers report that their goals for this difficult discussion are: to help the patient (and others) understand the diagnosis, to comfort and reassure appropriately, and to agree on the next step for further diagnosis and/or treatment.

The patients' goals may or may not be the same as your goals. Severity of the STI diagnosis is an important factor. In workshops in which a variety of health problems were represented, participants were asked, "Right at that moment, what did you want and need from your care provider?" They recalled an impressive variety of needs:

- Show me you empathize with how bad this is.
- Leave me alone and let me think and pull myself together.
- Tell me I will be all right.

- Tell me what should happen next.
- I have no idea what I want right now.
- Let me use your phone.
- Tell me I did not do anything wrong.
- Tell me where to go for repeat test.
- Tell me this is a bad dream.
- Tell my spouse/partner/parents for me.
- Tell me where to go to read about this infection.
- Tell me the worst thing that can happen.
- Tell me I can get treatment today.

Because the patient's goals may be different from your goals, you will need to ask what she or he needs at that moment. It is important not to guess; you might launch into education when she or he needs comfort, or offer comfort when she/ he wants privacy. Ask, "How can I be helpful right now? Do you want to know more?" When we do not ask what someone needs, we tend to assume his or her needs are the same as what we would need in similar circumstances. For example, if you are comforted by facts, a fuller scientific understanding (as clinicians often are), and your patient just wants to get to a telephone and call a spouse (or other support), your science will not feel helpful. Learn your personal crisis coping style. Then be careful not to assume your patient copes in exactly the same way.

Educating About an STI Diagnosis

Let the patient cue how much you teach in this initial discussion, and pace your teaching at a speed the patient can follow. Clinicians are ethically bound to teach patients about their diagnosis and proposed treatment in a manner consistent with full disclosure, informed choice, and informed consent. However, this initial discussion may or may not be the right time for teaching, because people experiencing strong emotions may not be able to absorb much information. Consider whether it is practical to give patients materials to read at home and share with others, and perhaps schedule a time to talk again in a few days.

Comfort and Reassurance

For most people, attending is comforting, so be present with your patient as long as you can. If it is not apparent what your patient is worried about, ask. "What are you most worried about right now? What concerns do you have?" Most patients want to know what to expect, at least to some extent. Spoken or silent questions can include:

- Is this curable?
- What will the treatment be like?
- Will it hurt?
- What will happen to me?
- How did I get it?

- How did I get this infection? I've only had sex with my boyfriend (or girlfriend, husband, or wife)? This can be an awkward moment for both the clinician and the patient. If the STI is known to be transmitted only via sexual contact, tell the patient so in plain language. Offer to assist in testing and treatment for the partner. If you can, also offer to facilitate a discussion.
- "Would it be helpful if you and your husband come in together so I can answer questions and help the two of you talk this over?"

Avoid false reassurance about serious infections, and follow the patient's lead on looking into the future. Share evidence-based general outcome data about her or his particular STI if it is available, cautioning that you cannot predict with certainty how things will go in this particular case. Some patients want to discuss the future right away, and others look no further ahead than telling the news to loved ones, and preparing for next-step medical procedures.

Some patients face a health crisis with hope; others do not. Workshop participants credited a healthy and intact personal support system, a strong faith community, and/or an optimistic personality when they were able to face a health crisis with a positive outlook.

Closing the Discussion

For most STI diagnoses, treatment will be provided on the premises, without a referral at the same time the diagnosis is conveyed to the patient. As clinician, you will move from the counselor mode into the educator mode to teach the patient about medication regimen details and advise her/him to seek testing and potential treatment for the partner(s).

Once you have conveyed the diagnosis, responded to immediate patient needs, provided comfort and support, and educated the patient on treatment procedures, bring the discussion to a close by assessing understanding of the diagnosis and treatment and assessing composure. Then seek a joint commitment to the next step in the care process.

Assess understanding of the diagnosis and treatment plan by asking the patient to explain what she or he has heard, in her own words. "Tell me what you learned today, as though you were telling your best friend." If the next step is a medical referral, be sure the patient can tell you in her or his own words where to go, when, what to take, and how to prepare for the appointment. Referred patients sometimes feel "handed off" and abandoned, so be sure that you close the referral loop and track care as much as possible. If you can, invite your patient to call or e-mail the office and keep you informed.

One way to assess patient composure is to ask, "What will you do when you leave here?" Responses will vary considerably. Workshop participants reported their immediate activities, roughly in this order: connecting with spouse, family, or others; going back to work or home and "going through the motions"; crying; going to the Internet, bookstore, or library to read about the infection; praying;

walking, exercising, or "anything to keep moving"; using food, alcohol, or another drug ("I went straight to Baskin-Robbins").

Red Flags and Special Concerns

Patients should not leave your office alone if you are concerned about their physical or emotional well-being after hearing bad news. Listen for suicidal or magical thinking ("Maybe this will go away on its own"), or inability to formulate a plan ("Where am I going from here? How should I know?") For these patients, consider more time in your facility with you or with another staff person, or offer to call a spouse or family member to come to your office.

When you tell a teenager she or he has an STI, remember that they may feel very isolated and alone, even if they live in a big family, so assess the support system carefully. Teens sometimes are unable to tolerate waiting for outcomes, and may struggle with your plan: "Why can't I get the treatment today?"

Be careful not to usurp autonomy from a patient who has just heard bad health news, even if you are invited to make decisions on the patient's behalf. Remember also that when the patient is a health care professional, she/he needs the same educational and emotional support as any other patient.

Breaking bad news is draining, and you will need to take care of yourself. Be prepared for occasional "blame the messenger" experiences, for patients with unrealistic expectations of medical problem solving, and for the frustrations of not knowing what has become of referred patients.

SUPPORTING BEHAVIOR CHANGE

Clinicians often face the daunting challenge of helping patients move from diagnosis, to treatment, to talking with a partner about treatment, to changing behavior to reduce the likelihood of future infections, all in one brief visit. This is a demanding task list, both for the provider and the patient. Consider a strategy that will encourage the patient to maintain her/his healthy momentum after leaving the clinic, using one or more of these tools:

- Try a "homework" assignment: a short brochure to read, a diary to record any risky behavior and what seems to prompt it, and/or a signed contract that spells out healthy goals to achieve. Set a follow-up visit, perhaps with a nurse or counselor, to measure progress.
- Give patients the addresses of two or three reliable Internet sites that address sexual health concerns, such as "Go Ask Alice," operated by Columbia University, or "Teenwire," operated by Planned Parenthood Federation of America, and suggest 20 minutes of surfing. For patients without Internet access, provide toll-free numbers for reliable national or local health hotlines.
- Give patients a short brochure or fact sheet written for partners of people recently diagnosed with an STI to assist in talking to her or his partner to encourage testing and/or treatment.

- Offer a follow-up phone call or e-mail message from a nurse or counselor in a week or so to assist with any questions or problems.
- Openly acknowledge the "whirlwind" nature of this sort of visit. "We've moved from telling you that you have a sexual infection, to discussing how we'll treat it, to telling your partner, to planning for the future. A lot of territory to cover in a few minutes, and I have done most of the talking. What is important to discuss from your point of view?"

Working toward behavior change with patients who will need or seek ongoing care has challenges as well. Adhering to a treatment plan, especially for chronic STIs, is an enormous challenge for some patients, and altering long-standing sexual behavior patterns can be even harder. Mental illness, addiction, or history of emotional trauma can impede adherence and behavior change. The primary care clinician can help patients clarify their personal obstacles to behavior change, and seek a commitment to incremental, concrete, and personalized steps toward healthful behavior.

Remember that behaviors that seem unambiguously healthful and valuable to you may seem very costly and bizarre to your patient. For example, you might view condom use as rational STI protection; the patient might fear losing a cherished sexual partner or even being vulnerable to partner violence.

Supporting adherence and other health behaviors is grounded in the theory that such change is incremental, and that clinician interventions must be tailored to the patient's own position along a continuum of change. One thoroughly studied model was developed in psychotherapy and smoking cessation research, *(6,7)* wherein behavioral scientists identified sequential steps along a behavior–change continuum. A model used to train HIV counselors *(8)* describes this incremental process of change and provides intervention strategies to use at various stages of change. Table 2 describes how patients at various stages of change might answer your question, "What do you do to protect yourself from AIDS?" The stages are described below:

Knowledge and awareness come first, because behavior change begins in understanding the consequences of a behavior. Respond to patients at this stage with facts and role model stories.

Significance to self, or ownership of the new knowledge and awareness, is critical for progressing to action. The patient realizes, "An STI doesn't only happen to other people; it can happen to me." At this stage, clinicians can help by assisting with personal goal setting, and asking questions to raise awareness of the impact of risk taking on those goals. "When would you like to have your first baby? Can we talk about how a sexual infection might affect those goals?" Listen carefully to the feelings that are expressed, verbally and nonverbally, about how hard it is to change sexual practices.

Self-efficacy determines the ability to put new insights into use. Once the patient sees her/himself as able to change and to be in control of a sexual situa-

Table 2
Identifying Patient Readiness for Behavior Change

Stage of change	How patient might answer, "what are you doing to protect yourself from AIDS?"
Knowledge, awareness	"There's not any AIDS around here."
Significance to self	"I guess I ought to be thinking about that."
Self-efficacy	"I wish my boyfriend would use condoms, but he doesn't want to."
Cost–benefit analysis	"Condoms are good and all that, but who wants to think about disease when you're getting it on?"
Capacity building	"We try to use condoms, but it's hard to talk about it."
Provisional tries	"I got some condoms at the health department but they felt weird and tight."
Sustained change	"I've been using condoms for years."

AIDS, acquired immune deficiency syndrome. Adapted from ref. 8.

tion, she or he can act on the new insights. People who have low levels of self-efficacy feel helpless to change. Your support as a clinician, with praise for steps toward better health behaviors, and expressions of respect for the patient as a person who is able to change, can foster genuine change in the patient's life.

As a clinician, you see a strong rationale for reducing sexual risk taking. However, from the patient's perspective, the status quo has both pros and cons. Be careful not to shortchange the pros of the status quo (such as having a partner) or the cons of the healthier behavior (such as having to face an awkward and sexually explicit conversation about condoms). Insisting on condom use could cost the patient the loss of an important relationship, loss of self-esteem from being in a relationship, loss of economic support from a partner, and even expose the patient to personal violence. Reducing the number of sex partners could cost the patient a loss of companionship and loss of social status. Each patient undertakes a cost–benefit analysis of the behavior change, so be sure you address and respect all the costs and all the benefits.

Change requires new skills. This capacity building might include help from you or another staff member on talking with a sex partner and coping with both the patient's and the partner's fears and discomforts. Communication is key in sexual behavior change. If you have 5 minutes to teach condom skills, use 1 minute to teach about putting on a condom, and 4 minutes to practice discussing condoms with a partner.

Behavior change is not like flipping an on-and-off switch. Most people need a series of provisional tries at new behavior. Help by framing all attempts as successes, not failures, by suggesting plan modifications, boosting self-efficacy

("I know you can do it"), appreciating the difficulty of change, and praising all efforts to change, large and small.

In addition to understanding the patient's position along a continuum of readiness for change, it is helpful to master counseling techniques that can be effective in a short amount of time. Motivational interviewing *(9)* is one such technique, an approach to helping patients overcome ambivalence that is preventing behavior change. Motivational interviewing was developed and tested in the field of addiction, and has wide application in other areas of healthful behavior change.

For example, one simple motivational interviewing tool might be used for beginning a discussion about condom use or other safer sex behaviors. First, show the patient a ruler on a piece of paper, a continuum marked off from 0 to 10. Ask, "How do you rate your condom use at present, with 0 being the lowest score and 10 the highest score?" Miller and Rollnick then suggest asking two questions: "Why are you a 4 (for example) and not a 0?" This question helps patients identify their positive, healthful behaviors. Then, "What would it take to get you to go from 4 (for example) to a 6 or an 8?" This question evokes the patient's own perceptions of barriers and other issues, and opens the door to a more fruitful and focused discussion. The authors caution against asking, "Why are you a 4 and not a 10?" because this tone is likely to put patients on the defensive, prompting them to defend and justify their present position.

This tool is fast and concrete, allowing you to evoke discussion of change without appearing to be oppositional or judgmental.

Changing Clinician Behavior

Patients may or may not change, but clinicians can and must be adept at change, matching interventions to patients needs. Remember that one or two questions such as "What are you doing to protect yourself from AIDS?" can help focus your counseling so that the few moments available for education will be grounded in the reality of the patient's life situation.

REFERENCES

1. National Institute of Allergy and Infectious Diseases. Workshop summary: scientific evidence on condom effectiveness for sexually transmitted disease (STD) prevention. Bethesda, MD: July 20, 2001.
2. Cates W Jr. The NIH condom report: the glass is 90% full. Fam Plann Perspect 2001; 33: 231–233.
3. Girgis A, Sanson-Fisher RW. Breaking bad news: consensus guidelines for medical practitioners. J Clin Oncol 1995; 13:2449–2456.
4. Ptacek JT, Eberhardt TL. Breaking bad news. A review of the literature. JAMA 1996; 276:496–502.
5. Buckman R. *How to Break Bad News: A Guide for Health Care Professionals.* Baltimore, MD: Johns Hopkins University Press, 1992.

6. Prochaska JO, DiClemente CC, Norcross JC. In search of how people change. Applications to addictive behaviors. Am Psychol 1992; 47:1102–1114.

7. Prochaska JO, Norcross JC, DiClemente CC. When you change. In: *Changing for Good: The Revolutionary Program That Explains the Six Stages of Change and Teaches You How to Free Yourself from Bad Habits*. New York, NY: William Morrow, 1994, pp. 36–50.

8. Garrity JM, Jones SJ. HIV prevention counseling: A training program. Atlanta GA: Centers for Disease Control and Prevention, 1993.

9. Miller WR, Rollnick S. Phase I: building motivation for change. In: *Motivational Interviewing: Preparing People for Change*, 2nd Ed. New York, NY: Guilford Press, 2002, pp. 52–84.

14

Cultural Competence in STI Care

Linda Dominguez

The germs usually do not change much over time but the human, social, economic and relational change for people is profound when they catch one.

Few medical issues challenge the most experienced clinician as much as the "foreignness" of different cultures, especially when compounded by the mystery surrounding sex and sexuality. Respecting cultural differences as well as the need for sexual sensitivity can be daunting. For the clinicians, the suspicion or diagnosis of a sexually transmitted infection (STI) is not about sex and relationships, but it is about disease. The patient's concerns are the opposite. STIs have always been part of the human condition. In most cultures, sex and sexual relationships are considered private and personal. However, when there is a diagnosis of an STI, that privacy is laid open to physical examination, inquiry, reporting, and expectations of disclosure. Complex feelings of betrayal, confusion, embarrassment, vulnerability, or shame are common when a patient is told he or she has an STI. These feelings transcend all cultures.

As a society, the United States is rapidly becoming more multicultural and multiracial. The US census for 2000 allowed for 66 different categories of racial and ethnic combinations with the world's 210 distinct nations represented in that mix. More than 32 million people speak a language other than English. These diverse cultures are being blended and merged and have a measure of influence on each other. Sex is one of the important ways in which they are merged and changed for better or worse. It could be argued that the United States is more like a stew than a melting pot. Cultures tend to retain, at least in the first generation, many of the features (foods, customs, and social practices) that help define the different groups.

Cultural competence in health care has emerged as an important goal for many reasons. Clinicians are increasingly seeing patients with different perspectives about health. Patients from different cultures may present with symptoms that are different from those generally recognized in textbooks, have different triggers for seeking care, and have different expectations about how health care will be

From: *Current Clinical Practice: Sexually Transmitted Diseases:*
A Practical Guide for Primary Care
Edited by: A. L. Nelson and J. A. Woodward © Humana Press, Totowa, NJ

administrated *(1)*. Health care professionals practicing in the area of reproductive health need to be comfortable and competent in multicultural issues so that they can communicate and practice effectively. They also must be very comfortable in dealing with the dynamics that surround sexuality in their own culture as well as those of the patients they serve. Yet there is little attention during academic and clinical training to equip the clinician to feel confident and competent in these areas of concern.

Of all the forms of inequality, injustice in health care is the most shocking and inhumane.

—Rev. Dr. Martin Luther King, Jr.

The Healthy People 2010 clearly states that it is necessary to eliminate disparities in health care provision and in health outcomes by 2010. The prevalence of every STI is higher within minority groups. Race and ethnicity are risk markers that are influenced by other health status determinants, such as poverty, health care access, and the availability of quality care, health care-seeking behavior, and living in communities with large reservoirs of STIs and high rates of illicit drug use.

There is an interdependence between the provider and the community. For instance, if the community is not educated about STIs, its members are not as likely to recognize symptoms and seek care. If the community does not trust the health care system or understand the health care provider's language, whether that be English or medicalese, its members will be less likely to seek evaluation and treatment.

Effective STI management includes the following elements:

- Effective prevention strategies.
- Patients must recognize that they are not well, and they must seek care promptly.
- Sites must be available to provide care.
- The correct diagnosis has to be made and appropriate treatment prescribed.
- Drugs must be available and be used correctly.
- Instructions about sexual activity during treatment must be followed.
- Patients must refer their partners *(2)*.

All of these elements must be offered in a culturally competent way, with language-appropriate materials, office hours that suit the needs of all (including the minority community), and clinicians and support staff who have some measure of patient language proficiency or translator support and awareness and respect for the beliefs and behaviors of the patient they serve.

CULTURAL CONTEXT

In the field of STI evaluation and treatment, the clinician will practice more effectively when a broader understanding of the patient's social and sexual contexts is obtained. Cultural issues may improve or impede successful outcomes, especially when dealing with infection transmission and contagion. Also, think of the patient's expectations of the encounter. In rural areas of developing countries, health care is provided by healers who have known the community members (their patients) for their whole lives. Medical records are not needed. Often physical touching or examinations are not needed. Decisions about health care (especially for a woman) are the responsibility of another person, or of the family as a whole. The Western concepts of patient confidentiality and autonomy are not embraced or even understood by the woman and her family. Suddenly she is faced by a white-coated professional and his staff asking her the most personal of questions. Even routine practices such as blood pressure measurement may confuse her. One study of Southeast Asians in central Ohio revealed that 94% of those surveyed did not know what blood pressure was *(3)*. The physical exam may expose parts of her body that have been seen only by the most intimate of her family members. Prior life traumas may make it difficult for the patient to tolerate physical examination. Many immigrants have witnessed or were subjected to physical or sexual torture during the instability of intensive civil strife and armed conflict in their home countries. The issues around posttraumatic stress disorder must be taken into account when what may be perceived by the clinician as an "over reaction" to a pelvic exam occurs. On the other hand, the reaction of the clinician, when the pelvic exam reveals the patient has undergone female circumcision, will be sensed by the patient and may adversely impact her sense of trust in her provider. As her visit continues, bodily fluids and samples are taken from the woman. These tests can be quite foreign to women *(4)*. Chinese women may be particularly disturbed by phlebotomy. In many cultures, blood is regarded as the source of life or energy for the entire body, the body's "chi" *(5)*. When blood testing is needed, experts recommend explaining that the amount taken is so small that the body will not be deprived *(6)*. After the exam is complete, the patient will be given a diagnosis (again in scientific terms in Western terminology), which she may not understand. She may then be given treatments, which may at best not make sense to her, or at worst may be contrary to her medical understanding. A classic example of such a conflict is a Hispanic woman from a rural community who presents with fever resulting from pelvic inflammatory disease. If she is given a penicillin-derived antibiotic, she will immediately lose all confidence in her clinician. She knows that hot diseases (she has a fever) should be treated with cold medicine. Penicillin is a hot medicine because it can cause fever with allergic reaction. It is quite likely she will not fill the prescription.

Communication is the key to success in patient–provider interaction. Even assuming both parties understand the same language, words have meanings beneath them that the provider may not recognize. Something as trivial as the number of pills prescribed can have a cultural impact. A Chinese Cantonese speaker will believe that the numbers three and eight are lucky. The number three sounds like the word for "life," the word for the number eight sounds like the word "prosperity." By contrast, the number four is the most unlucky number because it sounds like the word for "death." What will he think if you have to order four pills for antibiotic treatment? Native Americans rely on oral traditions and are more comfortable if note-taking is avoided (5). Another example of how cultural context can influence care would be the impact of a diagnosis of an STI in a Hispanic woman. In the Hispanic culture, each member depends on the relationship of family in times of trouble; to whom would the patient turn for advice or guidance when she is faced with such a diagnosis?

There is no field of medicine or nursing that has more need for good communication skills, understanding of interpersonal relationships, and nonverbal cues than the field of reproductive health. Some practical tips to improve communication are as follows:

- Let the patient take the lead. If the patient moves closer or touches you in a casual manner, you may do the same.
- Be cautious with the use of hand and arm gestures. Gestures can mean very different things in different cultures.
- Be careful not to over- or underinterpret facial expressions. This is also true regarding the presence or absence of expressions of pain, which are closely tied to a person's culture.
- Do not force a patient to make eye contact with you. The patient may be treating you with greater respect by not making eye contact.

Nonverbal communication is usually divided into several categories: facial expressions, movements of the head, gestures, physical space, touching, eye contact, and physical posture. There is potential for miscommunication in each of these areas unless the cultural background is understood.

Facial expressions:

- Smiling is an expression of happiness in most cultures but it can also signify other emotions. Some Chinese may smile when they are discussing something sad or uncomfortable.
- Winking is a romantic or sexual cue in Latin American cultures. Nigerians may wink at their children if they want them to leave the room. However, winking is considered rude to the Chinese.
- Blinking one's eyes conspicuously is a sign of disrespect and boredom in Hong Kong.
- Some Filipinos will point to something by shifting their eyes toward it or pursing their lips to point with their mouth instead of using their hands.
- Prolonged eye contact may be considered ill-mannered or an invasion of a person's privacy by Asians or Native Americans.
- Venezuelans consider pointing with a finger to be impolite and will use their lips to point at something.

Head movements:

- In Lebanon, the signal for "yes" may be a nod. To signal "no," the Lebanese may point the head sharply upward and raise the eyebrows.
- Saudis may signal "yes" by swiveling their head from side to side. The "no" signal would be to tip the head backward and click the tongue.

Gestures:

- The Japanese symbol for money is the "OK" sign because the circular shape of the fingers looks like a coin. In Argentina, Belgium, France, Portugal, Italy, Greece, and Zimbabwe, that sign means zero or nothing. In some eastern European countries and others, the gesture indicates a bodily orifice and is considered an offensive gesture.
- In the United States, to hold up crossed fingers is to wish good luck, but if the crossed fingers are held behind the back, the wish or thought is cancelled out. In Russia, this gesture is a way of rejecting or denying something. In Argentina and Spain, this sign is made to ward off bad luck. In China, it signifies the number 10.
- In Iran, the "thumbs-up" gesture has a vulgar connotation.
- In Columbia and other Latin countries, tapping the underside of the elbow suggests some one is a tightwad or stingy.
- Chinese people may point with their entire hand, because using one finger is viewed as rude. Similarly, in India, one may use the full hand but never only a single finger.
- In Latin America, a shrug with palms facing skyward is a vulgar gesture.

Personal space:

- Compared with people in the United States, Latin Americans are accustomed to sitting and standing close to people even if they are not well known to them.
- Middle Easterners may stand very close to each other while talking.
- In some Muslin cultures, a woman may be alarmed if a man, even a physician, sits or stands too close to her.

Touching:

- In some cultures, light touching of the arm or a light kiss or peck to the cheek is acceptable and common even for casual or new acquaintances, whereas people from many Asian cultures may consider this too personal.
- Touching another's head is offensive by some people from Asia as well as the Middle East. This includes patting a child on the head.
- Many Chinese may use a handshake to greet a Westerner but any other contact would seem inappropriate. This is especially true when dealing with respected elders or those in position of authority.
- Men in Egypt may be very touch-oriented. A handshake may be followed by a gentle touching of the recipient's elbow using the fingers of the left hand.
- A strong, warm handshake and embrace are traditional greetings between men in Latin America. Women may lightly brush their cheeks together.

- In the Middle East and in some African cultures, it is the custom to reserve the left hand for bodily hygiene and therefore the left hand is never offered for a handshake or to accept a gift or food.
- In India, a Western woman should not initiate a handshake with a man. Many Indian women will shake hands with a foreign woman, but not a foreign man (7).

Verbal messages:

- Native Americans prefer that conversations be conducted in lower tones than used by many Caucasians (5). They consider it rude to be asked to repeat answers.

EFFECTIVE APPROACHES

In the clinical dyad of provider and patient, each has concrete expectations of the other. The expectation of the providers is that they will make an accurate diagnosis and the expectation of the patients is that they must be successful and adherent to the treatment chosen. The accurate diagnosis is predicated on understanding the medical history and symptoms. This is impacted when the pair is not able to communicate, understand, or speak the same language, or the patient does not feel comfortable disclosing sensitive private information. The provider's approach should be friendly and relaxed, listening carefully, and asking more probative questions or reframing the question when the responses are not clear. Be sure to back off when it is apparent from the patient's body language, tone, or expression that he is tired or uncomfortable. The following series of questions are ethnic neutral but inclusive and can help the provider to illicit more patient-focused information and the patient's personal perception of the problem.

Tools for providers to elicit health beliefs (8):

- What do you call your problem?
- What do you think caused it?
- Why do you think it started when it did?
- What does it do to you?
- How severe is it? Do you think it will last a long time or a short time?
- What do you fear most about your problem?
- What kind of treatment do you think you should receive?
- What are the most important results you hope will happen from the treatment?

The issues surrounding successful completion or adherence to a treatment recommendation is fraught with more weighted judgment than the provider making a correct diagnosis. If the treatment does not make sense, or seem unrelated to the illness, or the patient is not clear about the cause of the illness and does not understand the diagnosis, the chances for successful treatment diminish. Adherence depends not only on the patient's acceptance of information about the health threat, but also on the provider's ability to persuade the patient that the treatment is worthwhile. The patient must also perceive the provider is credible, empathetic, interested, and concerned. The clinician must understand the feasibility of his recommendation. It is a taboo for some Hispanic women to discuss condom use with their partners; these women may risk physical or emotional abuse because their partners may assume that they are unfaithful or that they know more about sex than is desirable (3). These four activities can help to foster effective communication:

- Asking nonjudgmental questions that help the provider understand the patient's perspective on the illness, its causes, and its possible treatments.
- Listening carefully to the patient's replies, trying to gather clues to the patient's understanding as well as the patient's ability to be successful to the treatment recommendations.
- Working with the patient to set realistic goals for behavior change if needed.
- Involving the patient in active problem-solving (9).

All of our people all over the country—except the pure-blooded Indians—are immigrants or descendants of immigrants, including even those who came over here on the Mayflower.

—Franklin Delano Roosevelt
(Addressing the Daughters of the American Revolution)

A consortium of agencies has collaborated on the design and implementation of an electronic handbook to help providers develop and improve their skills toward cultural competence titled *The Provider's Guide to Quality & Culture (10)*. It defines cultural competence as a set of attitudes, skills, behaviors, and policies that support individuals and organizations to work more effectively in crosscultural settings. In this framework, it is recognized that understanding the healthcare beliefs, attitudes, communication patterns, and health practices are critical in improving the health of the individual, their communities and will allow for their participation. Cultural competence also affects broader population-specific issues such as the following:

- Health-related beliefs and cultural values (the socioeconomic perspective).
- Disease prevalence (the epidemiological perspective).
- Treatment (the outcome perspective).

The first and most important step in striving towards cultural competence is to evaluate oneself. It is hard to admit that we each harbor some judgments and even stereotypes about cultures other than our own. Cultural competence needs to be fueled by a desire to prevent these biases from treating individuals and communities with disrespect and disregard. Prejudicial thoughts usually are buried below our level of awareness and may be untested and unexamined. They operate on an unconscious and automatic level guiding us to react to what is "normal" or "strange." These prejudices and assumptions must be brought out to be examined in the light of fairness and personal development.

Some cultural competence pointers are at first view very broad. Nevertheless, it is from that broad view that people can begin to hone in on their own biases and entrenched positions.

- As clinicians, we need to "check our own pulse" and become aware of personal attitudes, beliefs, biases, and behaviors that may influence both consciously and unconsciously our care of patients as well as our interactions with other colleagues from diverse racial, ethnic, and socioeconomic backgrounds.
- Every clinical encounter is crosscultural. Developing true partnerships with our patients and maintaining "cultural humility" can help us to learn and better understand the historical, familial, community, occupational, and environmental context in which our patients live.
- It should be understood that there is no "one way" to treat any racial and ethnic group, given the great sociocultural diversity within these broad classifications. The framework of intervention needs to be individualized and applied in a patient- and family-centered fashion.
- Clinical and preventive care needs to be evidence-based, flexible, authentic, and ethical. We need to appropriately tailor our interventions to patients, families, and communities.
- Cookbook approaches about working with patients from diverse sociocultural backgrounds are not useful and instead risk potentially dangerous stereotyping and overgeneralization. In addition, it is important to not lose sight that there are influential intergenerational differences that exist in all cultures, and that diversity is often greater within groups than between them.
- It is important to understand not only patient and community barriers to care, but clinician and health care systems barriers to care. To eliminate racial and ethnic disparity, health care providers and organizations need to become both culturally and linguistically competent.
- We need to challenge and confront racism, sexism, classism, and other forms of prejudice and discrimination that occur in both clinical encounters and in society.

The Rabbi asked his students, 'How do you know when it is dawn?' They replied, 'When you can distinguish the difference between a sheep and a goat?, When you see the details in the leaf of a tree?, When you see the crest of the light breaking over the mountain?' The Rabbi replied, 'It is dawn when you look into the eyes of another and see your brother and sister.'

—Talmudic proverb

Communicating with a patient about STIs is difficult because we know that it impacts a person at the most personal and private level and can have far-reaching effects on relationships, both current and future. We are able to communicate most effectively when we recognize ourselves in the context of all humanity. To see the world through the eyes of another is to be truly illuminated.

To learn to respect and have regard for the different views and beliefs of others will help to shed light on what may seem to be mysterious ways of thinking or behaving. It broadens and enriches our own world, it stretches our boundaries and brings us to fuller understanding about those whom we have pledged to serve with our talents and skills. The impact of an improved and developed interest in cultural competence should result in more successful patient education, which can improve a patient's health care-seeking behavior, and more appropriate selection of testing and screening by the provider who knows more about a patient's genetic risks, health beliefs, and risk exposure. There should be fewer diagnostic errors because of more comprehensive and accurate medical histories and fewer drug complications because the provider can discover information about folk/home remedies. Most importantly, there will be a likelihood of great successful adherence to a treatment plan. For society, another positive outcome is that there will be an expanded pool of high-quality clinicians who will practice with a broader base of knowledge. Patients and their communities will have greater choices (11). The weaving and blending of science and art are powerful when technical, clinical, and communication skills are all utilized to their fullest and providers practice with an open heart and a clear view of who their patients really are.

REFERENCES

1. Betancourt JR. Cultural competence—marginal or mainstream movement? N Engl J Med 2004; 351:953–955.
2. Dallabetta GA, Field ML, Laga M, Islam QM. STDs: Global burden and challenges for control. In: Dallabetta GA, Laga M, Lamptey PR, eds., *Control of Sexually Transmitted Diseases: A Handbook for the Design and Management of Programs*. Durham, NC: The AIDSCAP Electronic Library (Family Health International/The AIDS Control and Prevention Project), 1996. Available from: http://www.fhi.org/en/HIVAIDS/pub/guide/stdhandbook/index.htm. Accessed Nov. 24, 2006.
3. National Iinstitutes of Health. Publication 98-4247. Women of Color Health Data Book: Asian Americans. Bethesda, MD: National Institutes of Health, 1998.
4. Andrews MM, Boyle JS. *Transcultural Communication in Health Care*, 3rd Ed. Philadelphia, PA: Lippincott Williams & Wilkins, 1999.
5. Spector RE. *Cultural Diversity in Health & Illness*, 5th Ed. Upper Saddle River, NJ: Prentice Hall Health, 2000.
6. Medical Education Collaborative video. *Culture, Women, and Healthcare: a Multicultural Approach to Patients*. Golden, CO: Medical Education Collaborative, 2002.
7. Morris D. *BodyTalk: The Meaning of Human Gestures*. New York, NY: Crown Trade Paperbacks, 1994.
8. Kleinman A. *Patients and Healers in the Context of Culture: An Exploration of the Borderland Between Anthropology, Medicine, and Psychiatry*. Berkeley, CA: University of California, 1980.
9. *Management Sciences for Health and World Health Organization. Managing Drug Supply: The Selection, Procurement, Distribution, and Use of Pharmaceuticals*, 2nd Ed. Hartford, CT: Kumarian Press. 1997, p. 428.

10. Management Sciences for Health, US Department of Health and Human Services, Health Resources and Services Administration, Bureau on Primary Health Care. The Provider's Guide to Quality & Culture. Electronic Resource Center. Available from: http://erc.msh.org. Accessed Nov. 24, 2006.
11. Brach C, Fraser I. Can cultural competency reduce racial and ethnic health disparities? A review and conceptual model. Med Care Res Rev 2000; 57:181–217.

15 Effectiveness of Barrier Methods for Sexually Transmitted Infection Prevention

Penelope M. Bosarge

INTRODUCTION

We are living in a world that is suffering a pandemic of human immunodeficiency virus (HIV) infection, continued high levels of other sexually transmitted infections (STIs), and an unsustainable population explosion. In the last 40 years, the number of humans on this planet has doubled. The youth of the world's population today ensures that all STIs will continue to increase unless concentrated, deliberate, and committed efforts are made to slow their spread. In the face of these critical crises, it is important to recognize the impact that different contraceptive agents may play in the spread or control of STIs.

Intrauterine contraception does not contribute to the spread of STIs because IUDs are used primarily by low-risk women. The role of hormonal contraception has been closely investigated. There are obvious tradeoffs, but on balance, hormonal birth control methods are thought to have a neutral effect on STIs. Estrogen may increase the susceptibility of cervical chlamydial infections, but progestins thicken cervical mucus to block the ascent of gonorrhea into the upper genital tract. DMPA and oral contraceptives have not been associated with increased risk HIV risk *(1)*.

The debate today focuses on determining what the relative contributions are that behavior and barrier methods of contraception can make to the efforts to combat the STI epidemics.

FAST FACTS

- There are no differences in the long-term infection rates of adolescents who take virginity pledges compared with those who do not.
- The United Nations and World Health Organization (WHO) recognize use of male latex condoms as the best defense in preventing STIs.

From: *Current Clinical Practice: Sexually Transmitted Diseases:*
A Practical Guide for Primary Care
Edited by: A. L. Nelson and J. A. Woodward © Humana Press, Totowa, NJ

- Using of male latex condoms more than 25% of the time may avert 315,000 new cases of herpes simplex virus (HSV)-2 infection among US women each year.
- Although condom slippage and breakage rates are 1.6–3.6%, the greatest cause of condom failure is nonuse.
- Effectiveness of condom use in preventing STIs varies with each STI. The more contagious an infection is, the more likely inconsistent condom use will not profoundly reduce its transmission.
- Contraception prevents 577,200 unplanned births to HIV infected mothers each year in Sub-Saharan Africa *(1a)*.

OVERVIEW

One of the primary objectives of sexually transmitted infection (STI) control and prevention is to persuade at-risk people to adopt safer sexual behaviors to reduce their chances of contracting an STI and subsequently transmitting it to someone else. Many people are unaware they are infected, have no recognizable symptoms, and do not perceive themselves at risk. They are, therefore, less motivated to change behaviors consistently, putting their partners at risk.

STI prevention programs must address the needs of individual people and society. Programs that address only the treatment needs of individuals will not be successful; prevention is needed at a societal level. STIs spread throughout networks; focusing only on individuals leaves gaps that perpetuate the infection.

Many factors (both biomedical and behavioral) cause the spread of STIs. These include characteristics of the infection's organism; the site of the infection; the health of the infected individual; the health, age, and genetic susceptibilities of the uninfected partner; the couple's sexual practices and behaviors; and the prevalence of the STI in different groups. Sexual practices including foreplay, types of contact (oral–genital, penile–vaginal, anal), abrasions, duration of contact, frequency of contact, and intercourse during menses all affect the risk of infection transmission. The duration and commitment to the relationship and gender roles and empowerment affect the use of condoms and choices regarding sexual monogamy. Measures to prevent spread of infection may counteract each other. For example, HSV-infected people on antiviral suppression therapies may discontinue condom use. Transmissibility also affects the effectiveness of barrier methods in decreasing the spread of individual STIs. With highly infectious organisms, such as *Neisseria gonorrhoeae*, failure to use a condom even once may result in infection; less highly contagious organisms (such as HIV) may be better protected against by inconsistent (real-world) condom use. Against this background, it is obvious that the effectiveness of barrier and behavioral methods in preventing STI spread may be difficult to quantify.

Faced with today's problems, some policymakers and thought leaders have concluded that there is no sex that is safe except abstinence before marriage to one lifelong (similarly previously abstinent, uninfected) partner *(1b)*. In an absolute sense, this position is clearly true; very little of the STI epidemic comes from perinatal or other nonsexual types of exposure. However, that position is not relevant for many people for a wide variety of reasons, such as the fact that some people cannot control their choice of partner or because their judgment is sometimes clouded by passion. It must be noted that abstinence must not only be vaginal–penile abstinence, but must include abstinence from all activities that permit STI transmission.

Given the diversity of human experiences, the seriousness of the infections, and the adverse impact that these infections can have on those not even involved in the decision to have risky sex (such as the fetus), it is important to have second-line defenses available in case less-than-perfectly-safe sex happens. The situation is very similar to the approach society takes to automobiles. Driving is known to be dangerous; 44,065 Americans were killed in motor vehicle traffic accidents in 2002. However, we do not advise against use of cars, because they provide so many benefits. Instead, we try to make the driving experience less dangerous by agreeing to rules of the road and installing seat belts and antilock brakes for safety.

MALE CONDOMS

Male condoms were developed and used from their inception to decrease unwanted fertility and prevent the acquisition and spread of STIs. Male condoms were used extensively in Europe during the centuries when syphilis was a large public health problem. The importance of condom use was reinforced during and after World War I when the United States paid the price of not protecting its soldiers from STIs; the thought leaders of the time refused to provide condoms or any treatments for STIs because they believed that those who engaged in immoral/risky behavior should suffer the consequences of their actions. This decision was followed by a generation of syphilis (*see* Chapter 9). By World War II, the lesson had been learned and soldiers were instructed in detail about condom use. The importance of male condoms was again emphasized in the 1980s–1990s when HIV/acquired immune deficiency syndrome (AIDS) was recognized.

How strong is the evidence that barrier methods protect individuals or reduce the spread of STIs? The most persuasive and definitive evidence in medicine comes from prospective, randomized, placebo-controlled double-blind studies (randomized clinical trials). This is neither possible nor ethical in the case of STI studies. At a practical level, subjects cannot be blinded to whether or not they are using condoms. More importantly, it is not ethical to withhold protection from an at-risk subject. No Institutional Review Board in the world would permit such research. Therefore, evidence of STI protection must be assessed from less than perfect study designs, which often leaves gaps in our knowledge and dilutes the strength of the study findings.

Table 1
Hypothetical Relative Risk Model of Condom Use

Condom use event	Semen exposure (volume, averaged over event probability)	Relative risk (compared to nonuse)
Failure to use a condom	3.3 mL	1
Condom used, but it breaks	1 mL × 2/100	0.006
Condom used, no break but has visibly detectable hole (by water leak test)	10^{-2} mL × 1/400	0.000008
Condom used, no break or visibly detectable holes, but still passes virus	6×10^{-6} mL × 0.023	0.00000004
Condom used, no break, no leak	0.0 mL	0

Source: From ref. 36.

In 2000, a National Institutes of Health (NIH) panel composed of experts from the NIH, Centers for Disease Control and Prevention (CDC), Food and Drug Administration, and the United States Agency for International Development undertook a comprehensive review of all the existing studies of male condom use and STIs. The panel specifically addressed the issue: "What is the scientific evidence on the effectiveness of latex male condom use to prevent STD transmission during vaginal intercourse?" The highlights of the NIH panel report are important to review:

1. Condom quality. Manufactured latex condoms are of high quality and meet manufacturing specifications. Laboratory tests have shown that latex condoms provide a "highly effective barrier to transmission of particle of similar size to those of the smaller STD viruses."

2. Condom breakage and slippage. Condom breakage rates range from 0.4 to 2.3%. Risk factors affecting slippage and breakage are related to user familiarity and knowledge, including user experience, selection of condom size (width), and proper use of additional (exogenous) lubricant (2–4). With increased education and improved experience, decreased condom slippage and breakage rates can be expected. Even in the face of such apparent failure, the risk of exposure to STIs is reduced. Table 1 shows the calculated relative risk of such events compared with the risk of not using a condom.

3. For HIV infection, meta-analysis of 12 studies of discordant couples showed that correct and consistent use of condoms was associated with a HIV seroconversion rate of 0.9 per 100 person-years. Never users of condoms had HIV seroconversion rates of 6.7 per 100 person-years. This represents an 85% reduction in HIV/AIDS transmission risk (5). The NIH concluded that these data provide strong evidence of the effectiveness of condoms for reducing HIV transmission.

4. For *N. gonorrhoeae*, the NIH panel found four studies in men and two studies in women that provided adequate information. The single prospective studies of US sailors and sex workers found that none of the men who always or sometimes used condoms became infected, whereas 10.2% of nonusers did, although the difference did not achieve statistical significance *(6)*. Two cross-sectioned studies and one case-involved study found a 49–75% reduction in risk of infection for men reporting condom use *(7–9)*. For women, one case–control study compared ever users for the previous 3 months to never users for the same time period and found a statistically significant reduction in risk of gonorrheal infection *(10)*. A cross-sectional study found a 39% reduction in gonorrheal infection among women in an STI clinic who used condoms compared with those who used no barrier method *(11)*. The relatively modest reduction of risk in women who practiced only occasional use of condoms is understandable, because even one exposure to an infected man causes a 60–80% risk of infection for the woman.

5. For pelvic inflammatory disease (PID; either gonorrheal or chlamydial), one case–control study demonstrated a 55% reduction in women who had used a condom even once in the previous 3 months compared with never users *(12)*. A second study of tubal infertility found no difference in constant use of condoms for 3 months previous vs nonusers *(13)*. The lack of significant decrease in infertility rates with current condom use is also understandable. Past and even remote infection, not recent infection, causes infertility. Recent condom use could only be credited for reduction in recent infection.

6. For chlamydia, the NIH panel determined that six studies were sufficiently informative for inclusion: three prevalence studies, two retrospective studies, and one prospective study. In women, two of the three studies failed to find that recent ever use of condoms by high-risk women reduced infection risk. Interestingly, only 14% of the commercial sex workers in one of the studies reported any condom use in the last week. The difference in infection rates for these women (10%) and the nonusers (13%) was not significant *(14)*. This is not surprising, given that even a single unprotected exposure to *Chlamydia trachomatis* causes a high risk of infection. In addition, many of the women may have been infected for more than 1 week, because chlamydial cervicitis is usually an asymptomatic infection. The cross-sectional study of women in an STI clinic found no differences in the prevalence of infection among women who reported using condoms as a method of birth control (1.27%) compared with the prevalence in women not using a barrier method (13.49%) *(11)*. The third study among new female military recruits found that women who reported consistent use of condoms had a statistically significant reduction in chlamydial infection compared with those with inconsistent or no use of condoms (OR = 0.6) *(15)*.

In men, three studies (one cross-sectional, one case–control, and one prospective study) evaluated the relationship between chlamydia and condom use. The cross-sectional study found no difference in chlamydial infection rates for at-risk men who reported consistent condom use compared with never use *(16)*.

The case–control study found a 33% risk reduction with consistent condom use compared with ever or never use, but this did not achieve statistical significance (9). The prospective study found that none of the consistent condom users became infected compared with 6.3% of the men who reported sometimes or never using condoms, which was statistically significant (17).Overall, the NIH panel concluded that the literature as a whole does not allow an accurate assessment of the degree of potential protection against chlamydia offered by correct and consistent condom usage. The report reminded readers that such a conclusion does not mean that condoms do not provide protection; it means that studies that can answer that question conclusively have not been completed.

7. For trichomoniasis, the NIH panel found only one study of sufficient quality to evaluate. This cross-sectional study found that women using condoms as a method of birth control were 30% less likely to have trichomonal infection than women who used no barrier method of contraception (11). However, the NIH panel concluded that lack of published data prevented an accurate assessment of the reduction of risk of trichomoniasis offered by condom usage.

8. For genital herpes, the NIH panel admitted that several technical problems are posed by HSV, which makes most conventional study designs inadequate. Because most people with genital HSV infection do not know they have herpes and because most people cannot distinguish between new and recurrent infections, serological tests and self-reports cannot determine if recent condom use had any impact on recent HSV acquisition. Other complications are that in most studies, men are more likely to use condoms with high-risk sexual contacts, so condom use is a marker for increase risk, which may not be adjusted for statistically. The panel found that no study specifically addressed the question, but five cross-sectional studies included information about HSV transmission. The NIH panel concluded that the limitations in epidemiological study design and the lack of primary outcome measures prevented it from forming any conclusions about the effectiveness of correct and consistent condom use in the reduction of risk of HSV infection.Since the NIH report, a vaccine study has been conducted in monogamous discordant couples (one partner was seronegative and the other was seropositive). This study demonstrated that condom use during more than 25% of sex acts was associated with protection against HSV-2 acquisition for women (adjusted HR 0.08; 95% confidence interval [CI] 0.01–0.67) but not for men (adjusted HR 2.02; 95% CI 0.32–12.50) (18).

9. Syphilis. The NIH panel found eight reports including case–control, cross-sectional, and ecological designs. The panel concluded that most of the studies suggested a protective effect, but all were hampered by design limitations. Because of these limitations, the panel found that no rigorous assessment of the degree of reduction in the risk of syphilis transmitted by correct and consistent condom use could be shown.

10. Human papillomavirus (HPV). The NIH panel found that the interpretation of studies of condom use and HPV infection/disease to be more difficult than for

other STIs. The panel concluded that there was no evidence from the literature at the time that condom use reduced the risk of HPV infection, but study results suggested that condom use might afford some reduction in the risk of HPV-associated diseases, such as genital warts in men and cervical neoplasia in women.

Based on the findings of the NIH panel, the CDC posted the following summary in black boxes on its Web site for public health personnel: "Latex condoms, when used consistently and correctly, are highly effective in preventing transmission of HIV, the virus that causes AIDS. In addition, correct and consistent use of latex condoms can reduce the risk of other STIs, including discharge and genital ulcer disease. While the effect of condoms in preventing human papillomavirus (HPV) infection is unknown, condom use has been associated with a lower rate of cervical cancer, and HPV-associated disease." Their statement continues: "Latex condoms, when used consistently and correctly, can reduce the risk of transmission of gonorrhea, chlamydia and trichomoniasis." The final black box states, "Genital ulcer disease and HPV infections can occur in both male and female genital areas that are covered or protected by a latex condom, as well as in areas that are not covered. Correct and consistent use of latex condoms can reduce the risk of genital herpes, syphilis and chancroid only when the infected area or site of potential exposure is protected." The fact sheet also includes an important reminder: "The surest way to avoid the transmission of sexually transmitted diseases is to abstain from sexual intercourse, or be in a long term mutually monogamous relationship with a partner who has been tested and you know is uninfected" (19).

Because the publication of the NIH panel report and the CDC recommendations, other information has been added that supports the protection condoms offer against STIs. Licensed commercial sex workers in Nevada who are required to use condoms with every act of sexual intercourse have low levels of professionally related STIs (20). Since 1988, when monthly HIV testing has been required for licensed commercial sex workers in Nevada, it has been noted that the workers are more likely to become infected from personal contact than from professional activities. Experience in Thailand provided evidence on a larger scale. In 1991, the Thai government implemented a "100% condom program" to encourage condom use in commercial sex facilities. The percent of commercial sex acts with condom use increased from 25% in 1989 to 94% in 1995. During that time, the incidence of curable STIs in government clinics decreased dramatically; HIV prevalence in Thai military recruits decreased (21).

Amidst all the polarization and politicization of the issue and the call for abstinence-only approaches to STI risk reduction, Cates cautions, "We must not in Voltaire's terms, let 'the best be the enemy of the good'" (22). He reminds us that our preventive approaches—not only to HIV, but other conditions as well, recognize that incremental "partially effective steps are necessary to mount collectively effective (but imperfect) prevention programs" *(23)*. Since the NIH conference, several important trials that have demonstrated the efficacy of male condoms in reducing the transmission and acquisition of STIs. Winer et al. reported that women whose partners used condoms consistently had a 70% reduction in acquiring HPV infection and 100% reduction in cervical dysplasia (compared to women whose partners used condoms less frequently *[23a]*). In a comprehensive review of articles published after the NIH consensus conference in 2004, Holmes et al. found that condom use is associated with statistically significant protection for men and women against chlamydia, HSV-2, and syphilis. The authors also reported that condoms may also be associated with protection against trichomoniasis in women *(23b)*.

Condom Materials

There is a growing appreciation of the extent and significance of latex allergies, which affect approximately 1% of Americans; the problem increases to 7–10% when considering health workers exposed to latex products *(24)*. Rates are even higher in workers in latex manufacturing plants. Complaints of decreased sensitivity and unpleasant smell (taste) make latex objectionable to some. Polyurethane condoms have been proven to be as effective as latex condoms in preventing pregnancy; however, they are associated with higher breakage and slippage rates than latex condoms. The impact of those increased failure rates on STI risk reduction has not been assessed.

Natural-membrane condoms or "skin" condoms are made of lamb's intestine. They are usually thinner than latex or polyurethane condoms and are said to allow for more sensation during intercourse. No empirical data exist on STI transmission rates with the use of natural-membrane condoms, but laboratory testing has demonstrated that they are permeable to hepatitis B virus, HIV, and HSV *(25)*. Therefore, natural-membrane condoms should not be recommended to reduce STI risk.

Spermicide-coated condoms offer no additional protection from either pregnancy or STI transmission/acquisition. The only benefit they confer is additional lubrication. Women at high risk for HIV acquisition should be cautioned to limit their exposure to nonoxynol-9 (N-9) spermicide (*see* the section "Spermicides and the Contraceptive Sponge"). Many manufacturers have stopped production and sale of spermicide-coated condoms in the United States.

Condom Sizes and Features

Successful condom use depends on selection of the correct size of condom. Slippage rates may be higher if an excessively large condom is used. Condom use may be discouraged altogether if an inadequately sized condom is applied. Table 2 lists the names of sample condoms by size and shape. Other features, such as ribbing or scents/flavors, may increase the attractiveness of condoms.

Table 2
Sizes and Shapes of Selected Condoms

Snug fitting

• Beyond Seven®	• LifeStyles® Snugger Fit	• Kimono® MicroThin
• Beyond Seven® Studded	• Iron Grip® Snugger Fit	• Kimono® Type-E

Larger size—more headroom

• Trojan® Ultra Pleasure	• LifeStyles® Ultrasensitive	• ONE Condom®-Roomier
• Trojan® Very Sensitive	• LifeStyles® Xtra Pleasure	• Pleasure Plus®
• Trojan® Her Pleasure	• Durex® Enhanced Pleasure	• Inspiral®
• Trojan® Twisted Pleasure	• Durex® Pleasuremax	• Contempo® Midnight Desire
• Trojan® Magnum Twister		

Larger size—roomy from top to bottom

• Trojan® Supra	• LifeStyles® Ultra	• Durex® XXL
• Trojan® Magnum	• LifeStyles® XL	• Durex® Maximum Love
• Trojan® Magnum XL	• Avanti®	• Crown® Skinless Skin
• Vivia® Large	• Kimono® Maxx	• ONE Condom®-Bigger

Benzocaine has been added to the inner surface at the tip of one brand of condoms to help those with premature ejaculation.

Condom Use

Consistent (every time) and correct use of condoms is required to provide maximal protection. Repeated education and counseling are crucial to enhance consistent and correct use of condoms. The risk of breakage and slippage of condoms when used correctly is low. The breakage rate for vaginal intercourse has been estimated at 0.4–2.3% for latex condoms *(26–35)* and somewhat higher (0.6–7.2%) for polyurethane condoms *(26–30,32,34)*. Breakage of a latex condoms leads to leakage of genital secretion. However, a lower amount of genital fluid (approximately one-third of the original volume) will be exposed in comparison to when no condom is used *(36)*. The slippage rate of latex condoms for vaginal intercourse has been reported to be between 0.5 and 1.3% *(26,27,32, 33,35)*, whereas polyurethane condoms range from 1.1 to 3.6% *(27,28,31,32)*.

The evidence about condom efficacy with anal intercourse is sparse, but available data confirm the protective properties of condoms during anal intercourse *(37,38)*. Anal intercourse is perceived as being associated with a higher breakage and slippage rate because of increased friction. Some European countries recommend use of thicker/stronger condoms for anal intercourse. This recommendation has been based only on expert opinion; little data to support use of thicker and stronger condoms available. A few small studies report a comparable breakage rate of standard and thicker condoms during anal intercourse *(39,40)*.

Table 3
Instructions for Correct Condom Use

- Handle the condom with care. Do not use sharp instruments such as scissors or teeth to open package.
- Apply the condom before any penetration (e.g., vaginal, rectal, or oral).
- Use a fresh new condom for each orifice contacted.
- Place the condom on the tip of the penis where it can be rolled down completely over the shaft. Leave a space at the tip of the condom to allow for movement to prevent breakage. Do not leave extra space in reservoir-tipped condoms. Only the reservoir needs to be left empty.
- Immediately following ejaculation, hold the condom at the base of the penis and withdraw from the partner. If the penis loses its erection before withdrawal, the semen may spill from the condom.
- If the condom breaks or slips off during the sex act, remove the penis immediately. The woman should use emergency contraception to prevent pregnancy, and each partner should consider the need for sexually transmitted infection prophylaxis if at risk.
- Do not turn the condom inside out and reuse; discard after one use. Use a new condom with each sexual act.
- If lubrication is needed, use commercial, water-based lubricants.
- Do not use oil-based lubricants; which can degrade latex; avoid using cooking oil, mineral oil, cold cream, petroleum, vaginal medications for yeast infections.
- Use good quality condoms, not those purchased at novelty shops; those have not been tested by the standards set by the Food and Drug Administration.
- Do not use condoms that have passed their expiration date.
- Store condoms at room temperature. Those kept in glove compartments or a billfold may deteriorate quickly.

The greatest risk of STD transmission is nonuse of condoms *(41)*. Incorrect use of condoms also contributes to failure. In one study of condom users who had personal breakage rates of more than 20% (their condoms broke or slipped more often than once in every five uses), it was discovered that these men had curious condom placement techniques. One man always stretched the condom before placement, and another always inflated it. One man did not even know that condoms needed to be unrolled. Recently, some condoms have been designed to minimize these errors. One new brand can be unrolled in either direction. To insure correct usage, it is helpful to review the instructions for condom use with every patient (*see* Table 3).

Female Barrier Methods

In recent years, an increased effort has been made to develop female-controlled STI-prevention methods. Female condoms were available in the 1920s and 1960s but they were not commonly used. In the 1980s, the AIDS epidemic renewed interest in female condoms. The female condom is a polyurethane sheath with an inner closed ring covering the cervix and outer open ring protruding visibly and covering the labia. The polyurethane material is impermeable to even the smallest viral particles. In clinical practice, the female condom appears to be as protective as the male condom in preventing HIV transmission with correct and constant use (every time). It is less likely to break or leak when compared with the male condom *(42)*. Slippage of the outer ring into the vagina, which then increases the probability of contact of semen with vaginal mucosa, is estimated to occur in 2% of users *(43)*. Acceptance of the female condom by women and their partners has been shown to be lower than acceptance of the male condom and the cost is considerably higher *(43)*. The Joint United Nations Program on HIV/AIDS promotes and supports female condoms in developing countries.

Diaphragms and sponges were not designed to prevent HIV transmission. Large areas of the vaginal remain exposed with these devices. Earlier research had suggested that women who used the diaphragm may experience reduced risk for cervical infections. Today, however, the WHO cautions that in women who are at high risk for HIV infection, the use of the diaphragm is not usually recommended unless more appropriate methods are not available or are not acceptable *(44)*.

Spermicides and the Contraceptive Sponge

N-9 is a nonionic detergent, which has been the active ingredient in most spermicidal products, such as foams, gels, films, and sponges for decades. N-9 has in vitro activity against STIs and HIV. It protected macaques against vaginal application of simian immunodeficiency virus *(45)*. Early observational studies suggested that spermicides were effective in reducing the risk of HIV transmission *(46)*. Initial enthusiasm for the protection that spermicides could offer against the spread of STIs (including HIV) prompted a major switch in the early 1990s from unmedicated condoms to spermicide-coated condoms. There was also a public health message that encouraged the use of spermicidal foam in conjunction with condoms.

Since that time, five major randomized clinical trials have demonstrated that N-9 use is associated with a statistically insignificant increase in the risk of HIV acquisition, and that women using N-9 have higher rates of genital ulcerations *(47)*. A double-blinded, randomized, placebo-controlled trial in female sex workers in Cameroon showed no protective effect of N-9 film against HIV infection *(48)*. The rate of HIV transmission was identical in the group receiving N-9 and in the placebo film group (6.7 vs 6.6 cases per 100 women-years, respectively). An unblinded study in Kenya compared the contraceptive sponge to a placebo sponge in commercial sex workers. The spermicidally medicated sponge use was associated with a 45% seroconversion rate compared with a 36%

acquisition rate among placebo sponge users. N-9 sponge users also reported a higher rate of genital ulcers (RR = 3.3, p <0.001) *(49)*. Another study among sex workers in Benin, Ivory Coast, South Africa, and Thailand comparing an N-9 gel (Advantage S) with a placebo vaginal moisturizer (Replens) showed a 48% higher risk of HIV transmission with the N-9 gel *(50)*. Again, the N-9 users reported a higher risk for genital ulceration. Other international studies using different concentrations of N-9 have confirmed that it is not protective against HIV and that high-frequency use of N-9 was associated with genital ulceration *(47)*.

As a result, although the WHO Medical Eligibility Criteria for Contraceptive Use rate spermicide use for women as risk for STIs as a "1" (use method in any circumstances), they rate spermicide use for women at risk for HIV as a "4" (method should not be used) *(44)*. The Cochrane collection has a more temperate conclusion that there seems to be little, if any, role for N-9 as an HIV prophylactic *(47)*.

CONCLUSION

Male condom use has been an important element in safer sex practices for centuries. Whenever that message has been lost, innocent as well as culpable victims have suffered, as has society. With improved materials and male condom designs, the potential contribution that male and female condoms can make to reduce spread of many STI epidemics cannot be overstated. Clearly, more research is needed to answer the remaining questions about individual STIs; to develop new, more effective barrier methods; and to learn how to encourage responsible sexual behaviors, including both abstinence and correct and consistent condom use by those who are sexually active.

REFERENCES

1. Morrison CS, Richardson BA, Celentano DD, et al. Hormonal contraception and risk of HIV-1 Acquisition (HC-HIV) study: background, results, and discussion. Presented at the 16th Biennial Meeting of the International Society for Sexually Transmitted Diseases Research (ISSTDR), Amsterdam, July 12, 2005.
1a. Reynolds HW, Steiner MJ, Cates W Jr. Contraception's proved potential to fight HIV. Sex Transm Infect 2005; 81:184,185.
1b. *Sex, Condoms & STDs: What We Now Know*. Austin TX: Medical Institute for Sexual Health, 2003.
2. Albert AE, Warner DL, Hatcher RA, Trussell J, Bennett C. Condom use among female commercial sex workers in Nevada's legal brothels. Am J Public Health 1995; 85:1514–1520.
3. Fleming DT, McQuillan GM, Johnson RE, et al. Related Articles, Herpes simplex virus type 2 in the United States, 1976 to 1994. N Engl J Med 1997; 337:1105–1111.
4. Messiah A, Dart T, Spencer BE, Warszawski J. Condom breakage and slippage during heterosexual intercourse: a French national survey. French National Survey on Sexual Behavior Group (ACSF). Am J Public Health 1997; 87:421–424.

5. Davis KR, Weller SC. The effectiveness of condoms in reducing heterosexual transmission of HIV. Fam Plann Perspect 1999; 31:272–279.

6. Hooper RR, Reynolds GH, Jones OG, et al. Cohort study of venereal disease. I: the risk of gonorrhea transmission from infected women to men. Am J Epidemiol 1978; 108:136–144.

7. Barlow D. The condom and gonorrhoea. Lancet 1977; 2:811–813.

8. Pemberton J, McCann JS, Mahony JD, MacKenzie G, Dougan H, Hay I. Socio-medical characteristics of patients attending a V.D. clinic and the circumstances of infection. Br J Vener Dis 1972; 48:391–396.

9. Schwartz MA, Lafferty WE, Hughes JP, Handsfield HH. Risk factors for urethritis in heterosexual men. The role of fellatio and other sexual practices. Sex Transm Dis 1997; 24:449–455.

10. Austin H, Louv WC, Alexander WJ. A case-control study of spermicides and gonorrhea. JAMA 1984; 251:2822–2824.

11. Rosenberg MJ, Davidson AJ, Chen JH, Judson FN, Douglas JM. Barrier contraceptives and sexually transmitted diseases in women: a comparison of female-dependent methods and condoms. Am J Public Health 1992; 82:669–674.

12. Kelaghan J, Rubin GL, Ory HW, Layde PM. Barrier-method contraceptives and pelvic inflammatory disease. JAMA 1982; 248:184–187.

13. Cramer DW, Goldman MB, Schiff I, et al. The relationship of tubal infertility to barrier method and oral contraceptive use. JAMA 1987; 257:2446–2450.

14. Joesoef MR, Linnan M, Barakbah Y, Idajadi A, Kambodji A, Schulz K. Patterns of sexually transmitted diseases in female sex workers in Surabaya, Indonesia. Int J STD AIDS 1997; 8:576–580.

15. Gaydos CA, Howell MR, Pare B, et al. Chlamydia trachomatis infections in female military recruits. N Engl J Med 1998; 339:739–744.

16. Zelin JM, Robinson AJ, Ridgway GL, Allason-Jones E, Williams P. Chlamydial urethritis in heterosexual men attending a genitourinary medicine clinic: prevalence, symptoms, condom usage and partner change. Int J STD AIDS 1995; 6:27–30.

17. Zenilman JM, Weisman CS, Rompalo AM, et al. Condom use to prevent incident STDs: the validity of self-reported condom use. Sex Transm Dis 1995; 22:15–21.

18. Wald A, Langenberg AG, Link K, et al. Effect of condoms on reducing the transmission of herpes simplex virus type 2 from men to women. JAMA 2001; 285:3100–3106.

19. Centers for Disease Control and Prevention. Fact sheet for public health personnel: male latex condoms and sexually transmitted diseases. Centers for Disease Control and Prevention, National Center for HIV, STD and TB Prevention, 2004. Available from: http://www.cdc.gov/nchstp/od/latex.htm. Accessed Nov. 24, 2006.

20. Albert AE, Warner DL, Hatcher RA. Facilitating condom use with clients during commercial sex in Nevada's legal brothels. Am J Public Health 1998; 88:643–646.

21. Rojanapithayakorn W, Hanenberg R. The 100% condom program in Thailand. AIDS 1996; 10:1–7.

22. Cates W Jr. The NIH condom report: the glass is 90% full. Fam Plann Perspect 2001; 33: 231–233.

23. Cates W Jr, Hinman AR. AIDS and absolutism—the demand for perfection in prevention. N Engl J Med 1992; 327:492–494.

23a. Winer RL, Hughes JP, Feng Q, et al. Condom use and the risk of genital human papillomavirus infection in young women. N Engl J Med 2006; 354:2645–2654.

23b. Holmes KK, Levine R, Weaver M. Effectiveness of condoms in preventing sexually transmitted infections. Bull World Health Organ 2004; 82:454–461.

24. Sussman GL, Beezhold DH. Allergy to latex rubber. Ann Intern Med 1995; 122:43–46.

25. Lytle CD, Carney PG, Vohra S, Cyr WH, Bockstahler LE. Virus leakage through natural membrane condoms. Sex Transm Dis 1990; 17:58–62.

26. Callahan M, Mauck C, Taylor D, Frezieres R, Walsh T, Martens M. Comparative evaluation of three Tactylon™ condoms and a latex condom during vaginal intercourse: breakage and slippage. Contraception 2000; 61:205–215.
27. Cook L, Nanda K, Taylor D. Randomized crossover trial comparing the eZ.on plastic condom and a latex condom. Contraception 2001; 63:25–31.
28. Frezieres RG, Walsh TL, Nelson AL, Clark VA, Coulson AH. Breakage and acceptability of a polyurethane condom: a randomized, controlled study. Fam Plann Perspect 1998; 30: 73–78.
29. Frezieres RG, Walsh TL, Nelson AL, Clark VA, Coulson AH. Evaluation of the efficacy of a polyurethane condom: results from a randomized, controlled clinical trial. Fam Plann Perspect 1999; 31:81–87.
30. Frezieres RG, Walsh TL. Acceptability evaluation of a natural rubber latex, a polyurethane, and a new non-latex condom. Contraception 2000; 61:369–377.
31. Macaluso M, Kelaghan J, Artz L, et al. Mechanical failure of the latex condom in a cohort of women at high STD risk. Sex Transm Dis 1999; 26:450–458.
32. Potter WD, de Villemeur M. Clinical breakage, slippage and acceptability of a new commercial polyurethane condom: a randomized, controlled study. Contraception 2003; 68: 39–45.
33. Rosenberg MJ, Waugh MS. Latex condom breakage and slippage in a controlled clinical trial. Contraception 1997; 56:17–21.
34. Walsh TL, Frezieres RG, Peacock K, Nelson AL, Clark VA, Bernstein L. Evaluation of the efficacy of a nonlatex condom: results from a randomized, controlled clinical trial. Perspect Sex Reprod Health 2003; 35:79–86.
35. Walsh TL, Frezieres RG, Peacock K, et al. Effectiveness of the male latex condom: combined results for three popular condom brands used as controls in randomized clinical trials. Contraception 2004; 70:407–413.
36. Workshop Summary. Scientific evidence on condom effectiveness for sexually transmitted disease (STD) prevention. National Institute of Allergy and Infectious Diseases, National Institute of Health, and The Department of Health and Human Services. Herndon, VA, June 12–13, 2000.
37. Saracco A, Musicco M, Nicolosi A, et al. Man-to-woman sexual transmission of HIV: longitudinal study of 343 steady partners of infected men. J Acquir Immune Defic Syndr 1993; 6:497–502.
38. Samuel MC, Hessol N, Shiboski S, Engel RR, Speed TP, Winkelstein W Jr. Factors associated with human immunodeficiency virus seroconversion in homosexual men in three San Francisco cohort studies, 1984–1989. J Acquir Immune Defic Syndr 1993; 6:303–312.
39. Golombok S, Sheldon J. Evaluation of a thicker condom for use as a prophylactic against HIV transmission. AIDS Educ Prev 1994; 6:454–458.
40. Golombok S, Harding R, Sheldon J. An evaluation of a thicker versus a standard condom with gay men. AIDS 2001; 15:245–250.
41. Steiner MJ, Cates W Jr, Warner L. The real problem with male condoms is nonuse. Sex Transm Dis 1999; 26:459–462.
42. Mitchell HS, Stephens E. Contraception choice for HIV positive women. Sex Transm Infect 2004; 80:167–173.
43. Kulczycki A, Kim DJ, Duerr A, Jamieson DJ, Macaluso M. The acceptability of the female and male condom: a randomized crossover trial. Perspect Sex Reprod Health 2004; 36: 114–119.
44. World Health Organization (WHO) Reproductive Health and Research. Medical Eligibility Criteria for Contraceptive Use, 3rd Ed. Geneva: WHO, 2004. Available from: http://www.who.int/reproductive-health/publications/mec/index.htm. Accessed Nov. 24, 2006..

45. Miller CJ, Alexander NJ, Gettie A, Hendrickx AG, Marx PA. The effect of contraceptives containing nonoxynol-9 on the genital transmission of simian immunodeficiency virus in rhesus macaques. Fertil Steril 1992; 57:1126–1128.
46. Wittkowski KM, Susser E, Dietz K. The protective effect of condoms and nonoxynol-9 against HIV infection. Am J Public Health 1998; 88:590–596.
47. Wilkinson D, Ramjee G, Tholandi M, Rutherford G. Nonoxynol-9 for preventing vaginal acquisition of HIV infection by women from men. Cochrane Database Syst Rev 2002;4: CD003936.
48. Roddy RE, Zekeng L, Ryan KA, Tamoufe U, Weir SS, Wong EL. A controlled trial of nonoxynol 9 film to reduce male-to-female transmission of sexually transmitted diseases. N Engl J Med 1998; 339:504–510.
49. Kreiss J, Ngugi E, Holmes K, et al. Efficacy of nonoxynol 9 contraceptive sponge use in preventing heterosexual acquisition of HIV in Nairobi prostitutes. JAMA 1992; 268:477–482.
50. Van Damme L, Ramjee G, Alary M, et al. Effectiveness of COL-1492, a nonoxynol-9 vaginal gel, on HIV-1 transmission in female sex workers: a randomised controlled trial. Lancet 2002; 360:971–977.

16 The Future Role of Vaccines and Microbicides

Patricia A. Lohr

INTRODUCTION

Infection with sexually transmitted pathogens, including human immunodeficiency virus (HIV), continues to be a major public health problem despite conventional prevention methods, such as mutual monogamy, condom use, and treatment campaigns. This is most evident among women, who are being infected with HIV in increasing numbers in every region of the world, primarily through heterosexual contact. In addition to biological factors, such as the increased susceptibility of the uterine cervix to sexually transmitted infections (STIs), social, cultural, and economic inequalities limit women's ability to protect themselves. Conventional prevention strategies, such as abstinence, mutual monogamy, condom use, and treatment of existing STIs, are not feasible for many women *(1,2)*. For couples who desire to conceive, condom use to prevent or decrease the risk of HIV transmission is counterproductive. As a result, scientists, public health organizations, and advocacy groups have searched for effective adjuncts to traditional methods of prevention.

Vaccines for STIs have been under investigation for decades as an alternative method of primary and secondary prevention. Vaccines offer the benefits of being noncoitally dependent, cost-effective, and widely distributable. Early vaccination attempts included auto-inoculation. Advances in genetics and the elucidation of the immunopathogenesis of many infectious agents have lead to the development of more specific vaccine candidates.

Currently, only vaccines for hepatitis A and B and some types of HPV are available for the primary prevention of STIs. Other vaccine candidates are in development, and some may attain regulatory approval within the next several years.

In addition to availability, widespread acceptance of vaccines for STIs is necessary to ensure their use. Because many of these vaccines will be adminis-

From: *Current Clinical Practice: Sexually Transmitted Diseases:*
A Practical Guide for Primary Care
Edited by: A. L. Nelson and J. A. Woodward © Humana Press, Totowa, NJ

tered before the onset of sexual activity, the support of parents, health care providers, third party payors, and professional organizations will be needed to promote distribution. From the standpoint of physicians, organizational support is important but may not be sufficient. For example, even after the American Academy of Pediatrics recommended universal vaccination against hepatitis B, only 21% of pediatricians and 12.5% of family practitioners surveyed in Cincinnati, OH reported routine vaccination of all infants *(3)*. Physician recommendation in addition to school requirements may be the two most important factors encouraging parents to accept vaccination *(4)*. Education will also play a crucial role. Seventy-five percent of parents and guardians of young adolescents surveyed would allow vaccination against human papillomavirus after education as compared with 55% beforebefore education *(4)*. Belief in vaccination, low cost, and perceived risk and repercussions such as social stigma are other factors affecting vaccine acceptance *(5)*.

Although the development of an HIV vaccine remains a priority, another important avenue of research being pursued is the development of microbicides. Microbicides are agents that are used at the time of coitus to reduce the risk of acquiring HIV and selective STIs. Some may also have contraceptive properties. At present, no proven microbicide agent is available for use outside of research protocols. However, several have entered into the late stages of clinical testing, with the potential for a marketable product visible on the horizon *(6)*.

This chapter reviews the status of vaccines for each of the STIs and discusses the potential for microbicides as a class and the microbicidal candidates currently under investigation.

HEPATITIS B VIRUS VACCINES

Peripartum vertical transmission, early childhood exposure, and contaminated needles are the predominant modes of hepatitis B virus (HBV) infection in the developing world *(7)*. In contrast, in the United States, most infections occur in young adults and 50% are thought to be a result of sexual contact *(8)*. Groups at increased risk of sexual transmission include men who have sex with men (MSM), sex workers, prisoners, persons with multiple sexual partners, and those with other STIs. Injection drug users, particularly females, are at exceptionally high risk from needle sharing and trading sex for drugs or money *(9)*.

The hepatitis B vaccine has been available since 1982 for the prevention of hepatitis B infection and subsequent hepatocellular carcinoma. Comprised of recombinant hepatitis B surface antigen, it is available in multiple formulations. Some preparations include more than one vaccine, such as diphtheria-tetanus-pertussis and inactivated poliomyelitis, so that immunization can be easily incorporated into the dosing schedule for infants and children. The vaccine is typically administered in three doses, with the second dose given at 1 month and the final dose given at 6 months. Along with the first dose of the vaccine, hepatitis B immunoglobulin can be given for prevention up to 14 days after sexual exposure *(10)*.

Hepatitis A can also be transmitted sexually and cyclic outbreaks have been reported among MSM *(11)*. Childhood vaccinations against hepatitis A are available and a vaccine that combines hepatitis A and B is available for persons over the age of 18 who require both immunizations.

Ninety percent of adults and 95% of infants, children, and adolescents develop immunity after completing the vaccine series *(10)*. The efficacy of the vaccine is nearly 100% if an adequate, long-lasting antibody response is generated. Failure to respond can be the result of obesity, immunocompromise, or age. This can often be overcome by providing a booster or higher dose vaccination *(12)*. DNA-based vaccines are also being evaluated as an option for nonresponders *(8)*.

Targeted vaccination of high-risk groups, which included health care workers, began soon after the licensing of the hepatitis B vaccine. Only health care personnel had a demonstrable improvement in the rates of HBV immunization and infection *(13)*. Since that time, universal immunization of infants and routine vaccination of adolescents has been the focus of HBV vaccination in the United States. This has resulted in 90% of infants and 67% of adolescents receiving the vaccine, and a decline in the incidence of HBV infection by 89% among persons 19 years of age or younger *(14)*. Global campaigns have also been very successful. Sixty-six percent of World Health Organization member states report universal infant or childhood vaccination programs *(15)*.

High-risk adults continue to account for more than 75% of new cases of HBV infection each year *(16)*. For example, among 3422 MSM under 30 years of age, only 9% were immunized and nearly one in five had acquired HBV by age 22 *(17)*. Poor series completion rates; missed opportunities for vaccination in prisons, STD clinics, and drug treatment centers; lack of funding, and education all remain barriers to immunization in these groups *(18)*. The difficulty of immunizing these groups is not limited to the United States. An increasing number of sexually acquired HBV infections have been reported in Japan, Thailand, Brazil, and Uruguay *(8)*.

HBV infection is an important cause of cirrhosis, liver failure, and hepatocellular carcinoma worldwide. Universal immunization reduces infection rates and is cost-effective *(19)*. Challenges remain to increase worldwide immunization of infants and children, as well as high-risk groups who are likely to be infected by sexual contact.

HUMAN PAPILLOMAVIRUS VACCINES

The hepatitis B vaccine was the first vaccine available for an STI and a cancer. The quadrivalent human papillomavirus (HPV) vaccine is the second class of vaccines directed against an STI that also causes cancer. The prevalence of HPV infection worldwide is estimated at 440 million *(20)*. HPV is accepted as a necessary cause of cervical cancer with more than 99% of specimens containing the virus *(21)*. Large-scale screening with Papanicolaou (pap) smears has drastically reduced the incidence of cervical cancer in the developed world. However, in the absence of routine screening, the average incidence remains 30 per 100,000 women *(22)*. Even with screening, the sensitivity of Pap cytology to detect cervical intraepithelial neoplasia or invasive cervical cancer is 51% with a specificity of 98% *(23)*. The high false-negative rate of the pap smear, the burden of cervical cancer in low-income countries, and an understanding of the oncogenic role of HPV have lead to research into an HPV vaccine as a method of primary prevention. Therapeutic vaccines that induce regression of precancerous lesions or remission of cervical cancer are also under study.

Research into vaccines for anogenital warts began in the 1920s with wart extracts. This work continued in the 1960s and 1970s with various wart materials, but none demonstrated a benefit over placebo *(24)*. Since that time, HPV has been genotyped, with 15 types being related to precancerous and cancerous anogenital lesions. Two oncogenes, *E6* and *E7*, are responsible for cervical carcinogenesis, and two late proteins, L1 and L2, are important capsid proteins that self assemble into virus-like particles and facilitate the entry of viral DNA into cells. Therapeutic vaccines target *E6* and *E7*. Prophylactic vaccines focus on neutralizing antibodies to L1 and L2 *(25)*.

Although there are many oncogenic HPV types, some are more common than others. Therefore, a vaccine directed against the two most common types (16 and 18) would theoretically prevent 71% of cervical cancers worldwide and a vaccine that included the seven most common HPV types (16, 18, 45, 31, 33, 52, and 58) would prevent 87.4% *(21)*. The current vaccine against types 16 and 18 and 6 and 11 has the potential to prevent 70% of cervical cancer and 90% of genital warts *(26–28)*.

This vaccine is intended for prevention of persistent HPV infection. It has been approved by the FDA and CDC for use in women age 11–26, but girls as young as 9 may be vaccinated if they are at risk. It is expected that approval to vaccinate young men will soon follow. A bivalent vaccine against 16, 18 is also being evaluated by the FDA. Each of these vaccines induces antibody formation targeted against proteins in the capsule. (No DNA is in the vaccine, so it not possible to acquire viral infection from the vaccine.) In all of the reports, the vaccines were 100% effective against persistent infection with their target viruses, although the activity against HPV-18 was not seen until 24 months *(31)*. The efficacy of these vaccines in immunocompromised individuals is an important, unanswered question.

Chimeric therapeutic and prophylactic vaccines are also being investigated. These vaccines candidates are based on L2 or L2 recombinant proteins that are fused to the E7 or E2 antigens. Safety trials have successfully been completed but efficacy remains to be determined (20).

HERPES SIMPLEX VIRUS VACCINES

Research into a vaccine for herpes simples virus (HSV) has been conducted since the 1920s. Therapeutic and prophylactic strategies have included auto-inoculation of live HSV, and vaccines containing whole-inactivated or attenuated live virus, modified live and cell-culture derived subunits, recombinant glycoproteins, disabled infectious single cycle virus, or HSV DNA (29). A complete understanding of the necessary determinants for effective immunity against HSV is not yet established, which has interfered with development of a prophylactic vaccine (29).

In the course of acute infection, an immune response is generated that inhibits viral replication and promotes recovery, but does not prevent latent infection of the sensory ganglia. These virions can subsequently re-activate leading to symptomatic or asymptomatic disease and shedding. The ideal vaccine would provide sterilizing immunity at all portals of entry (genital, facial, and ocular) before the establishment of latency (30). However, a vaccine that can increase the titer of virus needed to cause primary infection or latency, or prevent clinical disease and shedding may also be beneficial (30). Therapeutic and prophylactic vaccines are in development, but only the latter is addressed in this chapter.

Recombinant HSV glycoprotein vaccines were the first to show partial prophylactic efficacy against genital herpes. The first product tested in double-blind, placebo-controlled trials was a vaccine that contained the recombinant HSV glycoproteins gB2 and gD2 with an adjuvant (31). Although the vaccine failed to prevent infection with genital HSV, the acquisition rate was lower during the first 5 months of the trials and was more potent in females. Another vaccine consisting of truncated glycoprotein gD and alum with an adjuvant was well-tolerated and demonstrated humoral and cell-mediated immune response in phase I and II trials (32). Two phase III studies followed (33). The vaccine was 73–74% protective against genital herpes disease in HSV-seronegative women, but not in men or women who were seropositive for HSV type 1. There was a trend toward protection against infection, but it was not statistically significant. A third phase III trial (HERPEVAC) is underway. Other prophylactic vaccines currently in the early stages of development include products containing live genetically attenuated virus, disabled infectious single cycle and DNA vaccines (34).

Both therapeutic and prophylactic vaccines can reduce the impact of genital and nongenital herpes. The currently ongoing HERPEVAC trial may provide the evidence needed for regulatory approval of a vaccine for HSV-seronegative women. Work remains to be done to uncover a vaccine that will include protection for HSV-1-seropositive women and men.

HIV VACCINES

Given the increasing number of HIV infections worldwide, the development of a vaccine against HIV is considered a priority. Unlike traditional methods of prevention, an HIV vaccine would be more cost-effective, reach large numbers of people who do not have regular access to health care, and would not require consistent behavioral changes to prevent disease transmission *(35)*. The challenges to vaccine development have been substantial. The virus demonstrates extremely rapid evolution: viruses can differ by as much as 10% after 10 years of infection in a given person, and 30% between individuals *(36)*. Other limitations include inducing sterile immunity, stimulating B- and T-cell responses at mucosal sites, and using HIV subunits rather than live or attenuated viruses because of the concern of inadvertent infection through immunization *(37)*.

The history of HIV vaccine development began in 1987 *(37)*. The first vaccine candidates were designed to induce neutralizing antibodies to viral envelope proteins. Difficulty stimulating antibodies that could conform to the trimeric envelope proteins, antigenic variation, and mechanisms of immune system evasion all impeded the development of these vaccines. From 1996 to the present, the strategy has shifted. Vaccines that raise a cytotoxic T-lymphocyte response using DNA, viral, or bacterial vectors were developed in the mid-1990s. Currently, research is focused on vaccine candidates that prime boost and induce neutralizing antibodies as well as a cytotoxic T-lymphocyte response against multiple HIV genes and subtypes. Prime boosting is a method of inducing a robust immune response by administered the same antigen in two vectors successively. The first antigen "primes" the immune system, and the second "boosts" the immune response *(38)*.

Two phase III trials have been completed, both testing recombinant HIV-1 envelope glycoprotein subunit (rgp120) aimed at different subtypes. Neither trial demonstrated vaccine efficacy *(39)*. A third trial is currently ongoing in Thailand of prime boost model with a canarypox prime and an envelope glycoprotein boost *(37)*.

To date, more than 60 phase I/II trials of more than 30 vaccine candidates have been conducted worldwide and 13 phase I/II trials are ongoing *(40)*. It is hoped that among this group is the vaccine that can successfully halt the forward march of HIV infection.

Haemophilus ducreyi (CHANCROID) VACCINES

Chancroid is a common genital ulcer disease among people residing in the resource-poor countries of Africa, Latin America, and Asia. It is thought to affect approximately 6 million individuals annually *(41)*. Although described as infrequent in the United States, it is likely that chancroid is underreported because of the difficulty of clinical diagnosis, lack of commercially available culture media, and differing state requirements for confirmatory testing *(42)*. The disease has been found to be more prevalent among commercial sex workers and their clients, crack cocaine users, and those infected with HIV *(43)*.

Research into a vaccine for *H. ducreyi* has increased since the discovery that chancroid is a cofactor for HIV transmission and the documentation of antimicrobial resistance *(44)*. In addition, treatment of chancroid is commonly delayed for up to 3–6 weeks after inoculation, which allows for prolonged periods of disease transmission *(44)*.

Infection with *H. ducreyi* evokes a delayed-type (type IV) hypersensitivity reaction *(45)*. Although T cells are recruited to the lesion and a humoral response is stimulated, these antibodies do not lead to protective immunity and seem to have no role in bacterial clearance *(46)*. Bacterial survival appears to be dependent on HS evasion of phagocytosis. It has been suggested that vaccines that induce bactericidal antibodies or promote opsonophagocytosis, therefore, may be the most promising *(45)*.

Like humans, swine do not achieve protective immunity after a single infection with *H. ducreyi*. However, a reduction in disease severity as indicated by reduced recovery of viable *H. ducreyi* cells from lesions, can be achieved after repeated infection *(46)*. Partial protection has also been demonstrated in animal studies after inoculation with virulence factors and bacterial components, such as recombinant D15 antigen, pili, hemolysin, and cell wall preparations *(48–50)*. Human studies have not yet demonstrated equivalent humoral immunoprotective effects, but the discovery of candidate vaccine antigens continues to be a focus of current research.

Chlamydia trachomatis (CHLAMYDIA) VACCINES

Chlamydia is the most prevalent bacterial sexually transmitted pathogen in the Western world *(51)*. In addition to pelvic inflammatory disease and its associated long-term reproductive tract morbidity, infection increases the risk of HIV transmission and may increase the risk of HPV infection complications *(52)*. Challenges to vaccine development against *C. trachomatis* include the existence of multiple *C. trachomatis* serovars, infection primarily of mucosal surfaces, biological and antigenic complexity, and an immune response that is both protective and pathological *(53)*.

Chlamydia vaccine research and development has a long history. Beginning in the 1950s, inactivated whole-cell preparations were found to provide partial short-term protection against ocular disease. The discovery that re-infection in vaccinated individuals lead to exacerbated disease resulted in suspension of human trials *(54)*. Since that time, subunit vaccines have been the focus of research. Multiple trials of major outer membrane protein candidate vaccines have been undertaken but none resulted in sterile immunity *(53)*. Elucidation of the *Chlamydia* genome has lead to the identification of other candidates, such as HSP60, YopD homolog, enolase, and polymorphic membrane protein D *(55)*. TRACVAX™, a recombinant outer membrane subunit vaccine has been developed by Antex Biologics. The company filed an investigational new drug application with the FDA in 2003 with plans for clinical testing *(54)*.

The difficulty of developing an effective subunit vaccine has lead to research into DNA vaccines, a return to cellular models—such as dendritic cell-based therapy, and live-attenuated vaccines.

Neisseria gonorrhoeae (GONORRHEA) VACCINES

For nearly 100 years scientists have lead a largely unsuccessful search for an effective vaccine against gonorrhea. *N. gonorrhoeae* is a challenging organism for vaccine development. The bacteria exhibit marked antigenic and phase variation, and employ several mechanisms for evading immune system detection *(56)*. In addition, it is an obligate human pathogen and, until recently, there was no viable animal model available for experimentation *(57)*. Nevertheless, emerging antibiotic resistance and an associated increased risk of HIV transmission in the presence of active infection continues to underscore the need for research in this area.

Observations of the natural course of untreated disease suggest that strain-specific immunity can be obtained. Early, uncontrolled studies reported partial immunity after inoculation with whole-cell preparations *(58)*. Recent research has been directed at purified antigens that mediate the interaction between gonococci and human cells *(56)*. Pili, outer membrane proteins such as porin (Por), opacity proteins (Opa), lipooligosaccharide (LOS), and transferrin binding proteins have all been explored as vaccine candidates.

Pili are surface appendages that are involved in the adherence of gonococci to epithelial cells and appear to be necessary for infection. Anti-pili antibodies block adherence and opsonize bacteria. A consistent and local antibody response can be demonstrated after immunization *(58,59)*. Despite this promising evidence, a large randomized, placebo-controlled, double-blind efficacy trial conducted in 3123 men failed to show any protective benefit of a pilus-based vaccine *(60)*. It is likely that the antigenic heterogeneity of pilus proteins interfered with the vaccine's efficacy. Some regions of the pilin subunit are relatively conserved and may be a focus of future vaccine development *(61)*. The opacity proteins (Opa) are also adherence ligands and potential vaccine targets whose development has been limited for similar reasons.

LOS is the only carbohydrate that could be considered as a gonococcal vaccine target. Antibodies against the terminal core sugars of LOS are bactericidal *(62)*. However, the bacteria have evolved several mechanisms for evading immune system attack against LOS. In addition to antigenic variation, LOS core sugars mimic host antigens, and the terminal sugars undergo sialylation leading to masking of LOS and nearby protein antigens such as Por *(63,64)*.

Por is the major outer membrane protein of *N. gonorrhoeae*. It consists of eight surface-exposed loops and a membrane-spanning region *(57)*. The membrane-spanning region is conserved across serovars, which confers an advantage to Por as a vaccine target over other gonococcal antigens. A recent analysis of *N. gonorrhoeae* strains collected over a 10-year period found that the variation between surface-exposed loops is limited, suggesting that a small number of Por protein epitopes could potentially protect against a majority of strains *(65)*. Antibodies against Por have been found to promote complement-mediated killing and opsonization, and to inhibit bacterial interaction with epithelial cells *(66)*. As mentioned, sialylation of LOS masks Por, which would interfere with the bactericidal capabilities of a Por-based vaccine. Studies suggest that this effect might be overcome if high titers or high-affinity antibodies could be raised through immunization *(58)*. Animal studies of purified Por have shown it to be highly immunogenic and capable of promoting bactericidal antibodies *(58)*. Human studies remain to be conducted.

The transferrin-binding proteins (Tbps) are an additional group of proteins under investigation. Tbps are highly conserved surface antigens that are required for human infection. In the closely related species *N. meningitidis*, murine vaccine studies using the Tbps found that immunized mice were protected after subsequent lethal challenge *(67)*. Natural gonococcal infection does not elicit Tbp-specific antibodies in the genital tract and stimulates only a mild humoral response, however, a more robust protective response could potentially be elicited by using purified antigen *(68)*.

Trichomonas vaginalis (TRICHOMONIASIS) VACCINES

The parasite *T. vaginalis* is an extremely common sexually transmitted pathogen. It has been linked to an increased risk of HIV transmission, preterm delivery, low birth weight, and preterm premature rupture of membranes *(69–71)*. Until recently, metronidazole was the only approved medication for the treatment of trichomoniasis in the United States. An increasing number of metronidazole-refractory cases lead to the licensing of tinidazole, a long-acting 5-nitroimidazole compound that is chemically related to metronidazole, as an effective alternative *(72)*. Nevertheless, given the potential complications from trichomoniaisis, a vaccine for this common infection is viewed as desirable.

Initial efforts at developing a vaccine for refractory trichomoniasis were undertaken in the 1960s. Women were inoculated intravaginally with heat-killed *T. vaginalis (73)*. Despite the finding that all 100 women enrolled in the study demonstrated a reduction in clinical symptoms, no further research into this method of vaccination was undertaken. In the 1970s, a vaccine called

SolcoTrichovac® (or Gynatren®) was produced. It consisted of altered lactobacilli isolated from the vaginal secretions of women infected with *T. vaginalis*. A satisfactory explanation for the mechanism of action of the vaccine and poorly designed and conducted studies cast doubt on its reported efficacy and the vaccine never achieved acceptance *(73)*.

Since that time, research into the host response, immunology, pathogenesis, and virulence of *T. vaginalis* has advanced greatly. In addition to nonimmunological and cell-mediated responses, serum and parasite-specific cervicovaginal immunoglobulin (Ig) A, IgM, and IgG, as well as T-cell recruitment, are detected at the time of infection. After natural infection, these Igs decrease rapidly with treatment, thereby failing to provide protective immunity.

Encouraging data comes from vaccines produced against *Tritrichomonas foetus*, a bovine vaginal pathogen that is similar to the human pathogen *T. vaginalis*. Partial protection is induced by whole-cell and membrane preparations of *T. foetus*. Immunization results in a reduction in pathogen transmission, duration of infection, and reduction in spontaneous abortion in heifers *(74)*. In addition, these vaccines stimulate a similar genital mucosal antibody response to *T. vaginalis* infections *(75)*. Murine models of *T. vaginalis* infection have produced similarly optimistic results. Immunogenic proteins, such as α-actin and other common antigenic epitopes, and adherence molecules, such as adhesins, mucinases, and cysteine proteinases, are other as potential targets for vaccine development *(73)*.

Treponema pallidum (SYPHILIS) VACCINES

Syphilis is a chronic infectious disease cause by the spirochete *T. pallidum*. Endemic syphilis was effectively controlled by penicillin mass treatment programs in the 1950s and 1960s. However, infections are now resurfacing in parts of Africa and Southeast Asia, sometimes in an attenuated form *(76)*. In the United States, the number of infections has also increased in the past 5 years *(76)*.

The immune response to infection with *T. pallidum* can clear millions of treponemes from sites of primary and secondary syphilis but does not provide protective immunity *(77)*. Antigenic diversity may be a contributing factor. Rabbit models have been shown to develop complete immunity when challenged with homologous strains of *T. pallidum* but not with heterologous strains *(78)*.

The genome of *T. pallidum* was sequenced in 1998 and since then various proteins from spirochetes have been identified as possible vaccine candidates *(79)*. Much research remains to be performed in this area.

MICROBICIDES

Microbicides are topical compounds intended to reduce the risk of STIs when applied in the vagina or rectum *(80,81)*. Although primarily developed to decrease the risk of HIV transmission, many may also protect against other pathogens, such as genital herpes, chlamydia, gonorrhea, or HPV. Some may also serve as a form of contraception.

Microbicides in current development come in a variety of forms, including gels, creams, suppositories, and films *(82,83)*. They are inserted in advance of sexual intercourse, often with an applicator. Future formulations may include rings or sponges that dispense a microbicidal agent over long periods of time allowing for use over multiple acts of intercourse.

The ability of a microbicide to be used rectally and vaginally has emerged as an important feature as the prevalence of anal intercourse (AI) is better understood *(84)*. Among heterosexuals in North America, Europe, and Australia the rates of AI range from 6–38% *(85)*. Heterosexual AI is more common in Latin America, particularly Brazil, and reportedly less common in Africa, although the practice may be underestimated because of the taboo nature of the act *(85)*. Among MSM, more than half report having AI in the past year *(86)*. Structural differences between the vagina and rectum, variants in epithelial sensitivity to chemical products, and distinctions in the mechanisms of HIV transmission between the two organs all pose challenges for a rectally administered microbicide *(86)*.

Successful development of an efficacious microbicide must combine current scientific understanding of STI transmission with market economics, social and cultural factors, and individual preferences *(87)*. In addition to preventing infection, the ideal microbicide will be affordable, easy to use, easy to produce, accessible, have a long shelf-life, and be stable at high ambient temperatures. Other key qualities include minimal tissue irritation, preservation of latex integrity for use with condoms or diaphragms, limited reproductive toxicology for those women desiring to conceive (safe in pregnancy), and an absence of systemic absorption or toxicity. Surveys of potential users reveal that an acceptable color, odor, taste, physical consistency, and method of application are desired *(88–93)*. It would also be helpful if it had a long effect window and did not require application immediately before sex.

Microbicides as a female-controlled method of preventing STI transmission has been a central theme in their development. Advantages include the ability to use the product without a partner's knowledge or consent. There are risks and benefits to covert use *(94)*. Women who perceive that they are at risk of STIs and have partners that refuse to use condoms may benefit from secretly using a microbicide. However, this may lead to a negative, even violent response from the partner if the convert use is discovered. Alternatively, women may overestimate the efficacy of a microbicide and abandon previously consistent use of condoms in favor of a less effective method of protection.

A substantial proportion of women surveyed worldwide express interest in vaginal microbicides when queried about hypothetical formulations or after participating in safety trials (93,94). This is particularly true if women perceived themselves to be at risk of acquiring STIs. Men surveyed in the United States, Mexico, and Zimbabwe are also supportive of microbicides, stating that they will be likely to accept their use if the products are proven to be safe, effective, and do not interfere with sexual pleasure (95,96).

Categories of Microbicides

The first products actively studied for microbicidal activity were detergent-based spermicides containing nonoxynol-9. Enthusiasm for these products emerged when they were found to exhibit in-vitro activity against HIV and other sexually transmitted pathogens. Several clinical trials followed, but none demonstrated a protective effect against HIV transmission in humans (103). These findings spurred research into alternative compounds and delivery mechanisms.

Approximately 60 microbicides have been studied; more than 30 candidates are in preclinical development and 16 are in clinical trials at this time. These products are largely categorized by their mechanisms of action (82,83,87). Although the term "microbicide" indicates that the product is designed to kill a sexually transmitted pathogen, many work in other ways to prevent transmission. Some preserve or enhance the natural defense mechanisms of the vagina, whereas others interfere at various steps of the viral or bacterial life cycle. Each category has strengths and weaknesses. The optimal microbicide may be one that employs more than one mechanism of action to achieve the desired protective effect.

VAGINAL DEFENSE BUFFERS

The normal vaginal environment is slightly acidic, a state that is maintained by resident lactobacilli, which generate hydrogen peroxide and lactic acid. The low pH (~ 4.0) of the vagina is detrimental to sexually transmitted viruses and bacteria, as well as sperm (99). Semen increases the vaginal pH to neutrality in order to protect sperm viability. However, this allows viruses to persist in the ejaculate and interferes with the vaginal natural defenses. Epidemiological evidence supports an increased risk of HIV acquisition in the absence of lactobacilli species in vaginal secretions (100,101). No role for either pH or resident microflora has been established in the rectal transmission.

Lactobacillus crispatus and Lactobacillus jensenii are the predominant vaginal species colonizing women of reproductive age (102). The Lactin Vaginal Capsule (Osel Inc.) is a suppository containing hydrogen peroxide-producing lactobacilli. Despite promoting active colonization, its clinical utility is unclear (82,103). Engineered L. jensenii, which secrete CD4 proteins that bind HIV, are efficacious in vitro, but further testing is needed to assess their in vivo utility (104).

Acid-buffering gels, such as BufferGel™ (ReProtect, LLC, Baltimore, MD) and Acidform™ (TOPCAD, Chicago, IL and GMP/CONRAD, Arlington, VA), maintain vaginal acidity and create a physical barrier that interferes with the passage of pathogens into vaginal or cervical cells *(105–108)*. They may also have contraceptive properties *(109)*. In a recent phase III prospective, double blind, randomized trial, BufferGel with a diaphragm was found to have contraceptive efficacy of nonoxynol-9 with a diaphragm.

Other products designed to enhance vaginal defense mechanisms, such as antibiotic micropeptides and monoclonal antibodies, are in development *(110, 111)*.

NONSPECIFIC VIRUCIDAL OR BACTERICIDAL AGENTS (SURFACTANTS)

Surfactants are detergents that kill or disable viral or bacterial pathogens by breaking down their surface membranes. These compounds are nonspecific in their mechanism of action and can be toxic to existing microflora and host tissue cells. These products are often spermicidal.

Nonoxynol-9-containing formulations represented the first generation of this class of agents; however, their usefulness is limited because of epithelial toxicity. Newer, less irritating products, such as C31G/Savvy™ (Biosyn Inc., Huntingdon Valley, PA), have been successfully evaluated for safety and tolerability and are currently in phase III clinical trials *(112,113)*.

ADSORPTION, ENTRY, AND FUSION INHIBITORS

For many viral and bacterial pathogens, the first step of infection involves binding to cell surface molecules called heparan sulfate glycosaminoglycans, which facilitate entry into the host cell *(114,115)*. Large polysulfated carbohydrates that mimic heparan sulfate or attach directly to specific cell surface proteins make up the majority of the microbicides in this category. Nonspecific adsorption inhibitors coat epithelial cells, viruses, or bacteria and provide a physical barrier between the pathogen and the host cell. The more specific entry and fusion inhibitors directly block cell surface receptor interactions. Three products in this category are currently in phase III clinical trials. In addition to demonstrating protective effects against HIV, they are active against other sexually transmitted pathogens and some have a contraceptive effect *(116,117)*.

Carraguard™ (Population Council, New York, NY), whose active agent is carrageenan (a seaweed derivative commonly used as a thickening agent and emulsifier in food products) is active against infection with HSV 2, HPV, chlamydia, and gonorrhea *(118–120)*. Early clinical studies demonstrated the safety of Carraguard and related pilot carrageenans when used vaginally *(121,122)*. A recent study found that it has little rectal toxicity *(123)*. A randomized, double blind, placebo-controlled trial of Carraguard began in early 2004. The goal is to assess the efficacy of Carraguard in preventing male-to-female HIV transmission as a result of vaginal intercourse over a 3-year period in more than 6000 HIV-negative women *(124)*.

Cellulose Sulfate/Ushercell™ (Polydex Pharmaceuticals, Toronto, Ontario, Canada, TOPCAD, and GMP/CONRAD) is efficacious against gonorrhea and HSV *(115,125)*. Ushercell also has contraceptive properties *(126)*. It is well-tolerated, although some irritative symptoms have been reported particularly among uncircumcised men *(124,128)*. In one phase III clinical trial, the 6-month pregnancy rate with cellulose sulfate gel alone was 10%. In a second comparative trial, this gel was as effective as nonoxynol-9.

Polynaphthalene sulphonate/PRO-2000/5 Gel™ (Indevus Pharmaceuticals, Lexington, MA) is a water-based gel that blocks the interaction of the viral envelope glycoprotein gp120 with the CD4 receptor that HIV employs to enter healthy cells *(129)*. In addition to HIV, this compound has in vitro activity against HSV and gonorrhea *(115,130)*. It is also contraceptive in a dose-dependent manner.

Other compounds in this class, which demonstrate even more specific protein-binding inhibitory activity, are CCR5 inhibitors and cyclodextrins and are in pre-clinical testing *(131)*.

REPLICATION INHIBITORS

Members of this class were initially developed as medications for the treatment of HIV infection. The efficacy of HIV reverse transcriptase inhibitors in postexposure prophylaxis lead to their consideration as preventive agents *(132)*. Through localized diffusion to target cells, they act by inhibiting viral replication and local spread of infection. The potential for development of antiviral resistance, dilution, and systemic toxicity are potential complications with this class of microbicides.

PMPA/Tenofovir™ (Gilead Sciences, Foster City, CA) is a nonnucleoside reverse transcriptase inhibitor. It is absorbed into epithelial cells, where it is activated and halts viral replication *(82)*. Safety and acceptability testing for vaginal use is complete, and the product has entered phase II testing *(6)*.

Other nonnucleoside reverse transcriptase inhibitors in preclinical development include UC-781 and TMC 120 (Dapivirine) *(133,134)*. WHI-07, a derivative of zidovudine, has shown potential as a vaginal and rectal microbicide with spermicidal activity in animal models *(135,136)*.

COMBINATION MECHANISMS

HIV transmission is a complex process, which occurs through multiple steps at many sites. Future generations of microbicides are likely to employ more than one mechanism to inhibit transmission and to increase efficacy. Cellulose acetate phthalate (CAP) (New York Blood Center, New York, NY) is an example of a compound in current development that uses two mechanisms to inhibit transmission of viral pathogens. CAP is a negatively-charged sulfated polymer used as a coating for capsules and tablets. As a microbicide, CAP maintains the acidic environment of the vagina leading to viral disintegration *(82)*. It also blocks the gp120-binding mechanism, thereby acting as an entry and fusion inhibitor *(137)*. In addition to HIV, CAP has also demonstrated efficacy against HSV types 1 and 2, cytomegalovirus, gonorrhea, trichomonas, *H. ducreyi*, and chlamydia *(138)*. Another compound, PC815, is a combination of Carrageenan and MIV-150 for use as a microbicide *(138a)*.

Uncharacterized Mechanisms

Several formulations currently in preclinical testing have undefined mechanisms of action. These include water-soluble organic salts of zinc, *Spirulina platensis* hot water extract, and Praneem™ polyherbal (M/S Reproductive Technologics, New Dehli, India). Praneem polyherbal is comprised of a purified extract from the dried seeds of Azadirachta indica (Neem) and an extract from the pericarp of the fruits of the Sapindus species. Tested in both pessary and cream formulations, Praneem polyherbal is spermicidal and demonstrates activity against HIV, HSV 2, chlamydia, several candidal cultures, and *Escherichia coli (139–141)*.

Efficacy of Microbicides

Although many microbicides show promise in vitro and in animal models, their efficacy in humans remains to be determined. These results will be borne out in phase III clinical trials comprised of HIV-positive and -negative women and men in various demographic groups. It is likely that the first generation of microbicides will be less effective at preventing HIV transmission than condoms. As with condoms, their efficacy will depend not only on the ability of the product to prevent infection, but on consistency of usage. This, in turn, will depend on the user's acceptance and access to the product, motivation, and ability to negotiate its use with each sexual act.

The results of a Cochrane review highlights the impact of consistent condom use in seroconversion in HIV-discordant couples *(142)*. In couples who always use condoms there were 0.9 seroconversions per 100 person-years. For those couples who never use condoms, there were 6.7 seroconversions per 100 person-years. Overall, condom efficacy is approximately 80%. It is estimated that the first generation of microbicides will be 50–60% successful at preventing HIV transmission and 75–85% effective at preventing pregnancy *(85)*. They will likely only be available for vaginal application, and will be recommended for use with condoms or other barrier devices, such as diaphragms, to improve efficacy.

Similarly, the first generation of microbicides will likely protect against other STIs in addition to HIV, but how well is not clear. Condom efficacy against STIs varies by pathogen and reflects the infectivity of the organism with each act of unprotected coitus. This has been termed the condom's "forgiveness factor" *(143,144)*. For example, HIV is less easily transmitted than gonorrhea during unprotected coitus. Therefore, the condom is more forgiving of imperfect use when it comes to HIV prevention than for gonorrhea prevention. This may also prove to be true for topical microbicides.

Future generations of microbicides are anticipated to have greater efficacy as stand-alone products against HIV and other STIs. They will be useful rectally and vaginally, and have high rates of contraceptive efficacy when desired.

Public Health Impact of Microbicides

In the absence of clinical data, epidemiological modeling and economic analyses have been performed to assess the public health impact of an effective microbicide. These estimates measure the number of averted HIV infections and the global economic benefits of prevention. They have focused on low-income countries and those populations likely to have access to microbicides. These groups include sex workers and injection drug users in contact with HIV-preventive services, sexually active adolescents in school, and women in regular partnerships receiving contraceptive services.

Three-year cumulative numbers of prevented HIV infections at 20% coverage ranges from 1.6 million for a microbicide with 40% HIV and 0% STI efficacy to 2.7 million for a microbicide with 60% HIV and 40% STI efficacy *(145)*. Direct cost savings for a lifetime of treatment including medication, palliative care, treatment of opportunistic infections, and home-based care ranges from $1.77 to $2.88 billion. Productivity benefits gained by avoiding absenteeism, retraining, and replacing workers range from $0.67 to $1.13 billion *(145)*. (Estimates are measured in US dollars from the year 2002.)

The Effect of Microbicides on Condom Usage

Because the microbicidal efficacy of first-generation microbicides is anticipated to be less than that of condoms, counseling will recommend use in conjunction with a barrier method. Faced with the desire to protect themselves but unable to negotiate condom use, concern has been raised that women may abandon condoms, preferring the easier-to-use and undetectable microbicide. This has been termed "condom migration." Similar to the modeling used to project the efficacy and cost–benefits of microbicides, mathematical modeling has been performed to project the impact of condom migration *(146)*. As with condom use, in addition to its inherent efficacy, consistent use will be the primary determinant of a microbicide's protective ability. Additionally, the consistency of condom use in a given population at the time of microbicide introduction will affect the overall reduction of transmission in the event of condom migration. If the initial use of condoms is low (25% or less), a microbicide with high efficacy (estimated at 50%) is not projected to lead to an increased risk of HIV and STI transmission if it is used in 50% or more of sex acts. However, in areas where condom use is high, condom migration and the substitution of an equally efficacious microbicide used less consistently could lead to an increase in the risk of disease transmission.

CONCLUSION

The positive impact of vaccination against STIs has been evidenced by the successes gained through universal immunization against hepatitis B worldwide. The reemergence of previously controlled infectious agents, antimicrobial resistance, and the impact of infection with STIs on the transmission of HIV continues to support vaccines as research priority. A successful vaccine for some types of HPV is now available and it is likely that others will soon follow. Widespread acceptance, availability, and funding continue to remain barriers to adequate vaccination efforts worldwide.

Vaginal and rectal microbicides represent a new method for preventing infection with HIV and other STIs in an era in which both are increasing in prevalence and incidence. An effective microbicide has the potential to greatly affect economic and public health. Many mechanisms of action for microbicides have been identified and several products are in various stages of testing. Results from large scale phase III trials are being anxiously awaited because a commercially available microbicide is greatly needed.

REFERENCES

1. Royce RA, Sena A, Cates W Jr, Cohen MS. Sexual transmission of HIV. N Engl J Med 1997; 336:1072–1078.
2. The Population Council and International Family Health. *The Case for Microbicides: A Global Priority*, 2nd Ed. New York, NY: Population Council, 2001.
3. Siegel RM, Baker RC, Kotagal UR, Balistreri WF. Hepatitis B vaccine use in Cincinnati: a community's response to the AAP recommendation of universal hepatitis B immunization. J Natl Med Assoc 1994; 86:444–448.
4. Davis K, Dickman ED, Ferris D, Dias JK. Human papillomavirus vaccine acceptability among parents of 10- to 15-year-old adolescents. J Low Genit Tract Dis 2004; 8:188–194.
5. Boehner CW, Howe SR, Bernstein DI, Rosenthal SL. Viral sexually transmitted disease vaccine acceptability among college students. Sex Transm Dis 2003; 30:774–778.
6. Alliance for Microbicide Development. Microbicide Research and Development Database. Available from: www.microbicide.org. Accessed Nov. 25, 2006.
7. World Health Organization. Media Centre Fact sheet no. 204. Hepatitis B. Revised October 2000. Available from: http://www.who.int/mediacentre/factsheets/fs204/en/. Accessed Nov. 25, 2006.
8. Atkins M, Nolan M. Sexual transmission of hepatitis B. Curr Opin Infect Dis 2005; 18: 67–72.
9. Kuo I, Sherman SG, Thomas DL, Strathdee SA. Hepatitis B virus infection and vaccination among young injection and non-injection drug users: missed opportunities to prevent infection. Drug Alcohol Depend 2004; 73:69–78.
10. Poland GA, Jacobson RM. Clinical practice: prevention of hepatitis B with the hepatitis B vaccine. N Engl J Med 2004; 351:2832–2838.

11. Bell BP, Shapiro CN, Alter MJ, et al. The diverse patterns of hepatitis A epidemiology in the United States-implications for vaccination strategies. J Infect Dis 1998; 178:1579–1584.

12. Poland GA. Hepatitis B immunization in health care workers. Dealing with vaccine nonresponse. Am J Prev Med 1998; 15:73–77.

13. Alter MJ, Hadler SC, Margolis HS, et al. The changing epidemiology of hepatitis B in the United States. Need for alternative vaccination strategies. JAMA 1990; 263:1218–1222.

14. Centers for Disease Control and Prevention. Incidence of acute hepatitis B—United States, 1990–2002. MMWR Morb Mortal Wkly Rep 2004; 52:1252–1254.

15. Centers for Disease Control and Prevention. Global progress toward universal childhood hepatitis B vaccination, 2003. MMWR Morb Mortal Wkly Rep 2003; 52:868–870.

16. Goldstein ST, Alter MJ, Williams IT, et al. Incidence and risk factors for acute hepatitis B in the United States, 1982–1998: implications for vaccination programs. J Infect Dis 2002; 185:713–719.

17. MacKellar DA, Valleroy LA, Secura GM, et al. Two decades after vaccine license: hepatitis B immunization and infection among young men who have sex with men. Am J Public Health 2001; 91:965–971.

18. Rich JD, Ching CG, Lally MA, et al. A review of the case for hepatitis B vaccination of high-risk adults. Am J Med 2003; 114:316–318.

19. Beutels P. Economic evaluations applied to HB vaccination: general observations. Vaccine 1998; 16 :S84–S92.

20. World Health Organization. Initiative for vaccine research. Viral cancers: human papilloma-virus. Available from: http://www.who.int/vaccine_research/diseases/viral_cancers/en/index3.html. Accessed Nov. 24, 2006.

21. Munoz N, Bosch FX, Castellsague X, et al. Against which human papillomavirus types shall we vaccinate and screen? The international perspective. Int J Cancer 2004; 111:278–285.

22. Franco EL, Harper DM. Vaccination against human papillomavirus infection: a new para-digm in cervical cancer control. Vaccine 2005; 23:2388–2394.

23. Nanda K, McCrory DC, Myers ER, et al. Accuracy of the Papanicolaou test in screening for and follow-up of cervical cytologic abnormalities: a systematic review. Ann Intern Med 2000; 132:810–819.

24. Rupp R, Stanberry LR, Rosenthal SL. New biomedical approaches for sexually transmit-ted infection prevention: vaccines and microbicides. Adolesc Med Clin 2004; 15:393–407.

25. Tjalma WA, Arbyn M, Paavonen J, van Waes TR, Bogers JJ. Prophylactic human papillo-mavirus vaccines: the beginning of the end of cervical cancer. Int J Gynecol Cancer 2004; 14:751–761.

26. Villa LL, Costa RL, Petta CA, et al. Prophylactic quadrivalent human papillomavirus (types 6, 11, 16, and 18) L1 virus-like particle vaccine in young women: a randomised double-blind placebo-controlled multicentre phase II efficacy trial. Lancet Oncol 2005; 6:271–278.

27. Koutsky LA, Ault KA, Wheeler CM, et al. A controlled trial of a human papillomavirus type 16 vaccine. N Engl J Med 2002; 347:1645–1651.

28. Harper DM, Franco EL, Wheeler C, et al. Efficacy of a bivalent L1 virus-like particle vaccine in prevention of infection with human papillomavirus types 16 and 18 in young women: a randomised controlled trial. Lancet 2004; 364:1757–1765.

29. Stanberry LR. Clinical trials of prophylactic and therapeutic herpes simplex virus vaccines. Herpes 2004;11:161A–169A.

30. Stanberry LR, Cunningham AL, Mindel A, et al. Prospects for control of herpes simplex virus disease through immunization. Clin Infect Dis 2000; 30:549–566. Available from: http://www.journals.uchicago.edu/CID/journal/issues/v30n3/981676/981676.text.html-fn1.

31. Corey L, Langenberg AG, Ashley R, et al. Recombinant glycoprotein vaccine for the prevention of genital HSV-2 infection: two randomized controlled trials. Chiron HSV Vaccine Study Group. JAMA 1999; 282:331–340.

32. LeRoux-Roels G, Moreau E, Desombere I. Persistence of humoral and cellular immune response and booster effect following vaccination with herpes simplex 9gD2t candidate vaccine with MPL. 34th Interscience Conference on Antimicrobial Agents and Chemotherapy, Orlando, FL. 1994, October.

33. Stanberry LR, Spruance SL, Cunningham AL, et al. Glycoprotein-d-adjuvant vaccine to prevent genital herpes. N Engl J Med 2002; 347:1652–1661.

34. World Health Organization. Initiative for vaccine research. Sexually transmitted diseases: herpes simplex virus type 2. Available from: http://www.who.int/vaccine_research/diseases/soa_std/en/index1.html. Accessed Nov. 24, 2006.

35. Collins C. Policy issues in AIDS vaccine development. Feb, 2001. In: Peiperl L, Coffey S, Voldberding P, eds., HIV InSite Knowledge Base. University of California San Francisco and San Francisco General Hospital. Available from: http://hivinsite.ucsf.edu/InSite?page=kb-08-01-11. Accessed Nov. 25, 2006.

36. Korber B, Gaschen B, Yusim K, Thakallapally R, Kesmir C, Detours V. Evolutionary and immunological implications of contemporary HIV-1 variation. Br Med Bull 2001; 58:19–42.

37. Burgers WA, Williamson C. The challenges of HIV vaccine development and testing. Best Pract Res Clin Obstet Gynaecol 2005; 19:277–291.

38. Peiperl L. Why prime-boost? The Pipeline Project. HVTN Vaccines in Development. UCSF Center for HIV Information and the HIV Vaccine Trials Network. Available from: http://chi.ucsf.edu/vaccines/vaccines?page=vc-05-01. Accessed Nov. 25, 2006.

39. Flynn NM, Forthal DN, Harro CD, et al. Placebo-controlled phase 3 trial of a recombinant glycoprotein 120 vaccine to prevent HIV-1 infection. J Infect Dis 2005; 191:654–665.

40. International AIDS Vaccine Initiative Database of AIDS Vaccines in Human Trials. Available from: http://www.iavireport.org/trialsdb/. Accessed Nov. 25, 2006.

41. Al-Tawfiq JA, Spinola SM. *Haemophilus ducreyi*: clinical disease and pathogenesis. Curr Opin Infect Dis 2002; 15:43–47.

42. Schulte JM, Martich FA, Schmid GP. Chancroid in the United States, 1981–1990: evidence for underreporting of cases. MMWR CDC Surveill Summ 1992; 41:57–61.

43. Mertz KJ, Trees D, Levine WC, et al. Etiology of genital ulcers and prevalence of human immunodeficiency virus coinfection in 10 US cities. The Genital Ulcer Disease Surveillance Group. J Infect Dis 1998; 178:1795–1798.

44. Ison CA, Dillon JA, Tapsall JW. The epidemiology of global antibiotic resistance among *Neisseria gonorrhoeae* and *Haemophilus ducreyi*. Lancet 1998; 351:8–11.

45. Spinola SM, Bauer ME, Munson RS Jr. Immunopathogenesis of *Haemophilus ducreyi* infection (chancroid). Infect Immun 2002; 70:1667–1676.

46. Spinola SM, Wild LM, Apicella MA, Gaspari AA, Campagnari AA. Experimental human infection with *Haemophilus ducreyi*. J Infect Dis 1994; 169:1146–1150.

47. Cole LE, Toffer KL, Fulcher RA, San Mateo LR, Orndorff PE, Kawula TH. A humoral immune response confers protection against *Haemophilus ducreyi* infection. Infect Immun 2003; 71:6971–6977.

48. Lewis DA. Chancroid: from clinical practice to basic science. AIDS Patient Care STDS 2000; 14:19–36.

49. Thomas KL, Leduc I, Olsen B, Thomas CE, Cameron DW, Elkins C. Cloning, overexpression, purification, and immunobiology of an 85-kilodalton outer membrane protein from *Haemophilus ducreyi*. Infect Immun 2001; 69:4438–4446.

50. Dutro SM, Wood GE, Totten PA. Prevalence of, antibody response to, and immunity induced by *Haemophilus ducreyi* hemolysin. Infect Immun 1999; 67:3317–3328.

51. World Health Organization. Initiative for vaccine research. Sexually transmitted diseases: *Chlamydia trachomatis*. Available from: http://www.who.int/vaccine_research/diseases/soa_std/en/index1.html. Accessed Nov. 24, 2006.

52. Anttila T, Saikku P, Koskela P, et al. Serotypes of *Chlamydia trachomatis* and risk for development of cervical squamous cell carcinoma. JAMA 2001; 285:47–51.

53. Igietseme JU, Black CM, Caldwell HD. Chlamydia vaccines: strategies and status. BioDrugs 2002; 16:19–35.

54. Rupp R, Stanberry LR, Rosenthal SL. New biomedical approaches for sexually transmitted infection prevention: vaccines and microbicides. Adolesc Med Clin 2004; 15:393–407.

55. Brunham RC, Rey-Ladino J. Immunology of Chlamydia infection: implications for a *Chlamydia trachomatis* vaccine. Nat Rev Immunol 2005; 5:149–161.

56. Barbosa-Cesnik CT, Gerbase A, Heymann D. STD vaccines—an overview. Genitourin Med 1997; 73:336–342.

57. Plante M, Jerse A, Hamel J, et al. Intranasal immunization with gonococcal outer membrane preparations reduces the duration of vaginal colonization of mice by *Neisseria gonorrhoeae*. J Infect Dis 2000; 182:848–855.

58. Sparling PF, Elkins C, Wyrick PB, Cohen MS. Vaccines for bacterial sexually transmitted infections: a realistic goal? Proc Natl Acad Sci USA 1994; 91:2456–2463.

59. Tramont EC. Gonococcal vaccines. Clin Microbiol Rev 1989; 2:S74–S77.

60. Boslego JW, Tramont EC, Chung RC, et al. Efficacy trial of a parenteral gonococcal pilus vaccine in men. Vaccine 1991; 9:154–162.

61. Hagblom P, Segal E, Billyard E, So M. Intragenic recombination leads to pilus antigenic variation in *Neisseria gonorrhoeae*. Nature 1985; 315:156–158.

62. Apicella MA, Westerink MA, Morse SA, Schneider H, Rice PA, Griffiss JM. Bactericidal antibody response of normal human serum to the lipooligosaccharide of *Neisseria gonorrhoeae*. J Infect Dis 1986; 153:520–526.

63. Mandrell RE, Griffiss JM, Macher BA. Lipooligosaccharides (LOS) of *Neisseria gonorrhoeae* and *Neisseria meningitidis* have components that are immunochemically similar to precursors of human blood group antigens. Carbohydrate sequence specificity of the mouse monoclonal antibodies that recognize crossreacting antigens on LOS and human erythrocytes. J Exp Med 1988; 168:107–126. Erratum in: J Exp Med 1988; 168:1517.

64. Elkins C, Carbonetti NH, Varela VA, Stirewalt D, Klapper DG, Sparling PF. Antibodies to N-terminal peptides of gonococcal porin are bactericidal when gonococcal lipopolysaccharide is not sialylated. Mol Microbiol 1992; 6:2617–2628.

65. McKnew DL, Lynn F, Zenilman JM, Bash MC. Porin variation among clinical isolates of *Neisseria gonorrhoeae* over a 10-year period, as determined by Por variable region typing. J Infect Dis 2003; 187:1213–1222.

66. Butt NJ, Virji M, Vayreda F, Lambden PR, Heckels JE. Gonococcal outer-membrane protein PIB: comparative sequence analysis and localization of epitopes which are recognized by type-specific and cross-reacting monoclonal antibodies. J Gen Microbiol 1990; 136:2165–2172.

67. West D, Reddin K, Matheson M, et al. Recombinant Neisseria meningitidis transferrin binding protein A protects against experimental meningococcal infection. Infect Immun 2001; 69:1561–1567.

68. Price GA, Hobbs MM, Cornelissen CN. Immunogenicity of gonococcal transferrin binding proteins during natural infections. Infect Immun 2004; 72:277–283.

69. Laga M, Manoka A, Kivuvu M, et al. Non-ulcerative sexually transmitted diseases as risk factors for HIV-1 transmission in women: results from a cohort study. AIDS 1993; 7:95–102.

70. Minkoff H, Grunebaum AN, Schwarz RH, et al. Risk factors for prematurity and premature rupture of membranes: a prospective study of the vaginal flora in pregnancy. Am J Obstet Gynecol 1984; 150:965–972.
71. Cotch MF, Pastorek JG 2nd, Nugent RP, et al. *Trichomonas vaginalis* associated with low birth weight and preterm delivery. The Vaginal Infections and Prematurity Study Group. Sex Transm Dis 1997; 24:353–360.
72. Schwebke JR, Burgess D. Trichomoniasis. Clin Microbiol Rev 2004; 17:794–803.
73. Cudmore SL, Delgaty KL, Hayward-McClelland SF, Petrin DP, Garber GE. Treatment of infections caused by metronidazole-resistant *Trichomonas vaginalis*. Clin Microbiol Rev 2004; 17:783–793.
74. Cobo ER, Cano D, Rossetti O, Campero CM. Heifers immunized with whole-cell and membrane vaccines against *Tritrichomonas foetus* and naturally challenged with an infected bull. Vet Parasitol 2002; 109:169–184.
75. Corbeil LB, Campero CM, Rhyan JC, BonDurant RH. Vaccines against sexually transmitted diseases. Reprod Biol Endocrinol 2003; 1:118–123.
76. Peeling RW, Mabey DC. Syphilis. Nat Rev Microbiol 2004; 2:448–449.
77. Engelkens HJ, ten Kate FJ, Judanarso J, et al. The localisation of treponemes and characterisation of the inflammatory infiltrate in skin biopsies from patients with primary or secondary syphilis, or early infectious yaws. Genitourin Med 1993; 69:102–107.
78. Morgan CA, Lukehart SA, Van Voorhis WC. Protection against syphilis correlates with specificity of antibodies to the variable regions of *Treponema pallidum* repeat protein K. Infect Immun 2003; 71:5605–5612.
79. Simon M, Milward F, Lefebvre R, et al. Spirochetes: vaccines, animal models and diagnostics. Res Microbiol 1992; 143:641–647.
80. Farrington A. Microbicides: what they are and why we need them. Health Sex 2002; 7: 2–4.
81. Rockefeller Foundation Microbicide Initiative. *Mobilization for Microbicides: The Decisive Decade*. New York, NY: Rockefeller Foundation, 2002. Available from: http://www.micro bicide.org/microbicideinfo/rockefeller /.shtml. Accessed Nov. 24, 2006.
82. D'Cruz OJ, Uckun FM. Clinical development of microbicides for the prevention of HIV infection. Curr Pharm Des 2004; 10:315–336.
83. Harrison PF, Rosenberg Z, Bowcut J. Topical microbicides for disease prevention: status and challenges. Clin Infect Dis 2003; 36:1290–1294.
84. Gross M, Holte SE, Marmor M, Mwatha A, Koblin BA, Mayer KH. Anal sex among HIV-seronegative women at high risk of HIV exposure. The HIVNET Vaccine Preparedness Study 2 Protocol Team. J Acquir Immune Defic Syndr 2000; 24:393–398.
85. Halperin DT. Heterosexual anal intercourse: prevalence, cultural factors, and HIV infection and other health risks, Part I. AIDS Patient Care STDS 1999; 13:717–730.
86. Roehr B, Gross M, Mayer K. Creating a research and development agenda for rectal microbicides that protect against HIV infection. Report from the workshop: Baltimore, MD, June 7–8, 2001. American Foundation for AIDS Research. Available from: http:// www.microbicide.org/microbicideinfo/reference/amfar.report.on.rectal.microbicides. pdf. Accessed Accessed Nov. 24, 2006.
87. Science Working Group Of The Microbicide Initiative. *The Science of Microbicides: Accelerating Development*. New York, NY: Rockefeller Foundation, 2002. Available from: http: //www.microbicide.org/microbicideinfo/rockefeller/science.of.microbicides.rockfound.pdf. Accessed Nov. 24, 2006.
88. Hardy E, de Padua KS, Jimenez AL, Zaneveld LJ. Women's preferences for vaginal antimicrobial contraceptives. I. Methodology. Contraception 1998; 58:233–238.

89. Hardy E, de Padua KS, Jimenez AL, Zaneveld LJ. Women's preferences for vaginal antimicrobial contraceptives. II. Preferred characteristics according to women's age and socioeconomic status. Contraception 1998; 58:239–244.

90. Hardy E, Jimenez AL, de Padua KS, Zaneveld LJ. Women's preferences for vaginal antimicrobial contraceptives. III. Choice of a formulation, applicator, and packaging. Contraception 1998; 58:245–249.

91. Hardy E, de Padua KS, Osis MJ, Jimenez AL, Zaneveld LJ. Women's preferences for vaginal antimicrobial contraceptives. IV. Attributes of a formulation that would protect from STD/AIDS. Contraception 1998; 58:251–255.

92. Hardy E, de Padua KS, Hebling EM, Osis MJ, Zaneveld LJ. Women's preferences for vaginal antimicrobial contraceptives. V: Attitudes of Brazilian women to the insertion of vaginal products. Contraception 2003; 67:391–395.

93. Hammett TM, Mason TH, Joanis CL, et al. Acceptability of formulations and application methods for vaginal microbicides among drug-involved women: results of product trials in three cities. Sex Transm Dis 2000; 27:119–126.

94. Woodsong C. Covert use of topical microbicides: implications for acceptability and use. Perspect Sex Reprod Health 2004; 36:127–131.

95. Darroch JE, Frost JJ. Women's interest in vaginal microbicides. Fam Plann Perspect 1999; 31:16–23.

96. van de Wijgert JHHM, Khumalo-Sakutukwa GN, Coggins C, et al. Men's attitudes toward vaginal microbicides and microbicide trials in Zimbabwe. Int Fam Plann Perspect 1999; 25: 15–20.

97. Coggins C, Blanchard K, Friedland B. Men's attitudes towards a potential vaginal microbicide in Zimbabwe, Mexico and the USA. Reprod Health Matters 2000; 8:132–141.

98. Wilkinson D, Ramjee G, Tholandi M, Rutherford G. Nonoxynol-9 for preventing vaginal acquisition of HIV infection by women from men. Cochrane Database Syst Rev 2002; 4:CD003936.

99. Klebanoff SJ, Coombs RW. Viricidal effect of *Lactobacillus acidophilus* on human immunodeficiency virus type 1: possible role in heterosexual transmission. J Exp Med 1991; 174:289–292.

100. Martin HL, Richardson BA, Nyange PM, et al. Vaginal lactobacilli, microbial flora, and risk of human immunodeficiency virus type 1 and sexually transmitted disease acquisition. J Infect Dis 1999; 180:1863–1868.

101. van De Wijgert JH, Mason PR, Gwanzura L, et al. Intravaginal practices, vaginal flora disturbances, and acquisition of sexually transmitted diseases in Zimbabwean women. J Infect Dis 2000; 181:587–594.

102. Antonio MA, Hawes SE, Hillier SL. The identification of vaginal *Lactobacillus* species and the demographic and microbiologic characteristics of women colonized by these species. J Infect Dis 1999; 180:1950–1956.

103. Patton DL, Cosgrove Sweeney YT, Antonio MA, Rabe LK, Hillier SL. *Lactobacillus crispatus* capsules: single-use safety study in the Macaca nemestrina model. Sex Transm Dis 2003; 30:568–570.

104. Chang TL, Chang CH, Simpson DA, et al. Inhibition of HIV infectivity by a natural human isolate of *Lactobacillus jensenii* engineered to express functional two-domain CD4. Proc Natl Acad Sci USA 2003; 100:11,672–11,677.

105. Zeitlin L, Hoen TE, Achilles SL, et al. Tests of Buffergel for contraception and prevention of sexually transmitted diseases in animal models. Sex Transm Dis 2001; 28:417–423.

106. Clarke JG, Peipert JF, Hillier SL, et al. Microflora changes with the use of a vaginal microbicide. Sex Transm Dis 2002; 29:288–293.

107. Garg S, Anderson RA, Chany CJ 2nd, et al. Properties of a new acid-buffering bioadhesive vaginal formulation (ACIDFORM). Contraception 2001; 64:67–75.

108. Amaral E, Faundes A, Zaneveld L, Waller D, Garg S. Study of the vaginal tolerance to Acidform, an acid-buffering, bioadhesive gel. Contraception 1999; 60:361–366.

109. Amaral E, Perdigao A, Souza MH, et al. Postcoital testing after the use of a bio-adhesive acid buffering gel (ACIDFORM) and a 2% nonoxynol-9 product. Contraception 2004; 70:492–497.

110. Zeitlin L, Cone RA, Whaley KJ. Using monoclonal antibodies to prevent mucosal transmission of epidemic infectious diseases. Emerg Infect Dis 1999; 5:54–64.

111. Cole AM, Ganz T. Human antimicrobial peptides: analysis and application. Biotechniques 2000; 29:822–826, 828, 830–831.

112. Mauck CK, Weiner DH, Creinin MD, Barnhart KT, Callahan MM, Bax R. A randomized Phase I vaginal safety study of three concentrations of C31G vs. Extra Strength Gynol II. Contraception 2004; 70:233–240.

113. Bax R, Douville K, McCormick D, Rosenberg M, Higgins J, Bowden M. Microbicides—evaluating multiple formulations of C31G. Contraception 2002; 66:365–368.

114. Rostand KS, Esko JD. Microbial adherence to and invasion through proteoglycans. Infect Immun 1997; 65:1–8.

115. Herold BC, Siston A, Bremer J, et al. Sulfated carbohydrate compounds prevent microbial adherence by sexually transmitted disease pathogens. Antimicrob Agents Chemother 1997; 41:2776–2780.

116. Rusconi S, Moonis M, Merrill DP, et al. Naphthalene sulfonate polymers with CD4-blocking and anti-human immunodeficiency virus type 1 activities. Antimicrob Agents Chemother 1996; 40:234–236.

117. Pearce-Pratt R, Phillips DM. Sulfated polysaccharides inhibit lymphocyte-to-epithelial transmission of human immunodeficiency virus-1. Biol Reprod 1996; 54:173–182.

118. Zeitlin L, Whaley KJ, Hegarty TA, Moench TR, Cone RA. Tests of vaginal microbicides in the mouse genital herpes model. Contraception 1997; 56:329–335.

119. Zaretzky FR, Pearce-Pratt R, Phillips DM. Sulfated polyanions block *Chlamydia trachomatis* infection of cervix-derived human epithelia. Infect Immun 1995; 63:3520–3526.

120. Spencer SE, Valentin-Bon IE, Whaley K, Jerse AE. Inhibition of *Neisseria gonorrhoeae* genital tract infection by leading-candidate topical microbicides in a mouse model. J Infect Dis 2004; 189:410–419.

121. Coggins C, Blanchard K, Alvarez F, et al. Preliminary safety and acceptability of a carrageenan gel for possible use as a vaginal microbicide. Sex Transm Infect 2000; 76:480–483.

122. Elias CJ, Coggins C, Alvarez F, et al. Colposcopic evaluation of a vaginal gel formulation of iota-carrageenan. Contraception 1997; 56:387–389.

123. Sudol KM, Phillips DM. Relative safety of sexual lubricants for rectal intercourse. Sex Transm Dis 2004; 31:346–349.

124. Population Council Microbicides Program. The Population Council's lead candidate microbicide: Carraguard®. New York, NY: Population Council, 2005. Available from: http://www.popcouncil.org/biomed/carraguard.html. Accessed June 5, 2005.

125. Cheshenko N, Keller MJ, MasCasullo V, et al. Candidate topical microbicides bind herpes simplex virus glycoprotein B and prevent viral entry and cell-to-cell spread. Antimicrob Agents Chemother 2004; 48:2025–2036.

126. Anderson RA, Feathergill K, Diao XH, et al. Contraception by Ushercell (cellulose sulfate) in formulation: duration of effect and dose effectiveness. Contraception 2004; 70:415–422.

127. Mauck C, Weiner DH, Ballagh S, et al. Single and multiple exposure tolerance study of cellulose sulfate gel: a phase I safety and colposcopy study. Contraception 2001; 64:383–391.

128. Mauck C, Frezieres R, Walsh T, Robergeau K, Callahan M. Cellulose sulfate: tolerance and acceptability of penile application. Contraception 2001; 64:377–381.

129. Rusconi S, Moonis M, Merrill DP, et al. Naphthalene sulfonate polymers with CD4-blocking and anti-human immunodeficiency virus type 1 activities. Antimicrob Agents Chemother 1996; 40:234–236.

130. Bourne N, Bernstein DI, Ireland J, Sonderfan AJ, Profy AT, Stanberry LR. The topical microbicide PRO 2000 protects against genital herpes infection in a mouse model. J Infect Dis 1999; 180:203–205.

131. Veazey RS, Klasse PJ, Ketas TJ, et al. Use of a small molecule CCR5 inhibitor in macaques to treat simian immunodeficiency virus infection or prevent simian-human immunodeficiency virus infection. J Exp Med 2003; 198:1551–1562.

132. Henderson DK. HIV postexposure prophylaxis in the 21st century. Emerg Infect Dis 2001; 7:254–258.

133. Van Herrewege Y, Michiels J, Van Roey J, et al. In vitro evaluation of nonnucleoside reverse transcriptase inhibitors UC-781 and TMC120-R147681 as human immunodeficiency virus microbicides. Antimicrob Agents Chemother 2004; 48:337–339.

134. Zussman A, Lara L, Lara HH, Bentwich Z, Borkow G. Blocking of cell-free and cell-associated HIV-1 transmission through human cervix organ culture with UC781. AIDS 2003; 17:653–661.

135. D'Cruz OJ, Waurzyniak B, Uckun FM. Antiretroviral spermicide WHI-07 prevents vaginal and rectal transmission of feline immunodeficiency virus in domestic cats. Antimicrob Agents Chemother 2004; 48:1082–1088.

136. D'Cruz OJ, Uckun FM. Contraceptive activity of a spermicidal aryl phosphate derivative of bromo-methoxy-zidovudine (compound WHI-07) in rabbits. Fertil Steril 2003; 79:864–872.

137. Neurath AR, Strick N, Li YY, Debnath AK. Cellulose acetate phthalate, a common pharmaceutical excipient, inactivates HIV-1 and blocks the coreceptor binding site on the virus envelope glycoprotein gp120. BMC Infect Dis 2001; 1:17–28.

138. Neurath AR. Microbicide for prevention of sexually transmitted diseases using a pharmaceutical excipient. AIDS Patient Care STDS 2000; 14:215–219.

138a. Fernandez-Romero JA, Thorn M, Turville SG, et al. Carrageenan/MIV-150 (PC-815), a Combination Microbicide. Sex Transm Dis. 2006; [Epub ahead of print].

139. Talwar GP, Raghuvanshi P, Mishra R, et al. Polyherbal formulations with wide spectrum antimicrobial activity against reproductive tract infections and sexually transmitted pathogens. Am J Reprod Immunol 2000; 43:144–151.

140. Garg S, Taluja V, Upadhyay SN, Talwar GP. Studies on the contraceptive efficacy of Praneem polyherbal cream. Contraception 1993; 48:591–596.

141. Raghuvanshi P, Bagga R, Malhotra D, Gopalan S, Talwar GP. Spermicidal & contraceptive properties of Praneem polyherbal pessary. Indian J Med Res 2001; 113:135–141.

142. Weller S, Davis K. Condom effectiveness in reducing heterosexual HIV transmission. Cochrane Database Syst Rev 2002; 1:CD003255.

143. National Institutes of Allergy and Infectious Diseases. Workshop summary: scientific evidence on condom effectiveness for sexually transmitted disease (STD) prevention. Herndon, VA, July 20, 2001. National Institutes of Health, Department of Health and Human Services, 2001. Available from: http://www.niaid.nih.gov/dmid/stds/condomreport.pdf. Accessed Nov. 24, 2006.

144. Cates W Jr. The NIH condom report: the glass is 90% full. Fam Plann Perspect 2001; 33:231–233.

145. Microbicide Initiative Public Health Working Group. The public health benefits of microbicides in lower-income countries: model projections. New York, NY: Rockefeller Foundation, 2002. Available from: http://www.rockfound.org/Documents/488/rep7_publichealth.pdf. Accessed June 6, 2005.

146. Foss AM, Vickerman PT, Heise L, Watts CH. Shifts in condom use following microbicide introduction: should we be concerned? AIDS 2003; 17:1227–1237.

Index

3